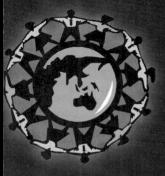

Essentials of
Public Health Research Methods

Richard A. Crosby, PhD
Endowed Professor of Public Health
University of Kentucky

Laura F. Salazar, PhD
Professor, Director of PhD Program
School of Public Health
Georgia State University

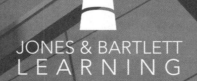

JONES & BARTLETT
LEARNING

World Headquarters
Jones & Bartlett Learning
5 Wall Street
Burlington, MA 01803
978-443-5000
info@jblearning.com
www.jblearning.com

Jones & Bartlett Learning books and products are available through most bookstores and online booksellers. To contact Jones & Bartlett Learning directly, call 800-832-0034, fax 978-443-8000, or visit our website, www.jblearning.com.

17606-3

Production Credits

VP, Product Management: Amanda Martin
Director of Product Management: Laura Pagluica
Product Manager: Sophie Fleck Teague
Product Specialist: Sara Bempkins
Project Specialist: Jennifer Risden
Digital Project Specialist: Angela Dooley
Senior Marketing Manager: Susanne Walker
VP, Manufacturing and Inventory Control: Therese Connell

Composition: Exela Technologies
Project Management: Exela Technologies
Cover Design: Michael O'Donnell
Senior Media Development Editor: Troy Liston
Rights Specialist: Liz Kincaid
Cover Image (Title Page, Chapter Opener):
    © science photo/Shutterstock
Printing and Binding: LSC Communications

Library of Congress Cataloging-in-Publication Data
Names: Crosby, Richard A., 1959- author. | Salazar, Laura Francisca, 1960- author.
Title: Essentials of public health research methods / Richard A. Crosby and Laura F. Salazar.
Description: Burlington, MA : Jones & Bartlett Learning, [2021] | Includes bibliographical references and index.
Identifiers: LCCN 2019050589 | ISBN 9781284175462 (paperback)
Subjects: MESH: Research Design | Public Health Systems Research–methods
Classification: LCC RA440.85 | NLM WA 20.5 | DDC 362.1072–dc23
LC record available at https://lccn.loc.gov/2019050589

6048

Printed in the United States of America

24 23 22 21 20   10 9 8 7 6 5 4 3 2 1

To the students for whom this book is intended. They are the future, and their passion and commitment to helping others will help put an end to health disparities.

—R. A. C. and L. F. S.

Brief Contents

Contents

Chapter 12 Data Management and Cleaning 161

Chapter 13 Parametric Data Analysis 187

with Anne Marie Schipani-McLaughlin

Chapter 14 Nonparametric Data Analysis 203

THE ESSENTIAL PUBLIC HEALTH SERIES

From the impact of AIDS to the cost of health care, this unique series will introduce you to the full range of issues that impact the public's health.

Current and Forthcoming Titles in the Essential Public Health Series:

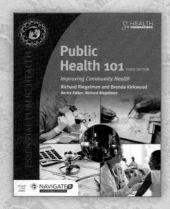

Public Health 101 THIRD EDITION
Improving Community Health
Richard Riegelman and Brenda Kirkwood
Series Editor: Richard Riegelman

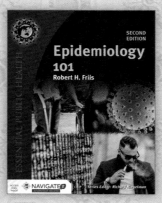

SECOND EDITION
Epidemiology 101
Robert H. Friis

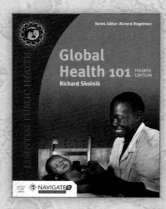

Series Editor: Richard Riegelman
Global Health 101 FOURTH EDITION
Richard Skolnik

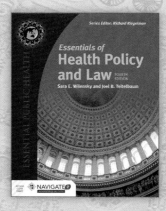

Series Editor: Richard Riegelman
Essentials of Health Policy and Law FOURTH EDITION
Sara E. Wilensky and Joel B. Teitelbaum

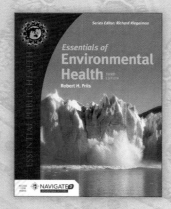

Series Editor: Richard Riegelman
Essentials of Environmental Health THIRD EDITION
Robert H. Friis

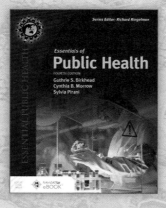

Series Editor: Richard Riegelman
Essentials of Public Health FOURTH EDITION
Guthrie S. Birkhead
Cynthia B. Morrow
Sylvia Pirani

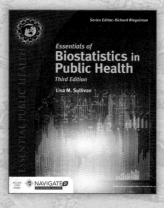

Series Editor: Richard Riegelman
Essentials of Biostatistics in Public Health Third Edition
Lisa M. Sullivan

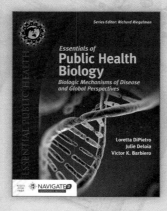

Series Editor: Richard Riegelman
Essentials of Public Health Biology
Biologic Mechanisms of Disease and Global Perspectives
Loretta DiPietro
Julie Deloia
Victor K. Barbiero

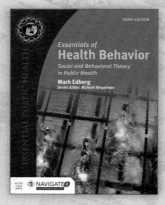

THIRD EDITION
Essentials of Health Behavior
Social and Behavioral Theory in Public Health
Mark Edberg
Series Editor: Richard Riegelman

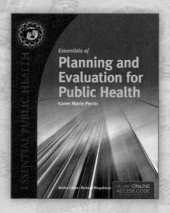

Essentials of Planning and Evaluation for Public Health
Karen Marie Perrin
Series Editor: Richard Riegelman

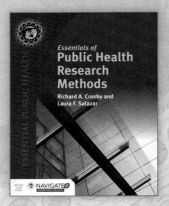

Essentials of
Public Health Research Methods
Richard A. Crosby and Laura F. Salazar

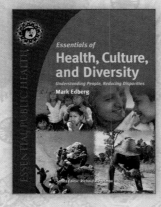

Essentials of
Health, Culture, and Diversity
Understanding People, Reducing Disparities
Mark Edberg
Series Editor: Richard Riegelman

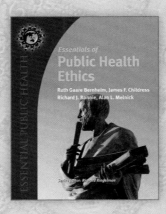

Essentials of
Public Health Ethics
Ruth Gaare Bernheim, James F. Childress
Richard J. Bonnie, Alan L. Melnick
Series Editor: Richard Riegelman

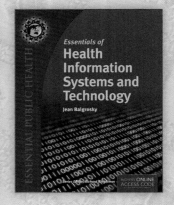

Essentials of
Health Information Systems and Technology
Jean Balgrosky

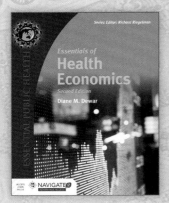

Series Editor: Richard Riegelman
Essentials of
Health Economics
Second Edition
Diane M. Dewar

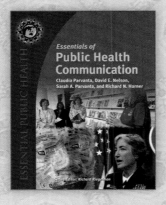

Essentials of
Public Health Communication
Claudia Parvanta, David E. Nelson,
Sarah A. Parvanta, and Richard N. Harner
Series Editor: Richard Riegelman

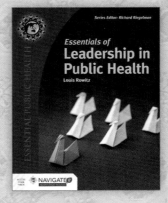

Series Editor: Richard Riegelman
Essentials of
Leadership in Public Health
Louis Rowitz

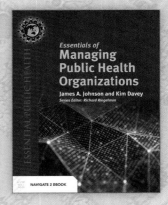

Essentials of
Managing Public Health Organizations
James A. Johnson and Kim Davey
Series Editor: Richard Riegelman

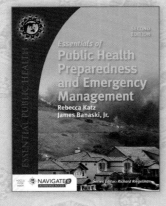

SECOND EDITION
Essentials of
Public Health Preparedness and Emergency Management
Rebecca Katz
James Banaski, Jr.
Series Editor: Richard Riegelman

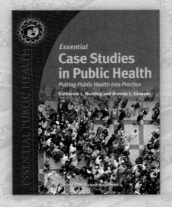

Essential
Case Studies in Public Health
Putting Public Health into Practice
Katherine L. Hunting and Brenda L. Gleason
Series Editor: Richard Riegelman

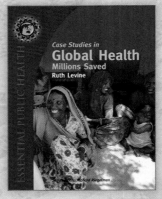

Case Studies in
Global Health
Millions Saved
Ruth Levine
Series Editor: Richard Riegelman

ABOUT THE EDITOR

Richard K. Riegelman, MD, MPH, PhD, is Professor of Epidemiology-Biostatistics, Medicine, and Health Policy, and Founding Dean of The George Washington University Milken Institute School of Public Health in Washington, DC. He has taken a lead role in developing the Educated Citizen and Public Health initiative which has brought together arts and sciences and public health education associations to implement the Institute of Medicine of the National Academies' recommendation that "…all undergraduates should have access to education in public health." Dr. Riegelman also led the development of The George Washington's undergraduate major and minor and currently teaches "Public Health 101" and "Epidemiology 101" to undergraduates.

www.EssentialPublicHealth.com

Foreword

Public health is often a career that is discovered after a first career is explored. A nurse, doctor, or other health professional may embrace the prevention and population dynamics in public health. A behavioral scientist may be attracted to the questions inherent in health maintenance, advocacy, and communication. Discovery of the cause of a given disease or condition lures biologists and social scientists alike to assess risk factors and etiologies. From a variety of backgrounds and interests, persons interested in environmental protection or in health equity and access to care may choose public health studies. When I did my own masters degree studies in public health almost 40 years ago, I was one of the youngest members of my class of 30, even though I had already completed my pediatrics training. For me, it is a source of immense satisfaction to see undergraduate programs in public and global health spring up, reflecting how students at colleges and universities are discovering the extraordinary preventive health challenges that need attention through the study of public health.

Not all undergraduate public health majors will become public health practitioners or researchers. But they come to their diverse careers in health care, policy, government service, or a variety of other fields with knowledge of social determinants of disease and how prevention can be more efficient and effective than application of a more limited, curative medical paradigm. They can apply their methodological expertise to a wide variety of topics, including that of the informed citizen and voter. As I write this foreword in 2020, we have entered a time of skepticism of science and its methods. "AntiVax" forces discourage childhood immunizations. Anti-regulatory forces lobby for the roll-back of environmental protection laws. Research into high-priority public health topics is inhibited or even blocked by special interests, as with gun violence or global climate change. It is more essential than ever that an informed citizenry study and interpret scientific data to make informed policy judgments.

This textbook now in your hands seeks to introduce population science methods to undergraduate public health students. Graduate students wishing a quick methods introduction will also find it useful. I predict that attorneys, journalists, healthcare workers, and policymakers will also find the introductory methodological material illuminating. Hence, its timely release helps empower us all to better dissect the fake news from the real science, the opinion from the fact, and the obfuscating from the elucidating.

I hope each reader will enjoy learning these methods. A value of methodological study is to see how one can distinguish a chance finding from one that may illustrate a causal relationship. The beauty of methods is to see how the same approaches might be applied across many topics and questions. The excitement of methods is to enable us to assess a question that might truly make a difference for humankind and Mother Earth. Top public health scientists have come together to present the core topics that underpin public health research and data interpretation. Your understanding of these topics will empower you for a lifetime, regardless of profession or avocation.

Sten H. Vermund, MD, PhD
Dean and Anna M.L. Lauder
Professor of Public Health
Yale School of Public Health
Professor of Pediatrics
Yale School of Medicine

Editor's Preface

Undergraduate public health education has grown exponentially during the first two decades of the 21st century. As majors and minors have developed, the need to introduce students to public health research methods has gained increasing importance.

Richard A. Crosby and Laura F. Salazar have written a unique book that fills this need. It provides an introduction to the full spectrum of knowledge and skills needed to research public health issues and apply them in practice. Their approach is based on what they call the *circular model of public health research*, which provides an organizing structure for their textbook, including framing the questions, identifying the study design, choosing methodology, data collection and analysis, and disseminating research findings

Using the metaphor of building a house, Crosby and Salazar systematically examine each component of the building process. They begin with an overview chapter that provides the framework for the textbook. The chapters follow a logical order, beginning with framing the research questions and ethical issues. The authors then examine the range of study types used in public health research, including community-based participatory research, qualitative research, observational research designs, experimental research designs, and quasi-experimental designs.

The chapters continue with a look at methods for data collection, including defining the study population, sampling techniques, and measurement. The data-analysis chapters start with data cleaning and management and continue on to introduce parametric and nonparametric approaches to data analysis. The text concludes with a chapter devoted to dissemination of research and defining follow-up research issues.

Crosby and Salazar bring their own research and experiences to writing the textbook, using extensive examples that bring the text to life. Their writing is approachable and does not require extensive quantitative coursework. Their creative mascots, Snow and Hamilton, help emphasize their key points.

The authors aim to provide students with what they refer to as a *working knowledge*. The use of this textbook provides the basis for an introductory public health research course that can stand on its own and provide the foundation for students to understand a comprehensive approach to public health research along with a solid grounding for more advanced education in research design and analysis.

Examples of research illustrating each component of the process are provided. The emphasis is on developing evidence-based practice, which requires practice-based evidence. Thus, Crosby and Salazar's text goes beyond the traditional approach to research, which stops with efficacy or how well an intervention works under research conditions. It goes on to address questions of effectiveness or how well interventions work in practice.

As the series editor of the *Essential Public Health* series, I am pleased that *Essentials of Public Health Research Methods* is now part of the series. It adds an increasingly important approach to teaching public health research not only as a technical skill but also as a way of looking at the connections between research and practice. I am confident that you will find the book provides an organized, thought-provoking, and widely applicable approach to public health research.

Richard Riegelman, MD, MPH, PhD
Professor and Founding Dean
Milken Institute School of Public Health
The George Washington University
Jones & Bartlett Learning
Essential Public Health Series Editor

Authors' Preface

As the idea of treating disease after it occurs slowly erodes and yields to the emerging paradigm of prevention, it becomes more important than ever to refine public health practice through rigorous research. This volume in the *Essential Public Health* series is designed to provide a road map to conducting basic research that can inform the practices, procedures, and policies of public health. Throughout the chapters, we embrace the concept that public health activities span the fields of epidemiology (the study of determinants, conditions, and patterns that influence health and disease), public health management (the design and oversight of healthcare systems), public health policy (leadership and regulation of public health practice and environmental influences on health and disease), and health promotion (the prevention of disease through the application of the social and behavioral sciences).

The explicit goal of learning the content presented in the following chapters is to build your professional acumen to understand the research you "consume" and to conduct your own research when opportunities arise. The implicit goal is to become inspired by the endless possibilities to constantly improve public health practice through the use of creative ideas that are tested empirically. As you read each chapter, please consider how the concepts apply specifically to work that you are (or will) take on as part of your role in protecting the health of the public. As noted in the *Framing the Future* initiative (as sponsored by the Association of Schools and Programs of Public Health), students preparing for careers in public health are expected to possess abilities relative to planning research, data collection, and data analysis and applying these research skills to evidence-based practice.

As a final suggestion before you begin learning about the various methodologies of public health research, please consider this volume as your guide to starting and completing a highly successful capstone, thesis, or honors paper. Indeed, in our experience, students often have trepidations about a culminating research experience, with their concerns typically focused on the question of "How do I conduct a research study?" In many ways, it is for this very reason that we have constructed the following chapters: We want you to be inspired by the importance of public health research and simultaneously empowered to take on a project that you can call your own.

Acknowledgments

First and foremost, we both wish to acknowledge and—more important—thank an incredible person and an amazing scholar who patiently mentored each of us during our postdoc years and then (almost imperceptibly) guided our careers as the years unfolded. His name is Ralph J. DiClemente, a name known widely in public health circles both domestically and abroad. His dedication to public health always inspired us, and his love of "getting it right" constantly kept us finding new and better ways to make a difference. Like so many other professors who work in public health practice and research, we are merely two people among hundreds who have been taught, inspired, and moved by this wonderful man.

We would also like to acknowledge our former editor at Jones & Bartlett Learning, Mike Brown, who has been our greatest supporter and a champion of this book. Also, we wish to acknowledge our new Jones & Bartlett Learning editor, Sophie Teague, who has been an enthusiast of our work and a true problem solver throughout this process and whenever issues arose. Sara Bempkins of Jones & Bartlett Learning has been an absolute delight to work with; we greatly appreciate her efficient and positive attitude and keeping things moving forward. Furthermore, we would like to extend our thanks to our main contributor, Dr. Anne Marie Schipani-McLaughlin, for her support while we wrote this textbook, her significant contributions on several chapters, and her humor and input on the memes of our beloved public health mascots Snow and Hamilton. We would also like to acknowledge our undergraduate public health interns, Allyson Salazar, Lily Baldwin, and Dori Balser for their due diligence and helpful and constructive feedback on our chapters. A special thanks to Lily Baldwin and Jhoan Dutton for their expertise in making many of our amazing and professional figures.

About the Authors

Richard A. Crosby, PhD, is an endowed professor of public health at the University of Kentucky. Dr. Crosby's research has been highly focused on promoting condom use for populations most at risk of HIV and STD acquisition. Dr. Crosby's PhD is from the School of Public Health at Indiana University (1998). After receiving his doctorate, he completed a 3-year postdoctoral fellowship (2001), funded by the American Association of Teachers of Preventive Medicine and occurring at the Centers for Disease Control and Prevention (CDC), as well as Emory University's Rollins School of Public Health. Since completing this postdoctoral fellowship, Dr. Crosby has been consistently funded by the National Institutes of Health (NIH) and by the CDC. In recent years, his research has expanded to include work with sexual and gender minority youth pertaining to food security, low-income rural women at elevated risk of cervical cancer, and pregnancy prevention among young minority males residing in urban foster care facilities. Having published more than 400 peer-reviewed journal articles and book chapters, Dr. Crosby's current passion lies in writing textbooks that greatly aid the teaching and learning process for students who have dedicated their careers to public health practice and research.

Laura F. Salazar, PhD, is a Professor and Director of the PhD Program at Georgia State University's School of Public Health. Dr. Salazar's research has been devoted to helping prevent and ameliorate violence against women and HIV and AIDS. She was trained as a community psychologist at Georgia State University (GSU) where she received her PhD (2001). She also completed a National Research Service Award postdoctoral fellowship in HIV and AIDS at Emory University's School of Medicine (2003). Before joining the faculty at GSU in 2011, Dr. Salazar was a member of the faculty at Emory University's Rollins School of Public Health. Her research has been funded by the NIH and the CDC and includes the use of educational entertainment in the form of serial drama episodes, social media marketing, and web-based approaches to expand the reach of public health efforts. Most recently, Dr. Salazar's research has expanded to focus on understanding the determinants of mental and physical health disparities experienced by sexual and gender minorities with an emphasis on contextual and structural-level factors. Dr. Salazar has published more than 150 journal articles in medical, public health, and social science journals and is the author of more than 30 book chapters and coauthor of four other public health textbooks. Dr. Salazar teaches advanced research methods and intervention development and evaluation for public health.

▶ Contributor

Anne Marie Schipani-McLaughlin, PhD, MPH, is a postdoctoral fellow in the Georgia State University School of Public Health as part of the Urban Drivers for Resilient Youth Initiative. She earned her PhD in Health Promotion and Behavior from the University of Georgia College of Public Health and her master's degree in Public Health from Emory University Rollins School of Public Health. Dr. Schipani-McLaughlin's research program focuses on interpersonal violence prevention and alcohol use and intervention development using innovative technologies.

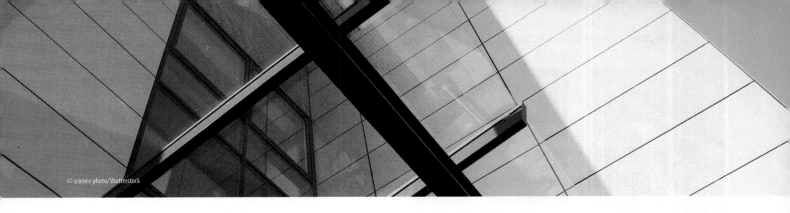
© science photo/Shutterstock

CHAPTER 1

Shaping Public Health Through Research and Practice

▶ Overview

The origins of public health practice extend back in time to iconic stories such as that of Dr. John Snow (1813–1858). Snow influenced a city council to remove the handle from the Broad Street pump that supplied cholera-contaminated water to people living in the Soho district of London, England, in 1854. Snow's seemingly simple solution to the cholera epidemic was far from just a hunch or bit of intuition. In fact, Snow created detailed maps of deaths in the area that were caused by cholera and then started looking for commonalities. His mapping not only informed the intervention (i.e., the disabling of the pump for these areas) but also provided a method for evaluating the intervention and became the premier research design (i.e., the **case-control design**) used in the public health discipline of **epidemiology**.

Another iconic figure in public health is Dr. Alice Hamilton (1869–1970). Hamilton is deemed the pioneer

of occupational epidemiology. She first led an investigation into a typhoid epidemic in Chicago in 1902 and then went on to have a long career in public health that started with her appointment as a medical investigator to the newly formed Illinois Commission on Occupational Diseases. Hamilton led the commission's investigations, which focused research on industrial poisons such as lead and other toxins and their effects. She also authored a groundbreaking report that documented the different industrial processes that exposed workers to lead poisoning and other illnesses. Hamilton's efforts resulted in the passage of the first workers' compensation laws in Illinois in 1911 and Indiana in 1915 and occupational disease laws in other states. The new laws required employers to take precautions to protect workers who were experiencing multiple workplace safety hazards. Both John Snow and Alice Hamilton (pictured in **FIGURE 1.1**) are considered pioneers in public health research and practice because their groundbreaking efforts resulted in

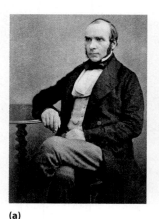 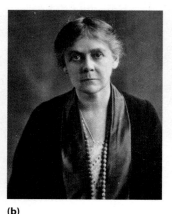

(a)   **(b)**

FIGURE 1.1 **(a)** John Snow; **(b)** Alice Hamilton.

(a) Wellcome Collection; (b) U.S. National Library of Medicine.

major improvements in public health. Their methods and policies remain relevant today.

The larger lesson here is that research (defined throughout this text as a systematic collection of data intended to inform public health practice) is the cornerstone of intervention policies and practices as applied to public health. To better illustrate the central nature of research in public health practice, consider the present-day example of taxing the sale of alcohol as a method of reducing its consumption. Raising taxes on alcohol may seem an intuitive approach to reducing consumption; indeed, a review of 72 empirical studies provides informed evidence of a robust correlation between the price of alcohol and purchase. This correlation is *inverse*—meaning that as one of these measures (i.e., the price) rises, the other measure (i.e., sales) falls. Collectively, these 72 studies further suggest that an effective method of preventing alcohol-related problems is to simply raise taxes on sales, with the caveat being that the

effect will play out differently, depending on people's level of disposable income and their willingness to spend more money on alcohol (see **FIGURE 1.2**) (Elder et al., 2010).

Whether research informs the removal of a pump handle, workplace safety policies, taxes on alcohol, efforts to promote uptake of vaccines, new programs designed to promote cardiovascular exercise, or social media marketing programs that promote breast and cervical cancer screening, it is inevitably the starting and ending point of all public health programs. Given the interdependence of public health research and practice, this chapter describes three primary strategies used to shape public health practice through the systematic collection of data: (1) research directed to practical implications for practice, (2) testing intervention programs to become evidence-based practices, and (3) testing policy-level changes designed for widespread dissemination.

▶ How Are Research and Practice Interdependent and Reciprocal?

FIGURE 1.3 displays what we have termed the "circular model of public health research." In addition to being a succinct visualization of the reciprocal nature of research and practice, this model is used to organize the subsequent chapters in this textbook. The model begins with the most crucial step: framing the research questions. Far from an easy-to-complete first step, this involves a thorough understanding of the field as it exists, including the gaps in knowledge and issues in practice. Once these gaps and issues are understood, the task becomes one of prioritizing

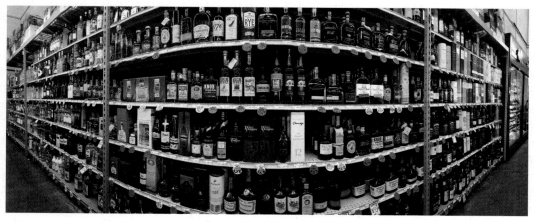

FIGURE 1.2 Bottles of Alcohol at Liquor Store.

© Mihai_Andritoiu/Shutterstock

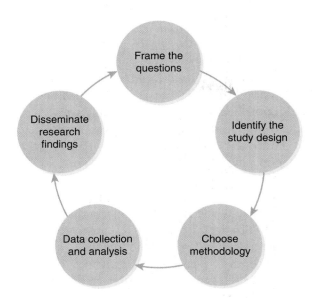

FIGURE 1.3 Circular Model of Public Health Research.

what can realistically be done to address these gaps through the systematic collection of data. Finding the gap in research that is critical to improving public health but also meets your own requirements (i.e., it is consistent with your expertise and it is within your abilities and resources to conduct the requisite research) is perhaps the most important step in the research cycle. Chapter 2 will guide you through the complete process of selecting and framing research questions designed to inform public health practice. For now, let us provide you with an example from our own research.

As the field of public health first began talking of "ending AIDS" in the United States, it was not clear how to achieve this goal because there were so many gaps in our understanding of what the disease was, who was affected, and how they were being affected. Once scientists discovered what was causing the condition (i.e., the newly discovered human immunodeficiency virus, or HIV), who was mostly affected, and what the risk factors were, prevention efforts were initiated, implemented, and tested for efficacy. Progress toward achieving goals of eradication, however, was focused on targeting those populations comprising the majority of new cases of HIV. Thus, research regarding behavioral and biomedical solutions to averting AIDS was intensified for key populations such as men having sex with men, injection drug users, and later, high-risk heterosexual women. Although this research was extremely valuable, it missed a tiny population: transgender women.

Transgender women experience disproportionate rates of HIV worldwide with estimates averaging

around 19% (i.e., nearly one of every five women) (Baral et al., 2013). Although we might expect this global estimate to be greater than the estimate specific for the United States, this is not at all the case. On the contrary, U.S. estimates range as high as 56.3%. So, doing a quick bit of mental math, you will see that the rate is three times greater than the global estimate. This should be alarming. What is even more alarming is that the value of 56.3% pertains to transgender women who identify as Black. Rates for those who identify as White or Hispanic are far lower—16.7% and 16.1%, respectively (Herbst et al., 2008). Somewhat later, the first *National HIV/AIDS Strategy* for the United States was published in 2010. This landmark document consequently prioritized HIV prevention for transgender individuals; however, it was not until 2015 when the strategy was updated that transgender women, specifically those identifying as Black (Office of National AIDS Policy, 2015), were prioritized. As we began to review the literature relative to HIV-prevention programming specific to Black transgender women, we found a surprising dearth of options. This was a gap, but we soon realized the gap extended far beyond HIV prevention.

As we continued to review the literature, we soon discovered that the context of daily life for transgender women, especially those identifying as Black, was all too often characterized by terms such as *chronic daily stress, victimization, discrimination, stigma, transphobia*, and *employment prejudice*, as well as *economic instability* and *housing instability*. We then learned that estimates suggested that approximately 1 million people living in the United States identified as transgender, with about twice as many being male to female rather than female to male (Crissman Berger, Graham, & Dalton, 2017). To make a bleak picture even worse, we then learned that discrimination and barriers to transgender-related healthcare were common in the United States. The barriers were further exacerbated by a lack of training on the part of clinical psychologists and healthcare providers relative to understanding and respecting gender diversity (Dickey, 2017).

At this point, we realized that the gap actually represented a lack of research designed to understand the context underlying the lives of most Black transgender women residing in the United States. To address this gap, we conducted a pilot study of 92 transgender women, most of whom identified as Black, living in Atlanta, Georgia (Salazar et al., 2017). What we found was rather stunning and incredibly sad. For instance, the majority of the sample was not employed full-time or in school (62.5%). A majority had engaged in commercial sex work (58.1%), did not have health insurance (52.7%), and had experienced multiple traumas: childhood sexual abuse (51.6%), intimate partner violence (55.9%), rape (52.7%), and jail or prison (57%). Further, homelessness in the preceding 12 months was reported by nearly one-half of the sample (48.9%). To make a dismal life context even less conducive to mental and physical health, nearly one-half of the sample reported being harassed by police because of being transgender women (46.8%) and was experiencing social or economic discrimination based on being transgender (48.4%). At this juncture in our careers, we began to escalate and prioritize the research attention we devoted to the mental and physical health and well-being of transgender women of color residing in urban areas of the southern United States. This work has since resulted in multiple publications of studies, all of which were designed around our identification of this initial gap (e.g., Crosby, Salazar, & Hill, 2016; Crosby, Salazar, & Hill, 2018; Crosby, Salazar, Hill, & Mena, 2018; and Hill et al., 2018).

Returning to the circular model, the second step of the model is one that demands a working knowledge of the varied options available with research designs. Much like the design of a house, research designs span a range from the fairly simple to the highly complex and to a host of hybrid designs that serve distinct purposes. The design itself is open to slight modifications—a necessary point given the vast array of possible research questions. Unlike the design of a house, research designs are not selected per se; instead, the task is to match the research question with the optimally appropriate design. Chapters 5 through 8 will provide you with the needed list of options to arrive at this match.

The third step in the model is to formulate the methodology needed to "move into the study design." In this sense, **methodology** refers to techniques required to fulfill the conditions of any given study design. For instance, study designs entail selecting a **sample** of the study population rather than all people or elements of that population. Chapters 9 and 10 offer a complete understanding of the techniques related to **sampling** from a **population**. Again using the metaphor of a house, study designs also offer a great deal of latitude in terms of the choices you make relevant to the measurement tools and measurement instruments you select (the "interior design of the home"). Chapter 11 will give you the basic skills needed to further refine your methodology through carefully selected measures and techniques of eliciting valid responses from study participants.

At this juncture, we hasten to add that measurement is often the single most critical aspect of methodology. Returning to our example from step one (our own story of how we embarked on a research trajectory of mental and physical health for transgender women of color), consider the health risk of chronic daily stress. Ample evidence implicates chronic daily stress in the deterioration of the human immune system and a general decline in physical and mental health (Bariola et al., 2015; Bockting, Miner, Swinburn Romine, Hamilton, & Coleman, 2013; Nuttbrock et al. 2014; Sevelius, 2013). The problem, as you might imagine, is that the experience of chronic daily stress presents a tremendous challenge to any researcher who intends to accurately assess its depth and frequency. Ultimately, we rejected the idea that self-reported measures could adequately capture a realistic portrait of how this experience might be lived on a daily basis across large numbers of study volunteers. We then explored the use of biological markers. **Biomarkers** are typically some type of chemical, antigen, hormone, or metabolite that will fluctuate as a function of changes to a given system in the human body. For instance, biomarkers for an enzyme that is only present in people who smoke have been widely used to validate self-reports of people quitting tobacco use.

We initially considered the use of telomeres to assess chronic daily stress. Telomeres are the end caps on strands of DNA; shortening caps signal cellular decay and ultimately death. One problem with the measure involved expense because the assay was difficult to conduct and therefore was quite costly. Next, we considered the use of elevated levels of catecholamines, a family of stress hormones, but later dismissed this option because of a lack of convincing evidence that elevation would fairly capture chronic daily stress. We finally entertained the biomarker of Epstein-Barr virus and constructed the following paragraph for a grant proposal to the National Institutes of Health.

> The dried blood spot test for Epstein Barr virus (EBV) will be incorporated as a time-varying covariate and included in two-way interaction terms with concurrent and subsequent time-varying risk factor measures. Because EBV is the most common herpes virus, with 90% of adults being infected, this is our selected biomarker for chronic daily stress. The assay uses 5 drops of whole blood collected through a finger-stick and placed on standard filter paper. The specimen can be stored at room temperature for up to 8 weeks and it is not considered a biohazard. The assay

determines the level of antibody titer to EBV. To keep assessment burden minimized, this assay will only be included in the baseline, 9-month, and 18-month assessments (yielding pre–post measures for two extended time periods of 9 months each).

Then, true to the intent to have more than one measure of chronic daily stress, we also included a self-reported measure in the baseline, 9-month, and 18-month assessments. This comprised a 24-item scale measure of chronic daily stress.

Ultimately, your selection of the best possible measures for the design and research question will dictate how you go about the soon-to-be planned process of systematically collecting data. Step four in the model comprises data collection and the subsequent task of data analysis. These related challenges are ongoing throughout a study and thus constitute the parallel of "living in the house" by use of our metaphor. Rather than being a planning step (as were the first three steps of this model), this fourth step is action oriented and defines the beginning and end of the study period.

To provide a flavor for the complexities and labor-intensive aspects of data analysis, although we cover this in-depth in Chapters 13 and 14, we highlight the step of data coding and data management because this step precedes data analysis. This process of data coding and management is often one that occupies a staff member on a full-time basis. It begins with the creation of what is known as a **codebook**. As its name implies, a codebook provides a key to naming study variables and, more importantly, to assigning a numerical value to each possible response to a given questionnaire item. This process is preliminary to data management because it establishes the method of translating people's responses on questionnaires into a data spreadsheet. **BOX 1.1** provides an excerpted example of a codebook used in a study that we conducted in Jackson, Mississippi. As you view Box 1.1, please note that each possible response to each question is assigned a numerical value. Also, please note that each entry has a variable name. For instance, "Q25Household__Members_A" is the variable capturing data informing us about the living arrangements of study participants (i.e., living alone, with a parent, with a family member who is not a parent, etc.).

BOX 1.1 Excerpt from a Study Codebook

Q1Initials_A Question for the RA: What are your initials (first and last name only)?
Q2IDQuestion for the RA: What is the participant's I.D. number?
Intervention Question for the RA: What is the participant's randomization code?

☐ MAC (1)
☐ PC (2)

Q3_1Age_A (please enter in number of years) _____
Q25Household__Members_A
Who do you live with?

☐ Alone (1)
☐ Partner (2)
☐ Parents (3)
☐ Other family members (4)
☐ Friends (5)
☐ Roommates (6)
☐ Other (7)

In the past 12 months, what were the different types of places that you lived? (please check ALL that apply)

☐ A house or apartment you paid for (1) Q26_1Housing_PrimaryFunding_A
☐ A house or apartment someone else paid for (2) Q26_2Housing_SecondFunding_A
☐ A motel, hotel, or boarding house (3) Q26_3Housing_Secondliving_A
☐ A car, on the street, or in a homeless shelter (4) Q26_4Housing_Homeless_A
☐ A halfway house or other transitional house (5) Q26_5Housing_TransitLiving_A
☐ A mental health facility (6) Q26_6Housing_MHFacility_A
☐ A sober living environment (7) Q26_7Housing_SLEnvironment_A
☐ A drug treatment facility (8) Q26_8Housing_DTFacility_A
☐ Other (9) _____ Q26_9Housing_Other_A

(continues)

BOX 1.1 Excerpt from a Study Codebook   *(continued)*

Q27Housing_Current_A
Currently, where do you live?

☐ A house or apartment you paid for (1)
☐ A house or apartment someone else paid for (2)
☐ A motel, hotel, or boarding house (3)
☐ A car, on the street, or in a homeless shelter (4)
☐ A halfway house or other transitional house (5)
☐ A mental health facility (6)
☐ A sober living environment (7)
☐ A drug treatment facility (8)
☐ Other (9) _____

Q28Housing_CrrntTime_A
How long have you been living there?

☐ Less than a month (1)
☐ At least 1 month, but less than 3 months (2)
☐ At least 3 months, but less than 6 months (3)
☐ At least 6 months, but less than a year (4)
☐ At least a year (5)
☐ None of the above (6)

Q29SexRelat_Status_A
Are you currently involved in a regular and ongoing sexual relationship that is important to you?

☐ Yes (1)
☐ No (2)

Step 5 is the one that is far too often neglected: actually sharing the findings with the people engaged in public health practice. Chapter 15 addresses the most effective methods of achieving this goal. We urge you to be as vigilant about the fifth step as you would be about any previous step in the model, bearing in mind that public health is indeed a public activity.

As shown in Figure 1.3, the model "ends" by a feedback loop to the research question itself. In this context, think of feedback as a type of news report, one that answers the original research question. Of course, this answer will be a matter of degree, meaning that you will have insights and ideas as to the answer, but during the research process, you may also come across aspects (albeit these may be small) of the research question that were not answered by your systematic collection of data. As opposed to seeing this as a shortcoming, any deficiencies in your answer deserve to be transformed into opportunities for the next cycle of research pertaining to the same question. Although this entire process may seem like you are running in circles, you are essentially building critical knowledge. This cycle, in fact, is the essence of research and accentuates the point that research is a shared endeavor—with any given research question being addressed by dozens, if not hundreds, of research-to-practice

scholars such as you. At the end of each cycle, findings are disseminated to the field; however, they are also used to inform the next cycle of research along the same lines of inquiry.

Now that you understand the circular nature of research, you can also easily imagine that it is best viewed as an evolution, not a revolution. Indeed, the stereotype of laboratory-confined researcher involves "breakthroughs" and "discoveries," neither of which occur in public health research. Instead, public health research can be viewed along an evolutionary continuum, one that begins with practice-based implications from basic research questions, progresses to tests of research-refined practice, and ultimately culminates in the positive evaluation of new practice methods applied to prevent disease and promote health.

As you progress through this text, it will become apparent that this evolutionary nature of research defines its place in practice. Without research, practice standards would be set by intuition and, even worse, potentially guided by preexisting values and beliefs held by practitioners. As long as public health practice is guided by science, it will remain a vital part of the global response to existing and emerging threats to the quality and quantity of human life.

What Type of Research Has Immediate and Direct Implications for Practice?

To begin, consider the point that millions of people do not have ready or affordable access to healthcare services. Inverting the paradigm of having "people see doctors," we can envision practices that include home-based screening for conditions such as pending heart disease, precancerous growths, and elevated levels of blood sugar signaling prediabetic conditions. A key question for public health practice is whether it is practical to have people self-collect specimens, at home or in other nonclinical settings, that can be sent to a laboratory for testing (averting the immediate need for people to attend a clinic). For example, a simple test exists that determines the presence of any precancerous growth in the colon (note that colorectal cancer is the second leading cause of cancer death in the United States). The test only requires that the user touch a smallish paint brush to a new stool specimen and then dab the stool sample on a pretreated cardboard flap that is sealed and thus ready for laboratory analysis. This is known as the *fecal immunochemical test* (FIT).

The research question here is, will people complete this kit at home and faithfully return it for processing by U.S. postal mail or by using a drop-off location? Consider the importance of knowing the answers to this question. What if, for example, the research found that only one-third of all people receiving a free kit actually self-collected the specimen, and that less than half of these people actually returned their completed kits. Further, suppose that 90% of the returned kits were collected from drop-off locations, with only 10% being sent by mail. So, what would these research findings tell us about practice? Perhaps, for example:

- Kits should only be given to people who are willing to be contacted repeatedly if they do not return them within 7 to 10 days;
- The expense of using prepaid postage for kits when they are given out in person may not be worth the yield in terms of return; and
- Increasing the number of drop-off locations may produce higher overall return rates of kits.

BOX 1.2 provides a more in-depth view of this example relative to FIT screening for colorectal cancer. Given this example, what do you think are the primary

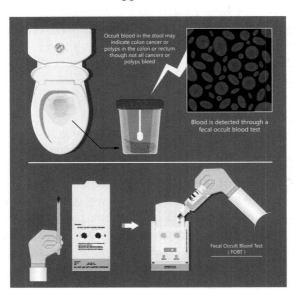

Fecal Immunochemical Test (FIT).

Rumruay/Shutterstock, Inc.

BOX 1.2 Summary of Study Investigating the Completion and Return of "Second" Test Kits for Early Detection of Colorectal Cancer

The fecal immunochemical test is designed to be used *annually*. Thus, one problem with implementing this new technology lies in the issue of how to best promote annual use of FIT as opposed to a single one-time use. For this reason, a study was conducted of 229 people who had completed an initial screening with FIT. The goal of the study was to then determine the number who completed a second test one year later. The study also investigated factors related to completing a second FIT. Of the 229, 10.8% completed and returned a FIT kit within approximately one year. Of 14 factors tested for association with completing a second annual test, 5 were significant at $P < 05$. These were:

1. Women were more likely to complete a second annual test than men, with the difference between them greater than fourfold.
2. Persons perceiving themselves as being overweight or obese were nearly three times as likely to complete a second annual test compared to those not indicating this perception.
3. A similarly large effect was observed relative to indicating whether the initial FIT was "easy to complete," with this difference favoring those who indicated ease of completion.
4. People indicating worry about colorectal cancer were more than twice as likely to complete a second annual test compared to those who were less worried.
5. Older age was associated with completing the second FIT test. Among those completing the second test, the mean age was 61.9 years, compared to 56.0 years among those not completing a second test ($t = 2.69$, $df = 227$, $P = .008$).

implications relative to public health practice? (Please read the box carefully before answering.) For instance, is it possible that completion rates of less than 11% are simply a product of people forgetting to take the test? If so, then what are the messages or incentives that may help people create an annual habit of completing a FIT kit? Of course, the range of possible answers to these questions, as well as the number of other questions that could be posed, is nearly infinite. The point here is that public health research should be designed to yield practical findings that can then serve as a basis for shaping practice. Indeed, this ethic of *research to practice* is one way in which public health research differs from research in fields such as psychology, sociology, and anthropology.

Another example of an at-home testing kit is the OraQuick test for HIV. The OraQuick test can be performed at home or in another discrete location (Hurt & Powers, 2014). This testing kit allows an individual to take a mouth swab and receive results within 20 to 40 minutes. One research question regarding OraQuick is, how likely is it that an individual will seek medical care after a positive test? Normally, a clinic can immediately start treatment if a patient attends an appointment and tests positive for HIV; however, those who test positive with the OraQuick testing kit must reach out to a clinic to receive further treatment. If results of a study show that individuals who test positive are not likely to subsequently see a physician for treatment, there may not be a net benefit to the at-home testing kit. This may provide evidence against the at-home version of the testing kit and guide our practices for HIV testing.

In these scenarios, the research-to-practice implications are both immediate and direct. The research findings guide practice, much like a map guides navigation. This form of research is typically easy to conduct and requires far fewer resources than the types of research described in the next two sections. Typical research designs that can be used to directly inform practice include the **cross-sectional design** and prospective design (see Chapter 6).

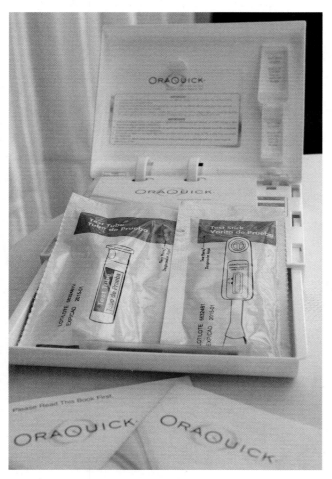

The OraQuick Test for Human Immunodeficiency Virus (HIV).

▶ What Is Evidence-Based Practice?

Often considered the hallmark of public health, evidence-based practice is formed through a somewhat regulated process of turning research from randomized controlled trials (see Chapter 7) into practice-based programs that function effectively in real-world settings. The process is one that can take more than a decade to complete, so it is best suited to public health problems that *do not require urgent responses*. Alternatively, the advantage of this often-lengthy process is that it builds a repository of tested programs that can be used with confidence in various practice settings. In fact, the Community Prevention Services Task Force (an independent panel commissioned by the U.S. Department of Health and Human Services) regularly updates and publishes *The Community Guide*, which is available in book form (see Community Prevention Services Task Force, n.d.).

As previously noted, the first step in the process of creating an evidence-based program is to conduct what many professionals consider to be the definitive form of research: a **randomized controlled trial (RCT)**. This process alone may take 5 or more years to complete. RCTs are labor intensive and thus costly. Further, numerous pitfalls and events may easily compromise the integrity of an RCT. Even when one is conducted "perfectly," there is absolutely no assurance that significant differences between groups (known as **effect size**) will be found.

Next, and only if the RCT yields significantly favorable findings, the program must be replicated in

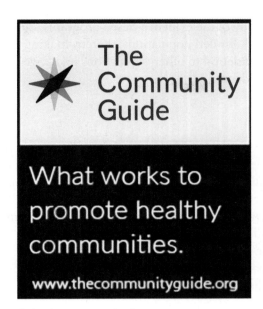

Cover of *The Community Guide.*

a nonresearch setting. This, of course, is the first step of removing the program from its rather artificial academic origins to settings that begin to mirror actual public health practice. This is known as an **effectiveness trial**. The primary difference between the RCT (known as an **efficacy trial**) and the effectiveness trial is that the latter does not necessarily use a control group and is most often conducted in real-world settings. (You will learn more about control groups in Chapter 7.) Again, however, even without a control group, an effectiveness trial can take 2 to 3 years to complete. It is, however, imperative that effectiveness trials take place because this is the only method to ascertain whether the intervention program really works when taken out of the context of the tightly controlled conditions of a randomized trial. **TABLE 1.1** provides a comparison of goals and methods of efficacy trials versus goals and methods of effectiveness trials. As the table readily reveals, it is as though we are comparing apples to oranges: The two modalities actually have little in common. So, again, we emphasize that you must do both types of trials. An efficacy trial that is not followed up by an effectiveness trial leaves the question of whether there are real-world application effects completely unanswered.

If the findings from the effectiveness trial are significantly favorable, the next step becomes one of *manualizing* the program, a process that includes developing guides for training the people who implement the program. With this process consuming as many as another 3 years, you can easily see how at least a decade of time passes before a new intervention idea becomes a practice-based reality. The start-to-finish process has been estimated to last as long as 17 years (Morris, Wooding, & Grant, 2011). Of course, as you

TABLE 1.1 A Comparison of Efficacy Trials to Effectiveness Trials	
Efficacy Trials	**Effectiveness Trials**
The goal is to establish effects in highly controlled conditions.	The goal is to show that an intervention program can work in practice settings.
The test population is highly homogenous.	The test population mirrors the diversity found in public health practice settings.
People enroll in a study and are typically paid to complete study assessments.	People are not enrolled in a study; instead they are real-world recipients of the program. Incentives for their participation are not provided.
The setting is largely artificial; it is a product of the ample resources that so often exist for efficacy trials.	The setting is a reflection for normal circumstances that surround the practice environment.
Project staff are specifically hired and trained to conduct the study, and the entire process has oversight from supervisors.	Project staff are typically "shared" with other employment positions such as medical providers, employees of a health department, and volunteers in agencies of community-based organizations.
Findings are analyzed in the context of rather sophisticated models that account for extraneous variables and potentially confounding factors.	The findings are typically not subjected to correction factors.

can easily imagine, public health changes quickly over 17 years, as does the way the public perceives and reacts to prevention messages, prevention programs, and medical recommendations. Consider, for instance, that citywide bike-to-work programs are a relatively recent microtransportation option. Although public health professionals may not have directly inspired these programs, they are nonetheless serving the goals of public health via the aerobic benefits reaped by those who faithfully bike to work on a daily basis and through the reduction in emissions from cars. In the 17 years or so it may have taken to translate an urban fitness program into public health practice, such a program may well be obsolete (given the existence of bike-to-work programs) by the time it is put into practice. The key point here is that public health "moves quickly," so it is imperative to begin testing programs that do not require a 17-year window between inception and practice. This imperative is especially applicable to the prevention of emerging infectious diseases.

Given that the development of evidence-based practices is a time-consuming process, their availability is limited, so *The Community Guide* (for example) constitutes a powerful force that shapes public health practice. However, it is important that you recognize the following strengths and weaknesses of adopting these programs.

Weaknesses

■ The time lag may mean that some programs are not consistent with the more recent social and political changes of a society.

■ Many of the evidence-based programs are tested with limited populations, thereby making their translation to other populations less driven by evidence.

Strengths

■ Evidence-based programs typically contain "core elements"; these can sometimes be adopted to other populations (those not included in the original RCTs).

■ Only a small percentage of all tested programs successfully progress through the entire translation process; this implies that those passing through the entire process have been thoroughly tested.

▶ How Does Research Inform Policy-Level Interventions?

Increasingly, public health practice relies on the quest to find modest changes in policy that can lead to large-scale changes in health behaviors. **TABLE 1.2** provides numerous examples of these types of intervention.

An eloquent advantage of these types of policy-level intervention programs is that they can be tested for effectiveness, bypassing the preliminary step of efficacy testing (as described in the previous

TABLE 1.2 Examples of Policy-Level Interventions Designed to Influence Health Behavior

Example	Description	Source
Promoting "walkable" environments	Programs were implemented to favorably alter use of existing space for walking.	Kerr et al., 2010
Taxes on soda to reduce consumption	A Berkeley, California, soda tax reduced soft drink consumption and increased sales of water.	Falbe at al., 2016
Averting violent crime through altering the physical environment	A Seattle-based project showed that strategic changes to urban space can reduce violent crime.	Sohn, 2016
"Take the Stairs" campaign	A university program increased activity levels of employees by making stair use more aesthetic.	Quick et al., 2015
Hands-free cell phone traffic laws	In 2001, New York became the first state to ban use of all handheld devices to promote safe driving.	McCartt et al. 2014
Sodium Reduction Communities Programs	Thirty Arkansas schools implemented food-preparation guidelines to reduce sodium content in meals.	Long et al., 2018

section). Accordingly, the time frame needed to demonstrate the value of a policy-level program is far shorter than that for evidence-based programs. As a rule of thumb, the time frame corresponds with the period of time needed for a tangible outcome to occur (or not occur) within the geographic area experiencing the policy change. Thus, for example, if the goal was to reduce body mass index (BMI) through a sweetened-beverage tax, a reasonable study period would be 1 year (because this would be ample time to observe whether the tax led to enough lowered sweetened-beverage consumption to produce significant drops in mean BMI levels within the area).

Although policy-level research has a time advantage over research used for evidence-based programs, the disadvantage involves a requirement to assess change across the entire area impacted by the policy change. This need implies that **quasi-experimental designs** should be applied (see Chapter 8). In this paradigm of experimental research, the area impacted by the policy change can be (1) studied for change within its population over time or (2) compared with a noncontiguous area of a similar demographic composition for differences before and after a sufficient period of time passes from the date of policy implementation. **BOX 1.3** provides an example of a study that used quasi-experimental design to evaluate new medical marijuana policies on adolescents.

As public health becomes progressively more important on a global scale, we suggest that an ever-expanding percentage of the interventions will be focused on the policy level. This shift will entail expanding the existing repertoire of research design options that can be applied to policy-level intervention programs. As such, many of the chapters in this text will provide you with direction, advice, and even inspiration relative to this third form of using research to shape public health practice.

As an example of the strength of policy-based programs, consider the widespread public health benefits of policy regulating the tobacco industry and the corresponding adoption of environmental tobacco smoke laws throughout the United States. This revolution in public health was a product, in part, of the tobacco settlement program, a rather historic event in modern public health practice.

To emphasize the importance of policy change as informed by research, using tobacco as our continued example, consider the following quote taken from a report issued by the *Institute of Medicine*.

At the request of the U.S. Food and Drug Administration, *Public Health Implications of Raising the Minimum Age of Legal Access to Tobacco Products* considers the likely public health impact of raising the minimum age for purchasing tobacco products. The report reviews the existing literature on tobacco use patterns, developmental biology and psychology, health effects of tobacco use, and the current landscape regarding youth access laws, including minimum age laws

---

BOX 1.3 Example of a Quasi-Experimental Study to Evaluate Medical Marijuana Laws

In recent years, some states have enacted new laws and policies regarding marijuana use. Because marijuana use carries mental and physical health risks for adolescents, it is essential to evaluate the effects of these recent marijuana policies. This study sought to delineate associations between state-level shifts in decriminalization and medical marijuana laws (MMLs) and adolescent marijuana use. The study used data collected on 861,082 adolescents (14 to 18+ years) from 1999 to 2015 by the Centers for Disease Control and Prevention's state Youth Risk Behavior Surveys. Statistical models were estimated to assess how decriminalization and MML policy enactment were associated with adolescent marijuana use, controlling for tobacco and alcohol policy shifts, adolescent characteristics, and state and year trends. It is interesting that results showed that MML enactment was associated with small significant *reductions* in current marijuana use, with larger significant declines for male, Black, and Hispanic adolescents. In addition, these effects increased significantly with each year of exposure. In contrast, decriminalization was not associated with significant shifts in use for the sample as a whole but predicted significant declines in marijuana use among 14-year-olds and those of Hispanic and other ancestry, but with significant increases among White adolescents. Neither policy was significantly associated with heavy marijuana use or the frequency of use, suggesting that heavy users may be resistant to such policies. This is the first study to concurrently assess the unique effects of multiple marijuana policies. The results should alleviate concerns over potential but detrimental effects of more liberal marijuana policies on youth use (Coley, Hawkins, Ghiani, Kruzik, & Baum, 2019).

and their enforcement. Based on this literature, the report makes conclusions about the likely effect of raising the minimum age to 19, 21, and 25 years on tobacco use initiation. The report also quantifies the accompanying public health outcomes based on findings from two tobacco use simulation models. According to the report, raising the minimum age of legal access to tobacco products, particularly to ages 21 and 25, will lead to substantial reductions in tobacco use, improve the health of Americans across the lifespan, and save lives. *Public Health Implications of Raising the Minimum Age of Legal Access to Tobacco Products* will be a valuable reference for federal policy makers and state and local health departments and legislators. (*Source*: Committee on the Public Health Implications et al., 2016)

Given this report, it should be clear to you that policy—and, by extension, practice—are each linked to an initial set of research studies. Research is exactly what you should be doing to optimally protect the public, which is your mandate as a public health professional. We encourage this endeavor by blatantly using our adorable public health mascots, Snow and Hamilton, to inspire you (see **FIGURE 1.4**). Also, look for Snow and Hamilton in subsequent chapters for important

WE NEED YOU

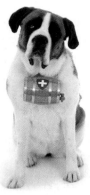 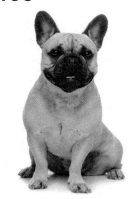

TO DO PUBLIC HEALTH RESEARCH!

FIGURE 1.4 Public Health Mascots Snow and Hamilton Put Out the Call.
© Eric Isselee/Shutterstock; © Svetography/Shutterstock

inspirational messages. At this juncture, even if you do not have a specific public health issue of interest, we wish to speculate that the policy challenges in the next decade and beyond will become increasingly (and by dire necessity) focused on turning back the tide of **climate change**. So, as you ponder what you are learning here initially and throughout the reading of our textbook, we ask that you begin to think about this in terms of what you can do in your career to help minimize climate change.

Think About It!

Without question, rigorous research is time consuming and often resource intensive. As a result, it is costly. Despite, for instance, the extremely high price tag on a study such as a randomized controlled trial, an unfortunate fate of trial outcomes that do not yield significant findings is that the data are never published. We call this unfortunate because when an intervention program, for example, does not work, the knowledge gained by substantiating this point is nonetheless of great value (i.e., it rules out a possibility that was otherwise logical). Given the difficulty that researchers often have in convincing journal editors to publish nonsignificant findings from costly studies, the term **publication bias** is one that you most likely encounter in your career. This bias is, of course, avoidable if journals were more open to publishing papers reporting null (i.e., not significant) findings. So, now you may ask, "Why do the

journal editors avoid papers with null findings?" The answer lies in understanding the motives of any one journal: These motives are based on ensuring that articles reflect the objectives of the journal, creating an expanded base of readers, and thus income, as well as increasing the **impact factor** and, therefore, the prestige for the journal. The impact factor is extremely important for journals. It is a measure of the frequency with which the average article in a journal has been cited in a particular year. It is used to measure the importance or rank of a journal by calculating the times its articles are cited. Consequently, the field is caught between two motives: the public health imperative to rule out ideas that do not work and the goals and objectives of scientific journals. How this inherent conflict of motives can be resolved is thus an important question for you as your career progresses.

Take Home Points

- Public health practice is shaped and refined by research.
- The process of shaping and refining is reciprocal and ongoing.
- The research process is defined as a series of steps; each is critical and none can be omitted.
- Research can have immediate practice implications if it tests a discrete aspect of an existing public health practice.
- Research is the basis for developing evidence-based programs, a staple of public health practice.
- Research can be applied to the evaluation of how much impact occurs from changes in public health policy.

Key Terms

Biomarkers	Effectiveness trial	Publication bias
Case-control design	Efficacy trial	Quasi-experimental design
Climate change	Epidemiology	Randomized controlled trial
Codebook	Impact factor	(RCT)
Cross-sectional design	Methodology	Sample
Effect size	Population	Sampling

For Practice and Discussion

1. Each year in the United States, the average person uses approximately 500 gallons of gasoline. By contrast, the average Canadian uses only 310 gallons. Clearly, U.S. citizens are overconsuming gasoline. In your role as an agent to help minimize climate change, you and three colleagues decide to conduct a survey of "average U.S. citizens" to learn more about their priorities and desires relative to the use of gasoline. The survey includes questions about gasoline for cars, boats, all-terrain vehicles, yard tools, and much more. In a group of four students or so, please answer the following questions.
   a. What aspects of this chapter best apply to this research proposed by you and your colleagues?
   b. What are the potential public health practice implications of the proposed research?
   c. How might the research inform interventions?

2. This chapter taught you that the research-to-practice gap may be quite lengthy (an average of 17 years), and you have wisely decided that this is simply unacceptable. You begin to think about how you might shorten this gap. Your area of focus is on teen pregnancy prevention, and you are painfully aware that policy-level changes are unlikely to be readily adopted. Thus, your end goal is to develop and test an intervention program. Working with one other student in this course, please develop a research-to-practice plan that will inform an intervention designed for rapid translation into practice. This implies that the plan must:
   a. Be low cost and low resource,
   b. Make it easy to train staff who implement and monitor the program,
   c. Be readily understandable to any organization wishing to adopt the program, and
   d. Be highly accessible to the average person.

3. You have graduated with your degree in public health and now you work for a large health department. You have been assigned the difficult task of designing a social marketing campaign that will promote record numbers of people being vaccinated for influenza in the coming fall season. You wisely remember reading Chapter 1 in this text and recall the key point that some types of research can have *immediate and direct implications* for public health practice. So, working with several students in this same course (as though they were your coworkers in

this new job), respond to the following questions regarding this pending research.

a. In a survey of 200 or more community members who were not vaccinated last flu season, what would you measure that would have immediate implications for practice?

b. In that same survey, which of the following items would be a *top priority*, a *medium prioroty*, or a *low priority* for inclusion in the survey given that it could only contain a limited number of questions? Please rank each item as top priority, medium priority, or low priority.

   Cost as a barrier
   Time to get the vaccine as a barrier
   Fear of side effects
   Mistrust of doctors
   Belief that the vaccine is useless
   Doctor recommends vaccination against the flu

References

Baral, S. D., Poteat, T., Strömdahl, S., Wirtz, A. L., Guadamuz, T. E., & Beyrer, C. (2013). Worldwide burden of HIV in transgender women: A systematic review and meta-analysis. *The Lancet Infectious Diseases, 13*(3), 214–222.

Bariola, E., Lyons, A., Leonard, W., Pitts, M., Badcock, P., & Couch, M. (2015). Demographic and psychosocial factors associated with psychological distress and resilience among transgender individuals. *American Journal of Public Health, 105*(10), 2108–2116.

Bockting, W. O., Miner, M. H., Swinburne Romine, R. E., Hamilton, A., & Coleman, E. (2013). Stigma, mental health, and resilience in an online sample of the U.S. transgender population. *American Journal of Public Health, 103*(5), 943–951.

Coley, R. L., Hawkins, S. S., Ghiani, M., Kruzik, C., & Baum, C. F. (2019). A quasi-experimental evaluation of marijuana policies and youth marijuana use. *American Journal of Drug and Alcohol Abuse, 45*(3), 292–303.

Committee on the Public Health Implications of Raising the Minimum Age for Purchasing Tobacco Products, Board on Population Health and Public Health Practice, & Institute of Medicine. (2016). In R. J. Bonnie, K. Stratton, & L. Y. Kwan (Eds.)., *Public health implications of raising the minimum age of legal access to tobacco products*. Washington, DC: National Academies Press.

Community Prevention Services Task Force. (n.d.). *The community guide*. Retrieved from https://www.thecommunityguide.org/

Crissman, H. P., Berger, M. B., Graham, L. F., & Dalton, V. K. (2017). Transgender demographics: A household probability sample of U.S. adults, 2014. *American Journal of Public Health, 107*(2), 213–215.

Crosby, R. A., Salazar, L. F., & Hill, B. J. (2016). Gender affirmation and resiliency among Black transgender women with and without HIV infection. *Transgender Health, 1*(1), 86–93.

Crosby, R. A., Salazar, L. F., & Hill, B. J. (2018). Correlates of not using antiretroviral therapy among transwomen living with HIV: The unique role of personal competence. *Transgender Health, 3*(1), 141–146.

Crosby, R. A., Salazar, L. F., Hill, B., & Mena, L. (2018). A comparison of HIV-risk behaviors between young black cisgender men who have sex with men and young black transgender women who have sex with men. *International Journal of STD & AIDS, 29*(7), 665–672.

Dickey, L. M. (2017). Toward developing clinical competence: Improving health care of gender diverse people. *American Journal of Public Health, 107*(2), 222.

Elder, R. W., Lawrence, B., Ferguson, A., Naimi, T. S., Brewer, R. D., Chattopadhyay, S. K., . . . & Task Force on Community Preventive Services. (2010). The effectiveness of tax policy interventions for reducing excessive alcohol consumption and related harms. *American Journal of Preventive Medicine, 38*(2), 217–229.

Falbe, J., Thompson, H. R., Becker, C. M., Rojas, N., McCulloch, C. E., & Madsen, K. A. (2016). Impact of the Berkeley excise tax on sugar-sweetened beverage consumption. *American Journal of Public Health, 106*(10), 1865–1871.

Herbst, J. H., Jacobs, E. D., Finlayson, T. J., McKleroy, V. S., Neumann, M. S., Crepaz, N., & HIV/AIDS Prevention Research Synthesis Team. (2008). Estimating HIV prevalence and risk behaviors of transgender persons in the United States: A systematic review. *AIDS and Behavior, 12*(1), 1–17.

Hill, B. J., Crosby, R., Bouris, A., Brown, R., Bak, T., Rosentel, K., . . . & Salazar, L. (2018). Exploring transgender legal name change as a potential structural intervention for mitigating social determinants of health among transgender women of color. *Sexuality Research and Social Policy, 15*(1), 25–33.

Hurt, C. B., & Powers, K. A. (2014). Self-testing for HIV and its impact on public health. *Sexually Transmitted Diseases, 41*(1), 10.

Kerr, J., Norman, G. J., Adams, M. A., Ryan, S., Frank, L., Sallis, J. F., . . . & Patrick, K. (2010). Do neighborhood environments moderate the effect of physical activity lifestyle interventions in adults?. *Health & place, 16*(5), 903–908.

Long, C. R., Rowland, B., Langston, K., Faitak, B., Sparks, K., Rowe, V., & McElfish, P. A. (2018). Reducing the Intake of Sodium in Community Settings: Evaluation of Year One Activities in the Sodium Reduction in Communities Program, Arkansas, 2016–2017. *Preventing chronic disease, 15*, E160–E160.

McCartt, A. T., Kidd, D. G., & Teoh, E. R. (2014). Driver cellphone and texting bans in the United States: evidence of effectiveness. *Annals of Advances in Automotive Medicine, 58*, 99–114.

Morris, Z. S., Wooding, S., & Grant, J. (2011). The answer is 17 years, what is the question: Understanding time lags in translational research. *Journal of the Royal Society of Medicine, 104*(12), 510–520.

Nuttbrock, L., Bockting, W., Rosenblum, A., Hwahng, S., Mason, M., Macri, M., & Becker, J. (2014). Gender abuse, depressive symptoms, and substance use among transgender women: A 3-year prospective study. *American Journal of Public Health, 104*(11), 2199–2206.

Office of National AIDS Policy. (2015). National HIV/AIDS strategy for the United States: Updated to 2020. pp. 1–65.

Quick, M., Jones, R., Spengler, E., & Rugsaken, D. (2015). Transforming elevator riders into stair climbers: Impact of a "Take-the-Stairs" campaign. *Academy of Educational Leadership Journal, 19*(3), 235.

Salazar, L. F., Crosby, R. A., Jones, J., Kota, K., Hill, B., & Masyn, K. E. (2017). Contextual, experiential, and behavioral risk factors associated with HIV status: A descriptive analysis of transgender women residing in Atlanta, Georgia. *International Journal of STD & AIDS, 28*(11), 1059–1066.

For Further Reading

Aarons, G. A., Green, A. E., Palinkas, L. A., Self-Brown, S., Whitaker, D. J., Lutzker, J. R., . . . & Chaffin, M. J. (2012). Dynamic adaptation process to implement an evidence-based child maltreatment intervention. *Implementation Science, 7*(1), 32.

Chambers, D. A., Glasgow, R. E., & Stange, K. C. (2013). The dynamic sustainability framework: Addressing the paradox of sustainment amid ongoing change. *Implementation Science, 8*(1), 117.

Feldstein, A. C., & Glasgow, R. E. (2008). A practical, robust implementation and sustainability model (PRISM) for integrating research findings into practice. *Joint Commission Journal on Quality and Patient Safety, 34*(4), 228–243.

Sevelius, J. M. (2013). Gender affirmation: A framework for conceptualizing risk behavior among transgender women of color. *Sex Roles, 68*(11–12), 675–689.

Sohn, D. W. (2016). Residential crimes and neighbourhood built environment: Assessing the effectiveness of crime prevention through environmental design (CPTED). *Cities, 52*, 86–93.

Øvretveit, J. (2011). Understanding the conditions for improvement: research to discover which context influences affect improvement success. *BMJ Quality & Safety, 20*(Suppl 1), i18–i23.

Shelton, R. C., Cooper, B. R., & Stirman, S. W. (2018). The sustainability of evidence-based interventions and practices in public health and health care. *Annual Review of Public Health, 39*, 55–76.

Stange, K. C., & Glasgow, R. E. (2013). *Contextual factors: The importance of considering and reporting on context in research on the patient-centered medical home*. Rockville, MD: Agency for Healthcare Research and Quality.

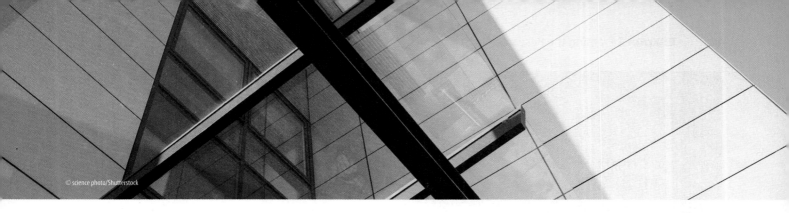

CHAPTER 2

Framing the Research Question

▶ Overview

Ultimately, the most vital aspect of any research study is its primary (and sometimes secondary) research question. Like a set constructed for a theater production, the research question sets the stage for the entire study and defines the boundaries and scope of the study. Boundaries are the limits of the question; setting these limits to a narrow focus keeps the study precise and optimizes generalizability. *Scope* refers to the actual breadth of the question within the stated boundaries and is typically a function of the existing "gap" in the professional literature that is being "filled" by the study. FIGURE 2.1 illustrates this concept figuratively of filling the gap by selecting the optimal research question. At the beginning, the options for choices are abundant; after refining boundaries and making decisions about the scope of a study, one cohesive research question can be selected that will fill the gap and contribute to the knowledge base in a meaningful way.

To better illustrate the vital nature of the research question, consider this statement: "The purpose of the study was to test the efficacy of a brief intervention program designed to help opioid-addicted women avert unplanned pregnancy." Reading this sentence carefully, you will find that it is has four main objectives:

1. *Testing efficacy* typically implies that a randomized trial will be conducted.
2. A *brief intervention* must be designed for this test.
3. The study population is *opioid-addicted women*.
4. The goal is to *avert unplanned pregnancy*.

In turn, these four implications dictate the research design, the study sample, and assessment of the study outcomes. Thus, as you can imagine, the breadth is quite large, given that all possible ages of women are included, as well as all women regardless of race or ethnicity; and that particular methods of averting unplanned pregnancy are not specified. The boundaries are somewhat narrow in what may be an overly ambitious study by restricting the public health program to a "brief" intervention and targeting only women deemed as being addicted to opioids.

Understanding that the final evaluation of a research study is directly tied to its research question is

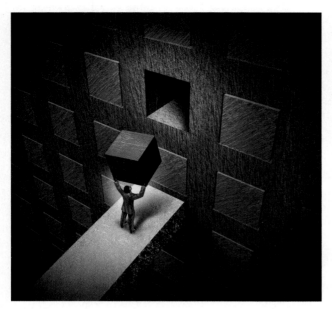

FIGURE 2.1 "Filling the Gap" in the Research Literature.
© Lightspring/Shutterstock

IT'S TIME FOR YOU

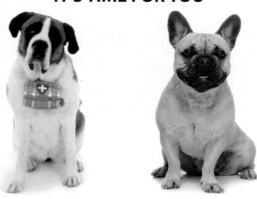

TO FILL THOSE GAPS!

FIGURE 2.2 Public Health Mascots Snow and Hamilton Provide Encouragement.
© Eric Isselee/Shutterstock; © Svetography/Shutterstock

vital. A rigorous study is one that has **internal validity**, meaning that it precisely addresses the research question and thus provides a definitive answer. So, as you might suspect, this precision becomes progressively less likely as the scope of the research question broadens. Consequently, a typical rule of conducting rigorous research is to "tighten the boundaries" of the research question and thereby enhance the odds of achieving high levels of precision. This chapter will teach you much more about this give-and-take between boundaries and breadth; it will also explain when secondary research questions are appropriate. The chapter begins by teaching you how to read the professional literature so that you will be motivated and able to identify critical gaps (see **FIGURE 2.2**) that, in turn, can be addressed by well-conceived research questions.

▶ What Is a Targeted Literature Review?

A common misconception (held by students and even professionals in public health) is that research begins with a specific interest held by the researcher. In reality, the researcher has an obligation to "slightly extend" the existing **chain of knowledge** relative to any given public health priority. Whether adding a new link to this chain of knowledge is consistent with the researcher's personal aspirations is merely an optional point. The alignment of personal aspirations and a research question is, instead, made possible by initially selecting a chain of knowledge that piques your curiosity. **FIGURE 2.3** illustrates the concept of the chain of knowledge and how research adds a link to this chain.

The topic represented here focuses on current knowledge of opioid addiction and treatment options. You will quickly notice that the first four links of the chain are complete and unbroken, indicating a significant amount of previous research and knowledge within the given concept area; however, the fifth chain is broken. This broken chain provides a starting point for new research in areas where there may be a gap within this umbrella topic of opioid-addiction treatment. This open fifth link is precisely where a researcher may try to target his or her research question.

At this juncture, the logical question becomes, how do I discover the chain of knowledge? The answer involves time and hard work on your part, all devoted to a **literature review**. First, please be aware that the term *literature* in this case refers only to peer-reviewed journal articles. This means that your searching is restricted to professional journals that accept manuscripts on a competitive basis,

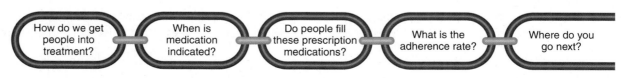

FIGURE 2.3 "Chain" of Knowledge Related to Opioid Addiction and Treatment.

normally from researchers funded to perform this type of work. The competition is based on having a small panel of experts (two to four people) review the manuscript for qualities such as innovation, rigor, and clarity of writing. Scores are typically provided, along with comments that support a decision to accept or reject the manuscript for publication. Journals commonly reject far more manuscripts than are accepted for publication, thus creating a competitive process based on peer review.

Now that you understand the term *literature*, let's move to the other term: *review*. A thorough review is one that summarizes the latest (past 10 years is typical) developments in a very specific area of inquiry. For example, consider the following paragraph:

> Broadly, nationally representative evidence suggests that food insecurity is causally related to a host of negative health outcomes such as diabetes, heart disease, hypertension, and mental illness.[1] Hunger is a specific form of food insecurity, one that has focus on the experience of ongoing lack of food as opposed to ample food of very poor quality.[2] Hunger has been associated with chronic disease and psychological distress.[1,3,4] Further, hunger has been associated with poor adherence to antiretroviral medications among persons living with HIV, including young Black males.[2,5–8] Emerging evidence suggests that hunger may be a risk factor for young Black males engaging in behaviors that lead to HIV acquisition.[9–11]

This paragraph is a succinct literature review regarding the issue of human immunodeficiency virus (HIV) risk and hunger for a specific population: young Black males. The superscripted numbers tell you that 11 peer-reviewed articles were synthesized to form this chain of knowledge. As you can see, the chain begins with rather broad points (e.g., hunger and its relationship to multiple types of health-related outcomes) and then progresses to the terminal point of citing evidence that hunger may be a risk factor for HIV. To give you further practice reading and understanding literature reviews, please look closely at the sample study provided in **BOX 2.1**. As you read this box, please pay close attention to how the literature review unfolds in a systematic fashion to "tell the story" (in this case, the story is one of need for a brief, clinic-based, condom-use promotion program specifically designed for women using highly reliable forms of contraception but who are nonetheless at risk of contracting sexually transmitted infections).

BOX 2.1 Sample of an Introduction Paragraph Leading Up to the Study

Recently, the United States has experienced unprecedented record-high incidence rates of sexually transmitted infections (STIs). These rates exceed all previous estimates, which were used to calculate the annual cost to the economy of $16 billion in healthcare.[1] Three STIs (trichomoniasis, chlamydia, and gonorrhea) are particularly common among women of color and exact a large toll among women in the form of infertility, pelvic inflammatory disease, and ectopic pregnancy.[2] Fortunately, evidence suggests that the consistent and correct condom use of male latex condoms is highly protective against these STIs and others that occur among women.[3]

The goal of the study was to test the efficacy of the condom-use promotion program designed for women. This is a single-session, clinic-initiated, and tailored program designed to promote male condom use among women using hormonal contraceptives and intrauterine devices, including those starting long-acting reversible contraceptives (LARCs). The program thus achieves the recommended dual use of male condoms and a highly effective contraceptive method.[4–6] Dual use augments contraceptive efficacy and is vital to the prevention of STIs. Condom use is especially vital among women relying on other methods of contraception that have no protective value in this regard. In fact, some reports indicate that women using LARCs are particularly unlikely to use male condoms for STI prevention[7–9] and have a higher incidence of STIs.[9] As a clinic-initiated but largely self-guided intervention program, this novel approach to prevention is planned as a personalized strategy that can accommodate changes with respect to partner involvement during the study. For women having sex with partners who have STIs or with multiple male partners, the program offers a component of clinical care that has been lacking in clinics that provide contraception. An eloquent advantage of brief single-session formats is that they do not involve group meetings; instead, these programs become an extension of clinical service.

Notes

1. Centers for Disease Control and Prevention. (2017). *Sexually transmitted disease surveillance, 2016*. Atlanta, GA: U.S. Department of Health and Human Services. Retrieved from https://www.cdc.gov/std/stats16/CDC_2016_STDS_Report-for508WebSep21_2017_1644.pdf
2. Finer, L., & Zolna, M. (2011). Unintended pregnancy in the United State: Incidence and disparities, 2006. *Contraception, 84*(5), 478–485. Retrieved from https://www.ncbi.nlm.nih.gov/pubmed/22018121
3. Williams, R. L., & Fortenberry, J. D. (2013, April 30). Dual use of long-acting reversible contraceptives and condoms among adolescents. *Journal of Adolescent Health, 52*(4), S29–S34.

(continues)

BOX 2.1 Sample of an Introduction Paragraph Leading Up to the Study *(continued)*

4. Crosby, R. A., DiClemente, R. J., Wingood, G. M., et al. (2001, May). Correlates of using dual methods for sexually transmitted diseases and pregnancy prevention among high-risk African-American female teens. *Journal of Adolescent Health, 28*(5), 410–414.
5. Eisenberg, D. L., Allsworth, J. E., Zhao, Q., & Peipert, J. F. (2012). Correlates of dual-method contraceptive use: An analysis of the National Survey of Family Growth (2006–2008). *Infectious Diseases in Obstetrics and Gynecology*, 717163.
6. Darney, P. D., Callegari, L. S., Swift, A., Atkinson, E. S., & Robert, A. M. (1999). Condom practices of urban teens using Norplant contraceptive implants, oral contraceptives, and condoms for contraception. *American Journal of Obstetric Gynecology, 180*, 929–937.
7. Steiner, R. J., Liddon, N., Swartzendruber, A. L., Rasberry, C. N., & Sales, J. M. (2016). Long-acting reversible contraception and condom use among female U.S. high school students: Implications for sexually transmitted infection prevention. *JAMA Pediatrics, 170*, 428–434.
8. Santelli, J. S., Davis, M., Celentano, D. D., Crump, A. D., & Burwell, L. G. (1995). Combined use of condoms with other contraceptive methods among inner-city Baltimore women. *Family Planning Perspectives, 27*, 74–78.
9. McNicholas, C. P., Klugman, J. B., Zhao, Q., & Peipert, J. F. (2017). Condom use and incident sexually transmitted infection after initiation of long-acting reversible contraception. *American Journal of Obstetric Gynecology, 217*(6), e1–e6.

Conducting a highly focused literature review is often expedited by locating a review article. In fact, frequently peer-reviewed journal articles will take the form of comprehensive reviews that eloquently synthesize existing literature around a given area of inquiry. **BOX 2.2** features an example of such a review article. The take-home point here is that you should make every effort to locate a recent and relevant article at the beginning of your literature review. The other bit of advice here is to conduct your literature review using key words taken from one or two articles. **Key words** are a standard feature of peer-reviewed journal articles because they serve as a convenient method of making searches efficient. Much like typing one or two words into the search bar of an online vendor (e.g., Amazon) and quickly obtaining "matches" that you can then use to make your final purchase, key words are indexed electronically, so "tagging" any given article with three to six words or phrases can make it a potential match for somebody doing a targeted literature review. Consider, for instance, the following key words:

- Latina
- Iron deficiency
- Medicaid
- Dietary supplements

Without knowing anything else about the article, you can most likely guess what it is about. If you guessed "Medicaid programs that provide nutritional supplements to Latinas experiencing iron deficiency anemia," you are indeed correct.

Thus, the lesson here is to use key words to your advantage when conducting literature reviews and to select key words with great care when writing a manuscript for a journal that is indexed online (as most are). Key words are typically included just after the abstract of an article: They will be labeled as such to make finding them quite easy.

One all-so-important skill is to learn how to put what you learn about into a few simple links in the chain of knowledge. In fact, it may help you to construct a visual much like Figure 2.3. Within that visual

BOX 2.2 Example of a Systematic Review of the Literature

This systematic review article described the use of social networking sites within HIV prevention. Specifically, this article reviewed studies describing how social networking sites have been used for recruitment, assessing the impact and reach of HIV-prevention interventions, and evaluating the efficacy of social media–based HIV-prevention interventions. The researchers conducted a literature review from June to July 2015 using PubMed, PsycINFO, ScienceDirect, and Google Scholar. The following key words were used in combination to identify relevant articles to include in the review: *HIV, prevention, intervention, social media, social networking sites, Facebook, Twitter, testing,* and *health promotion*. Article titles and abstracts were reviewed and screened for relevancy, and only articles that met the following inclusion criteria were included in the review: utilized social networking sites (e.g., Facebook and Twitter), was related to primary prevention of HIV, and described an intervention or prevention campaign. The initial search yielded a total of 39,771 records, but the research team narrowed it down to 21 articles after screening titles, abstracts, and articles. The final review included 16 articles that met inclusion criteria describing 12 distinct interventions. Findings reveal that social networking sites are critical for recruiting hard-to-reach populations and useful for expanding the reach of HIV-prevention social media marketing campaigns, and they played a significant role in reducing sexual risk behaviors and increasing HIV testing (Jones, & Salazar, 2016).

you can then label the links and arrange them in order; this exercise will lead you to see where the current knowledge relevant to your research questions begins to become sparse to nonexistent.

How Do I Systematically Look for Gaps?

Conducting the literature review should be an intense experience, one that occupies your time and thoughts for days or even weeks. This experience pays off by giving you ample information to take the critical step of identifying the research gap (see **FIGURE 2.4**). After you have mentally or even visually synthesized the research literature to date, you are on the verge of identifying a gap. These gaps may be obvious or quite subtle. For instance, returning to the hunger and HIV-risk example, you may find that published research has not described any study investigating associations between hunger and HIV-related risk behaviors. This is a clear and obvious gap. However, what if you found two studies, one investigating these associations among women and the other among White gay men. Is this a gap? The answer is "Yes" as long as you did not find a published investigation of a similar nature relevant to minority

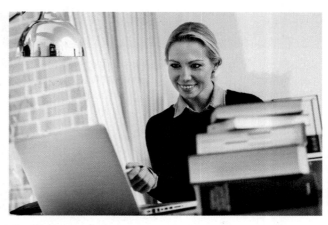

FIGURE 2.4 Researcher Looking for the "Gap" in the Literature.
© Kzenon/Shutterstock

men, or even White men, who do not identify as gay. The point here is that the population is critical to gap identification: One study of one population is far from adequate in the complex field of public health.

Another method of identifying critical gaps in the field skips the somewhat labor-intensive process of a literature review. You can do this by learning how to navigate a vital tool used in the funding world: NIH RePORTER. This is a public use system maintained by the National Institutes of Health (NIH). **FIGURE 2.5**

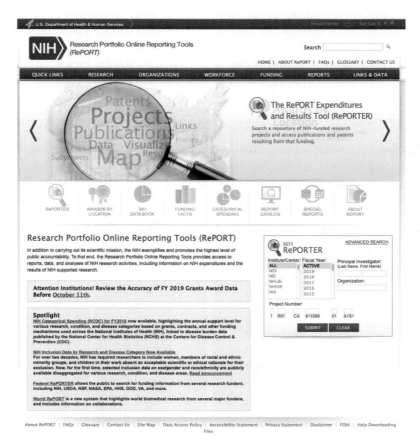

FIGURE 2.5 Screenshot of NIH Research Portfolio Online Reporting Tools (RePORTER).
NIH Research Portfolio Online Reporting Tools (RePORTER). Retrieved from https://report.nih.gov/

BOX 2.3 Example of Funded Grant That Addresses the Potential Influences of Relapse in Addiction

A 2018 study found on NIH RePORTER targeted the need for additional research into prevention of drug addiction relapse. Carried out by the National Institute on Drug Abuse treatment section, this study had two main goals in mind. First, the study wanted to investigate the influence of potential triggers such as stress or environmental factors in relation to relapse rates while also determining if pharmacological treatments are effective in relapse prevention. The following is a short excerpt with some of the most significant findings from the study.

In the rat reinstatement model of relapse, stress-induced seeking of heroin, cocaine, speedball (heroin-cocaine combination), alcohol, or nicotine is blocked by alpha-2 adrenoceptor agonists such as lofexidine, guanfacine, and clonidine. Thus, alpha-2 agonists may act on a final common pathway of stress-induced relapse, relevant to multiple drugs of abuse. In a randomized, placebo-controlled laboratory study, with non-treatment-seeking cocaine users, we have shown that clonidine was effective in reducing stress-induced (and, at a higher dose, cue-induced) craving in a pattern consistent with the findings from the reinstatement model. We have since shown, in a double-blind, randomized trial in abstinent opioid users receiving agonist maintenance, that adjuvant clonidine maintenance increases time to lapse and longest duration of abstinence.

By identifying the gaps within literature, studies such as this one can further work toward providing evidence to fill in the missing information. The study is titled "Prevention of Relapse in Addiction" and has a federally assigned funding number of DA000536-12. Use this information to search the NIH RePORTER system for additional information regarding this study or alternative studies within the topic of drug addiction.

provides a screenshot example of a homepage for this all-so-important service offered to researchers.

As part of being accountable to U.S. taxpayers, the NIH maintains searchable records of the research studies either recently or currently supported by NIH funds. Although this database is extremely useful to researchers as they prepare to "fill a gap" in the field of public health, it can be equally valuable to anyone (including you) who is searching for an unexplored niche in the world of research possibilities that exist relative to improving health and promoting the prevention of disease. **BOX 2.3** and **BOX 2.4** provide examples of records in this database that provide "clues" regarding the existence of gaps in the research literature via the overarching point that NIH preferably funds only innovative and so-called cutting-edge research studies. By learning as much as possible about studies that are funded (and typically several years away from producing published findings) you gain the ability to take advantage of other people's knowledge

BOX 2.4 Example of a Funded Grant from NIH RePORTER

As an example of how NIH RePORTER works, consider the following entry in the database. Funded to Butler Hospital in Providence, Rhode Island, for $218,842, this relatively modest study was based on meeting a need that had yet to be studied empirically. Funded by the National Institute on Drug Abuse, the gap addressed was simple yet important. Helping people overcome opioid addiction is often viewed in a medical paradigm, meaning that "good health" becomes defined as a lack of addiction. This project was designed to address a critical gap in the research literature by testing a physical activity program designed to augment health and recovery of persons overcoming opioid addiction through a methadone maintenance treatment program. An excerpt from the publicly available abstract follows. Key abbreviations are: (1) PA, physical activity; and (2) MMT, methadone maintenance treatment.

An increasing number of peer-facilitated PA interventions have been found to effectively increase and sustain physical activity levels, though none in substance abusing populations. Peers may play a particularly important role in increasing physical activity in MMT, as this population faces unique and significant barriers to PA (e.g., depression, smoking, triggers for drug use in environment). MMT peers who have successfully navigated through these barriers and are physically active can share information, help in problem solving barriers, act as role models, and offer support and encouragement, thereby helping inactive MMT patients increase self-efficacy and motivation for sustaining PA.

As this excerpt shows, a primary innovation was the use of peers to help promote positive behaviors, including physical activity. The project title is "Peer-Facilitated Physical Activity Intervention Delivered During Methadone Maintenance," and the federally assigned funding number is R33 DA041553. With this information, you can go online, enter the NIH RePORTER system, and learn much more about the impetus for the study as well as its design.

about important gaps in the field. As such, you can look closely at the study abstracts to glean the type of research questions considered highly innovative; these abstracts can give insight into what your unique and innovative research question may become as you clarify and refine this idea in your own way.

One more method of finding out where the gaps may lie is one that will require you to travel. We strongly encourage you to think about attending professional meetings as a way to learn as much as possible about cutting-edge research even before it is published. Typically, national organizations such as the American Public Health Association hold annual meetings that predominately focus on research findings that are not yet known in the field because they have not yet been published. This novelty seems to almost permeate the air in conference halls, with attendees (and often members of the news media) eager to learn about the most recent set of research findings relative to their own research interests. Beyond the novelty, the sheer eloquence of conferences is that you can (and should) meet and interact with the speaker after the presentation ends. For those who are not socially shy, we also encourage you to ask thoughtful questions during the presentation. Either way, your questions can include this one: "What is missing from the chain of evidence relative to the research you have presented today?" Finally in this regard, please note that most national conferences offer greatly reduced registration fees for students; some conferences even provide students with a "work option" that can be used in place of a registration fee (we also note here that food is often provided throughout the conference).

▶ What Is the Four-Step Method All About?

Much like a chef follows a recipe to make the perfect meal, we urge you to do the same to create the perfect research question (with "perfect" being defined as providing optimal clarity) thus leading to the perfect research study. Our recipe is one that is time-tested and relatively easy to make. It begins with the point that the entire research question must be so clear and succinct that it fits into a single sentence. That sentence must have four elements:

1. Several words that name the research design.
2. A succinct phrase that implies the study **hypothesis**.
3. A few words that name the study population.
4. A statement regarding the overall goal of the study.

Each element can be sequenced into a sentence that best suits you and makes the research question simple to understand. Let's take a look at how this process might work.

Building from the gap identified in Box 2.4 (physical activity for recovering drug addicts), imagine that you want to draft a research question about a study you think should follow the one described in Box 2.4. Your idea is that diet is as important as physical activity, so you want to learn more about the food consumption habits of recovering addicts. Generally thinking, you suspect that diets may be excessively laden with highly processed foods, many of which have the potential to negatively impact mental and physical health. Similarly, you suspect that health-protective foods (mainly vegetables and other single-ingredient foods) may be lacking in the diets of addicts. Your interest is in persons currently taking methadone treatment designed to eventually eliminate their dependence on opioids. You understand, however, that teens and homeless people are unlikely to have control over their dietary choices. As such, you decide to focus only on people who are stably housed adults. Overall, you want to do this study because you understand the value to public health of keeping former addicts mentally and physically healthy for the rest of their lives.

Given all of your ideas, your task is now to apply the recipe so the basic ingredients can be combined into that important single sentence. This is what you have now:

- Your research design does not require testing an intervention; you only want to know about dietary behaviors—and how these relate to mental and physical health; this can be done with a simple one-time assessment.
- Your working hypothesis is that recovering addicts who consume greater amounts of vegetables and unrefined foods will have better mental and physical health compared with those who primarily eat refined or processed foods.
- The study is to occur among people taking methadone treatment who are stably housed adults.
- The study can produce findings to help inform public health practice relative to promoting quality of life among recovered drug addicts.

Now the task becomes one of artfully blending these four bullet points into that single sentence. We suggest that you include information from all four bullet points (i.e., state the design, the working hypothesis, the study population, and the reason or goal for the study) in a sequence that streamlines the sentence for ease of reading. A reasonable first draft might look something like this:

> To determine the relationship of diet to the continued health of recovering drug addicts, the study will conduct in-person interviews eliciting dietary habits and assessing indicators of health of stably housed adults receiving methadone treatment.

Looking carefully at the draft sentence, you can see that it has all four ingredients.

1. Several words that name the research design [*conduct in-person interviews*]
2. A succinct phrase that implies the study hypothesis [*determine the relationship of diet to the continued health*]
3. A few words that name the study population [*stably housed adults receiving methadone treatment*]
4. A statement regarding the overall goal of the study [*continued health of recovering drug addicts*]

Of course, we do not pretend that this process of making the perfect research question is as simple as shown here; however, it is a process that always pays off in the long run. Again, a clear statement of the research question keeps you (and others working with you) tightly focused and on task. To help you master the art of using this four-step model, we have provided numerous examples of complete research statements in **TABLE 2.1**.

▶ What Is Secondary Research and When Is It Appropriate?

Secondary research is defined by the use of a preexisting data set for a study that was not planned at the time the data were collected. Far from being a fallback position, a large portion of the most important studies in public health are predicated on secondary data analysis. This is because federal funding is often allocated for the collection of nationally representative data, often in the context of ongoing studies. A good example is the National Survey of Family Growth (NSFG). Through the use of probability sampling, this nationally representative survey has been conducted over several cycles, thereby allowing researchers to make inferences about trends over time. Data are collected relevant to contraceptive practices, abortion, beliefs, and attitudes pertaining to a wide range of behaviors such as condom use, premarital sex, marriage, divorce, and reproductive health. Interviews are conducted in person with more than 10,000 adults in each cycle of this project. As you may imagine, this wealth of data is capable of being used over and over again to address a nearly infinite number of research questions. For instance, a recent publication from the NSFG (Daniels & Abma, 2018) documented national estimates of contraceptive use among women, ages 15 to 44. The estimates are that 64.9% used a method, with the most common being sterilization (18.6%), oral contraceptives (12.6%), long-acting reversible contraception (10.3%), and condoms (8.7%). This same study also found a relationship

---

TABLE 2.1 Examples of Research "Purpose" Statements That Follow the Four-Step Model

The purpose of this cohort study was to determine whether excessive sitting at work leads to adult-onset diabetes among middle-aged executives working in the technology industry.

To help rectify disparities in teen-related gun violence, this cross-sectional study tested the hypothesis that scores on a seven-item measure of impulsivity would be significantly associated with having engaged in gun violence among youth in juvenile detention facilities.

Given the urgency of addressing climate change, this trend study identified patterns in the use of recreational gasoline to determine whether consumption levels have declined in any of the past 10 years among a sample of middle-class adults.

To help promote improved preventive care, the purpose of the study was to qualitatively explore reasons why low-income White women living in rural areas have high levels of distrust for medical care providers.

This survey study responded to the U.S. need for a greater attention to understanding the unmet dental health needs of people residing in rural Appalachia; associations with lack of income were investigated.

With national attention being devoted to the epidemic of childhood obesity, the purpose of this study was to determine whether television viewing and snacking are correlated among a sample of low-income adolescents.

This study investigated the awareness of middle-aged males relative to their risks for developing prostate cancer, and it determined whether awareness was associated with having a primary care provider.

Because the city of Baltimore, Maryland, has recently created a built environment to promote walking and running, this study of residents over age 60 tested the hypothesis that peak use of trails would occur in the early evening hours.

To develop a measure of willingness to have a mammogram, this study tested the reliability and validity of a 12-item scale created specifically for low-income rural women who have never had mammograms.

between education level and contraceptive practices, with sterilization being less likely as education level increased, and oral contraception being more likely as education level increased. In another example, NSFG data were used to assess practices and attitudes toward cohabitation in the United States (Nugent & Daugherty, 2018). This study estimated that, of persons 18 to 44 years of age, 17.1% of females and 15.9% of males were currently cohabitating. Of interest, the study found that cohabitating couples were significantly more likely to report an unintended pregnancy compared with married couples.

To give you a sense of how ubiquitous secondary research is, **BOX 2.5** provides an example from the National Longitudinal Study of Adolescent Health. As

you will learn when reading this box, secondary data analysis was taken to a whole new level by this ongoing study funded by the U.S. government.

Now that you know a little bit about the NSFG and the National Longitudinal Study of Adolescent Health (known also as "Add Health"), consider once again the title of this chapter: "Framing the Research Question." Up until now in this chapter, we have treated the practice of formulating your research question as being based on the freedom to construct and subsequently implement a study. With data already collected; however, the tables are turned. This means that your research question must "fit" the study design, assessment methods, study population, and selection of measures that have already been set

---

BOX 2.5 Introduction to the National Longitudinal Study of Adolescent Health

The National Longitudinal Study of Adolescent Health (Add Health), has existed since 1995. Since then, the longitudinal study (i.e., study volunteers are followed over time) has involved home-based interviews with thousands of young people and many of their parents. Funded by the U.S. government, Add Health is a virtual treasure trove of data pertaining to every imaginable aspect of health (ranging from substance use and violence to HIV, diabetes, suicidal ideation, victimization, sexual assault, bullying, and binge drinking). The Add Health data can be accessed by qualified researchers, and this service is complete with a host of technical support relative to how the data can best be used to create nationally representative samples and thus highly generalizable findings. Counting book chapters, conference presentations, journal articles, and unpublished manuscripts, more than 7000 secondary studies have been conducted using these data. Just for fun, this box provides only a small sample of the journal articles from Add Health that were devoted specifically to the obesity epidemic in the United States.

Sample Journal Articles as Cited on the Add Health Website

Ajilore, Olugbenga; & Asiseh, Fafanyo. (2018). Ethnic differences in the influence of peers on weight-related behavior. *The Review of Black Political Economy, 45*(1), 69–90.

Becnel, Jennifer N.; & Williams, Amanda L. (2019). Using latent class growth modeling to examine longitudinal patterns of body mass index change from adolescence to adulthood. *Journal of the Academy of Nutrition and Dietetics.*

Belsky, Daniel W.; Caspi, Avshalom; Arseneault, Louise; Corcoran, David L.; Domingue, Benjamin W.; Harris, Kathleen Mullan; Houts, Renate M.; Mill, Jonathan S.; Moffitt, Terrie E.; Prinz, Joseph; Sugden, Karen; Wertz, Jasmin; Williams, Benjamin; & Odgers, Candice L. (2019). Genetics and the geography of health, behaviour and attainment. *Nature Human Behaviour.*

Boone-Heinonen, Janne; Sacks, Rebecca M.; Takemoto, Erin E.; Hooker, Elizabeth R.; Dieckmann, Nathan F.; Harrod, Curtis S.; & Thornburg, Kent L. (2018). Prenatal development and adolescent obesity: Two distinct pathways to diabetes in adulthood. *Childhood Obesity, 14*(3), 173–181. PMCID: PMC5910034

Carter, Jocelyn Smith. (2018). Stress and self-esteem in adolescence predict physical activity and sedentary behavior in adulthood. *Mental Health and Physical Activity, 14,* 90–97.

Cawley, John; Han, Euna; Kim, Jiyoon; & Norton, Edward C. (2019). Testing for family influences on obesity: The role of genetic nurture. *Health Economics, 28*(7), 937–952.

Do, Elizabeth K.; Haberstick, Brett C.; Williams, Redford B.; Lessem, Jeffrey M.; Smolen, Andrew; Siegler, Ilene C.; & Fuemmeler, Bernard F. (2019). The role of genetic and environmental influences on the association between childhood ADHD symptoms and BMI. *International Journal of Obesity, 43*(1), 33–42.

Fang, Di. (2019). Obesity: Transition from adolescence to adulthood and feedback partial GMM logistic model with time-dependent covariates. *Epidemiology Biostatistics and Public Health, 16*(1).

Fong, T. C. T. (2019). Indirect effects of body mass index growth on glucose dysregulation via inflammation: Causal moderated mediation analysis. *Obesity Facts, 12*(3), 316–327.

Hayibor, Lisa Ama; Zhang, Jianrong; & Duncan, Alexis. (2019). Association of binge drinking in adolescence and early adulthood with high blood pressure: Findings from the National Longitudinal Study of Adolescent to Adult Health (1994–2008). *Journal of Epidemiology and Community Health, 73*(7), 652–659.

He, Jinbo; Chen, Xinjie; Fan, Xitao; Cai, Zhihui; & Huang, Fang. (2019). Is there a relationship between body mass index and academic achievement? A meta-analysis. *Public Health, 167,* 111–124.

Inoue, Y.; Howard, A. G.; Stickley, A.; Yazawa, A.; & Gordon-Larsen, P. (2019). Sex and racial/ethnic differences in the association between childhood attention-deficit/hyperactivity disorder symptom subtypes and body mass index in the transition from adolescence to adulthood in the United States. *Pediatric Obesity.*

Irimata, Kyle M.; Broatch, Jennifer; & Wilson, Jeffrey R. (2019). Partitioned GMM logistic regression models for longitudinal data. *Statistics in Medicine, 38*(12), 2171–2183.

Nagata, Jason M.; Braudt, David B.; Domingue, Benjamin W.; Bibbins-Domingo, Kirsten; Garber, Andrea K.; Griffiths, Scott; & Murray, Stuart B. (2019). Genetic risk, body mass index, and weight control behaviors: Unlocking the triad. *International Journal of Eating Disorders, 52*(7), 825–833.

Niu, Li; Hoyt, Lindsay Till; & Pachucki, Mark C. (2019). Context matters: Adolescent neighborhood and school influences on young adult body mass index. *Journal of Adolescent Health, 64*(3), 405–410.

Shakya, Holly B.; Domingue, Ben; Nagata, Jason M.; Cislaghi, Beniamino; Weber, Ann; & Darmstadt, Gary L. (2019). Adolescent gender norms and adult health outcomes in the USA: A prospective cohort study. *The Lancet Child & Adolescent Health.*

Sokol, Rebeccah L.; Ennett, Susan T.; Gottfredson, Nisha C.; Shanahan, Meghan E.; Poti, Jennifer M.; Halpern, Carolyn T.; & Fisher, Edwin B. (2019). Child maltreatment and body mass index over time: The roles of social support and stress responses. *Children and Youth Services Review, 100,* 214–220.

Sokol, Rebeccah L.; Gottfredson, Nisha C.; Poti, Jennifer M.; Halpern, Carolyn T.; Shanahan, Meghan E.; Fisher, Edwin B.; & Ennett, Susan T. (2019). Does a parsimonious measure of complex body mass index trajectories exist? *International Journal of Obesity, 43*(5), 1113–1119.

Testa, Alexander; & Jackson, Dylan B. (2019). Food insecurity, food deserts, and waist-to-height ratio: Variation by sex and race/ethnicity. *Journal of Community Health, 44*(3), 445–450.

in place by other people. This creates a need to frame the question only after you have a complete working knowledge of what it is—exactly—that you can and cannot do within the limitations of the preexisting data set. It does not mean that your study is being compromised, only that your ideas and goals may require rethinking.

As an example of this rethinking, consider the following scenario. For the first research project of your career you had envisioned this research question:

> To identify whether adolescent males born after the year 2000 and living in the United States from single-parent homes report greater levels of alcohol and drug use compared to those from homes with two parents.

From this question, you know you will need data from adolescent males living with only one parent and also those living with two parents. Clearly, collecting these data could be expensive, especially if you want the results to be a fair reflection of U.S. adolescent males (of all racial and ethnic backgrounds). Rather than abandon your idea because of cost, you do some research and find the website described in Box 2.5. You know from reading this chapter carefully that the National Longitudinal Study of Adolescent Health is highly reputable and has the capacity for national implications. On the Add Health site, you find that public use data are available relative to your research question. Your disappointment, however, is that the

adolescent males in the most recent survey were born before the year 2000. At first, you are saddened by the idea of losing out on all of the literature you summarized relative to adolescent males born after 2000, but you soon recover from this loss and embrace the same research question (minus the caveat about males born after 2000) as a secondary analysis of this nationally representative data set.

As the preceding scenario illustrates, using publicly available data sets comes at a cost to your initial research question, but it is well worth the cost because of added benefits from having a representative sample. In fact, a stunning number of valued empirical studies are based on secondary analyses of publicly available data. **TABLE 2.2** provides several examples of studies that have used publicly available data sets.

Beyond the use of large publicly available data sets, secondary analysis of smaller studies is also an important and appropriate use of existing data. For example, randomized, controlled trials often collect large amounts of data over multiple points in time. The data needed for the actual analysis of the trial typically represents less than 50% of the entire data collected because measures are taken in the event that the randomized groups are not truly equivalent, thereby allowing for statistical control of otherwise problematic differences. **BOX 2.6** provides an example of a study based on secondary analyses of data collected as part of a large randomized, controlled trial funded by the National Institutes of Health (Crosby, Salazar, Mena & Geter, 2016).

TABLE 2.2 Examples of Studies That Have Used Publicly Available Data	
Study Name	**Summary**
Youth Risk Behavior Survey	This study by the Centers for Disease Control and Prevention (CDC) monitors high school youths' behavior through assessing factors contributing to youth disease, illness, and mortality.
Population Assessment of Tobacco and Health	This study explores associations between alcohol and marijuana use and e-cigarette use in a U.S. nationally representative sample of young adults. The data collected through 2013–2014 were used to analyze a possible link between use of alcohol and marijuana in e-cigarette use.
Framingham Heart Study	Since 1948, this long-term study has focused on the development of cardiovascular disease in residents of Framingham, Massachusetts.
Nurses' Health Study	Three cohort long-term studies have been examining nutrition, lifestyle habits, and stress in relation to health outcomes for residents in the greater Boston area.
The Peruvian Demographic and Health Surveys (2005–2012)	Examining within-country migration and obesity dynamics, this analysis used data from 94,783 women in Peruvian demographic and health surveys. This public data set was then used to analyze the possible relationship between rural-to-urban moving and an increase in obesity.

BOX 2.6 Example Study Based on Secondary Data Analysis of a Randomized Trial

Abstract

Objective: To assess internalized homophobia (IH) and its relationship to sexual risk behaviors and prevalence of sexually transmitted infection (STIs) in a clinic-based sample of young Black men who have sex with men (YBMSM).

Methods: A convenience sample of 600 YBMSM was recruited for participation from a randomized controlled trial of a safer sex intervention program designed specifically for this population, which was funded by the National Institutes of Health. *This study involved secondary data analyses of only baseline data* (collected before randomization and intervention) from that randomized controlled trial, thus allowing for a comparison of risk behaviors unconfounded by intervention. YBMSM completed a self-interview and provided specimens for testing. A 7-item scale assessed IH, and 19 sexual risk behaviors were assessed.

Results: In adjusted models, compared with men with less IH, those with greater IH were *more likely* to report any condomless anal receptive sex ($P = 0.01$) and sex with women ($P < 0.001$). Alternatively, men with greater IH were less likely to discuss acquired immune deficiency syndrome prevention with sex partners ($P = 0.009$), disclose their same sex sexual behavior to providers ($P = 0.01$), be tested for human immunodeficiency virus in the past 12 months ($P = 0.04$), report condomless oral sex ($P = 0.049$), and test RPR positive ($P = 0.01$).

Conclusions: With some exceptions, IH among YBMSM attending STI clinics may influence their sexual risk behaviors; however, STI prevalence was not associated with this construct.

As you can see in Box 2.6, the fact that the study is a secondary analysis of other data is made clear in the methods section of the abstract. This type of *declaration* (*full disclosure* is another term) is traditionally made in both the methods sections of the abstract and the methods section of the manuscript itself, usually in the opening paragraph. Once this declaration has been made, the manuscript becomes a freestanding contribution to the knowledge base in public health, because it has been published in a peer-reviewed journal.

Although the practice of using a primary data set to generate multiple secondary studies has been criticized as being too fragmented, we suggest that the obligation of any good (and ethical) researcher is to maximize what can be learned from the primary data sets, particularly those data sets that are derived from taxpayer dollars, which is most often the case. The ethical aspect here involves a frequent promise that is made to potential research volunteers before they provide written informed consent. The wording of that promise typically looks something like this:

> We do not know if you will get any benefit from taking part in this study. However, it is possible that what we learn from your participation will help us develop programs that will benefit other people like yourself.

You will learn much more about the ethics of public health research in the next chapter.

▶ Sticking with the Research Question: The Ethics of a Study

We close this chapter by offering a new term, *HARKing*, which is an acronym for *hypothesizing after the results are known* (Kerr, 1998). The all-so-tempting circumstance faced by far too many researchers involves a carefully planned and executed study that sadly results in a complete lack of significant findings. Thus, the "hunch" of the researcher (stated as a working hypothesis) is not supported. Rather than admit defeat, the "work-around" often taken is to capitalize on *tangential findings*—that is, findings that were not planned as part of the study. For instance, consider a study that tested the following hypothesis:

> Infant car seat installations will be easier for people to do on their own after watching a 15-minute video emphasizing the techniques of proper installation to ensure optimal safety of infants.

Further, imagine that this study assessed "perceived ease of installation" both before watching and after watching the video, and then it assessed "actual ease of installation" within the next 30 days. Unfortunately, despite having a small team of statisticians, differences among the three time points of assessment were not found; thus, the hypothesis was not supported. However, one statistician noted that, "I have learned from these data that men who attempt installation are far less likely (significantly so) to read the instructions." Now, at this point, the person in charge of the study has the apparent option of recasting the hypothesis to read something like:

> Men will be significantly less likely than women to report reading the instructions before attempting to install infant car seats.

So, consider three points here.

1. **Null findings** are also important. The study was somewhat successful because it demonstrated that a 15-minute video is *not* an adequate level of intervention relative to this complex task faced by parents of infants. Thus, not reporting these findings is a disservice to public health and infant safety.

2. The "men versus women" finding is significant, but is it important? Are there any practical implications for the field of infant safety by knowing about this finding?

3. If—and only if—the answer to the previous question is "Yes," the finding should be reported as a secondary analysis and should not be cast as a test of a previously established hypothesis.

Think About It!

An essential paradox in public health research is that people conducting the research may be inspired to do so based on a close connection with the population being studied or a particular affinity for the topic based on personal experience. For instance, let's say a student (we can call this person Jhoan) wants to conduct research solely devoted to the prevention of Lyme disease, a bacterial infection carried to humans via ticks that has lifelong debilitating consequences if not diagnosed early. Jhoan's motivation is based on a parent who is living with the effects of this disease. Given that research to prevent this disease from affecting other people is fulfilling to Jhoan, it becomes a central focal point of all future research efforts. This future leads Jhoan to work primarily in the northeastern United States (where Lyme disease is endemic) and to focus the prevention efforts primarily on rural persons living in tick-infested areas. Having been raised in rural New England, Jhoan can easily understand the target audience and manages to always engage with people from that population in a highly effective manner.

The question to consider with Jhoan is twofold: First, does having a personal stake in a research topic matter regarding the quality of the research? For example, is it possible that Jhoan will have any preconceived bias that may be too difficult to overcome? Also, if you think that having a personal stake is helpful and important, what about researchers doing the same kind of work who have never been personally affected by the disease or condition under study? Are these scientists somehow less committed to "the cause" even though they may be more objective?

The second question is actually larger in scope: Is being part of a population important to conducting research with that population? Consider, for example, an outbreak of hepatitis C among Hispanic males in Chicago. The city declares this "urgent" and allocates funds on a competitive basis to a researcher willing to devise an effective intervention program. The final two applications are both excellent, but only one of these is submitted by a Hispanic male. So, the question then becomes whether this personal identification with the target population is worthy of added credibility regarding the potential for high-quality research. We suggest that arguments here can be made for both sides of this issue. For instance, despite being important relative to language, heritage, culture, and perhaps shared experiences of discrimination, does being Hispanic and male truly make the researcher part of this population of people who inject drugs? Further, if you endorse the idea of "similarity," does this mean that the ideal researcher would also be one who currently (or formerly) injected drugs? Just to take this one step further, if a national epidemic of hepatitis C occurred among Hispanic male injection drug users, would you want to see highly qualified researchers address the epidemic even if they were White middle-class females with absolutely no personal connection to the disease or the population?

Take Home Points

- Framing the research question in a single sentence is a critical step in setting the scope and limits of a good study.
- Learning the skill of placing your research study into the broader chain of knowledge is a prerequisite to success.
- Research from the past is searchable through extensive literature reviews. A great deal of current or ongoing research can be accessed through a system known as NIH RePORTER.
- Four elements make up the final research question, which should be framed as a single sentence.

- Secondary analysis of data sets is a valuable and highly practical method of enhancing the knowledge base in public health. Your research question, however, must fit within the restrictions of the primary study and its corresponding data set.
- Depending on the research question and outcomes of the analysis, null findings can sometimes be equally important to publish and disseminate.

Key Terms

Chain of knowledge
Hypothesis
Internal validity

Key words
Literature review
Null findings

Secondary research

For Practice and Discussion

1. Working alone, go online to find the following peer-reviewed journal article and then answer the following questions based on a careful review of that article.
    Armitage, C., Connor, M., Cowap, L., Flett, K., Grogan, S., Meads, D., . . . , & Torgenson, C. (2019). Evidence that an intervention weakens the relationship between adolescent electronic cigarette use and tobacco smoking: A 24-month prospective study. *Tobacco Control.* Retrieved from https://tobaccocontrol .bmj.com/content/early/2019/06/28 /tobaccocontrol-2018-054905
    a. What are the boundaries and scope of this study? For example, what's the question, target population, testing efficacy, time frame, and so on?
    b. What are some key words you feel can identify the research study?
    c. Imagine that you have extensive knowledge in this field and address a potential gap in this study.
    d. Using the potential gap you addressed previously, devise a question that contains the four essential elements to a "perfect" research question. Make sure that you can phrase the question into a single sentence.

    e. Does your research question fall under a primary or secondary research category? Explain your reasoning.

2. Working in a group of three to four people, develop what your group believes to be "the ultimate research question," meaning that it perfectly fits the requirements of the four-step model. Be prepared to present and defend your ultimate research question to the rest of the class, whose members have also done this assignment in small groups.

3. Read the following original research question: "Given the urgency of climate change, this study identified beliefs held by people employed in hourly jobs about the maximum amount of time they should spend driving to and from work each day." The researcher proposing this study had intended to use data from the General Social Survey (GSS) to address this question. To the researcher's dismay, however, the GSS did not have any measures regarding this belief. Working alone or with a partner, go online and learn as much as you can about the GSS codebook (remember that a codebook shows all of the questionnaire items) and then recast the researcher's research statement into one that is possible as a secondary analysis of GSS data.

References

Crosby, R. A., Salazar, L. F., Mena, L., & Geter, A. (2016). Associations between internalized homophobia and sexual risk behaviors among young Black men who have sex with men. *Sexually Transmitted Diseases, 43*(10), 656–660.

Daniels, K., & Abma, J. C. (2018). *Current contraceptive status among women aged 15-49: United States, 2015–2017.* Washington, DC: U.S. Department of Health and Human Services, Centers for Disease Control and Prevention, National Center for Health Statistics.

Jones, J., & Salazar, L. F. (2016). A review of HIV prevention studies that use social networking sites: Implications for recruitment, health promotion campaigns, and efficacy trials. *AIDS and Behavior, 20*(11), 2772–2781.

Kerr, N. L. (1998). Hypothesizing after the results are known. *Personality and Social Psychology Review, 2,* 196–217.

Nugent, C. N., & Daugherty, J. (2018). A demographic, attitudinal, and behavioral profile of cohabiting adults in the United States, 2011–2015. *National Health Statistics Reports,* (111), 1–11.

For Further Reading

Bluestein, M., Kelder, S., Perry, C. L., & Pérez, A. (2019). Exploring associations between the use of alcohol and marijuana with e-cigarette use in a U.S.A. nationally representative sample of young adults. *International Journal of Health Sciences, 13*(1), 30–39.

Hinds, P. S., Vogel, R. J., & Clarke-Steffen, L. (1997). The possibilities and pitfalls of doing a secondary analysis of a qualitative data set. *Qualitative Health Research, 7*(3), 408–424.

McCall, R. B., & Appelbaum, M. I. (1991). Some issues of conducting secondary analyses. *Developmental Psychology, 27*(6), 911.

Najera, H., Nandy, S., Carrillo-Larco, R. M., & Miranda, J. J. (2019). Within-country migration and obesity dynamics: Analysis of 94,783 women from the Peruvian demographic and health surveys. *BMC Public Health, 19*(1), 263.

Smith, A. K., Ayanian, J. Z., Covinsky, K. E., Landon, B. E., McCarthy, E. P., Wee, C. C., & Steinman, M. A. (2011). Conducting high-value secondary dataset analysis: an introductory guide and resources. *Journal of General Internal Medicine, 26*(8), 920–929.

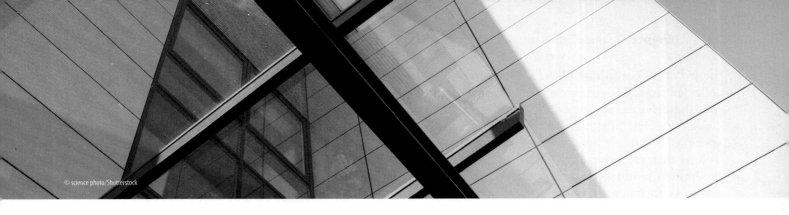

CHAPTER 3

Ethical Standards and Practice for Public Health Research

▶ Overview

Unlike research in the "hard sciences" (e.g., chemistry, physics, microbiology) public health research typically involves the study of populations of people. The qualifier of "typically" is used here because it is not uncommon for public health research to also investigate "systems" such as Medicaid-covered services to people of limited income. However, people are the "target" of the vast majority of public health research agendas. Consequently, our research relies on volunteers or are sometimes referred to as human subjects within the medical field. Before any research with volunteers begins, it must first be reviewed by what is deemed an **institutional review board (IRB)**. The IRB is an administrative body established to protect the rights and welfare of human research subjects who have been recruited to participate in

research activities conducted under the auspices of the affiliated institution. The IRB is responsible for reviewing all research (whether funded or not) involving human participants before it begins. The IRB is concerned with protecting the welfare, rights, and privacy of human subjects for its risks, benefits or value, integrity, and ethical nature. All qualities are important given that volunteers are being asked to donate their time or energy to a cause that is most often framed as benefiting science, although in some cases it may benefit them directly.

To prepare your proposed study for IRB review, you must possess a comprehensive understanding of the rules and guidelines that govern research with volunteers. The rules and guidelines are set and governed by the **United States Office for Human Research Protections (OHRP)** and are a product of several decades of evolving efforts to better protect the **privacy**, **confidentiality**, and **security** of data collected from study volunteers. As you might imagine, these issues are especially important when it comes to public health research questions involving sexuality, substance use, violence, and health conditions that are private by nature (e.g., living with the human immunodeficiency virus or HIV, being a victim of intimate partner violence, being addicted to opioids). Thus, one of your most sacred obligations in the process of conducting research is to first construct a set of safeguards designed to protect the volunteers who will eventually enroll in your study. This chapter will provide you with the information needed to fully understand the exact nature of these obligations.

▶ Why Is History Important in This Chapter?

You may be familiar with the famous quote by philosopher George Santayana: "Those who do not learn history are doomed to repeat it." So, now it is time to learn. Your first lesson is from a small town in Alabama known as Tuskegee. In 1966, a private physician used penicillin to treat an African American man for neurosyphilis, an advanced stage of syphilis, a common sexually transmitted disease (see **BOX 3.1** for an overview). It was later discovered that the man had enrolled in a research study that began in 1932 to observe the natural history of syphilis (meaning that investigators wanted to learn how the untreated bacterial infection progressively damaged the body). Although penicillin was available for use in 1942, this man was not given the antibiotic that could have cured him until 1966. Even more horrifying was that the private physician, who treated this case in 1966, was subsequently chastised by the regional medical society for "spoiling one of our subjects" (Meyerson, Martich, & Naehr, 2008). Although this one case is tragic in its own right, the history lesson here is that the study had been initiated by a branch of our government, the U.S. Public Health Service, using deception. (The agency was later relocated to the Centers for Disease Control and Prevention in 1957.) The study ultimately included 600 poor African American men before it was terminated in 1972 (6 years after the discovery by the aforementioned private physician).

As a result of Tuskegee and other atrocities of research studies using volunteers (see **BOX 3.2** for another example), federal protections were mandated to protect others enrolling in subsequent research studies. The National Commission for the Protection of Human Subjects in Biomedical and Behavioral

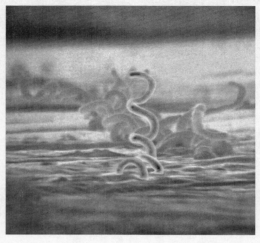

Dr. David Cox/CDC

A spirochete
Known throughout history as one of the most devastating sexually transmitted diseases, syphilis is caused by a bacterium called a spirochete (see image). True to its name, this bacterial infection begins by spiraling into the body through the skin near or on the genitals. This entrance into the body leaves a mark known as a *chancre*. The chancre typically heals within 7 to 10 days, often leaving people with the false impression that they "must be okay."

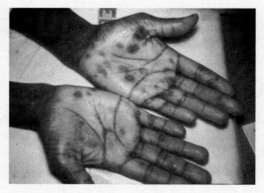

Courtesy of Centers for Disease Control and Prevention

Syphilis rash on palms of hands
If treated at this early stage, the syphilis does minimal damage to the body. However, syphilis may lie dormant from months and reappear as secondary syphilis, which is characterized by rashes of various forms throughout the body, but especially the palms of the hands (see image) and soles of the feet. This stage also resolves on its own, and the spirochete may then begin a year-by-year assault on the internal organs of the body, eventually leading to brain and spinal cord destruction (i.e., neurosyphilis). Although easily treated even in its secondary stage, syphilis has been termed the "great pretender," meaning that it mimics a host of other infections and is often misdiagnosed.

BOX 3.2 Summary of *Tearoom Trade: Impersonal Sex in Public Places*

One of the most infamous examples of ethical issues involving volunteer consent can be found in a book titled *Tearoom Trade: Impersonal Sex in Public Places* authored by Laud Humphreys and published in 1970 (Humphreys, 2017). The book worked to increase knowledge of homosexual male-to-male sexual encounters within the city of St. Louis, Missouri. Unlike other studies at the time, Humphreys was one of the only researchers at the time to focus his work on men engaging in public sexual acts in restrooms—*tea rooming* in gay slang. His ethnographic study involved him being a complete participant, meaning he was covert in his role as researcher and did not reveal this to the men he was observing and interacting. His rationale at the time was that he was concerned with response bias because homosexual activities held such stigma. He observed and also collected information from men by gaining their trust by offering to be a lookout during the sexual encounters. The book not only describes his observations of the public sexual interactions but also provides data regarding one-year follow-ups with these unknowing participants. Humphreys, in fact, wrote down license plate numbers of the men engaging in these public sexual encounters and tracked them down one year later. The unaware participants did not provide consent to be in a study and were under the impression that Humphreys was a health worker, so they agreed to the interviews. Humphreys conducted the interviews and asked men personal demographic questions about their home lives and additional male-to-male sexual encounters. All of the data were collected under a false pretense that he was a health worker. The book raised significant ethical discussions about personal privacy and researcher disclosure that ultimately guided newer ethical practices within research as a whole.

Research was formed and wrote the *Belmont Report*. This report has since become the key document in research ethics and has created many of the current federal regulations on research.

At this juncture, we wish for you to understand that the history leading to the ethical regulation of studies with volunteers has largely been shaped by medical research. Moreover, the current regulations are designed primarily with the intent of protecting volunteers of medical studies. It is from this legacy of medical research that policies have been applied to the behavioral and social science studies that constitute the bulk of public health investigations. The "harm" for public health studies is less of an issue of physically observable problems than of psychosocial harms. This makes the protection of volunteers far more complex.

▶ What Are the Key Issues Defining Ethical Recruiting Practices?

Although many recruitment issues are important, we will focus briefly on just four: (1) coercion, (2) deception, (3) the use of social media, and (4) literacy. First, researchers should inform participants of their right to refuse to participate or withdraw from research, and there should be no coercion or undue influence of research participants to take part in the research. **Coercion** or undue influence occurs whenever any form of incentive or pressure exists to enroll in a study. It is considered unethical to offer extreme financial

(relative to the targeted population) or nonfinancial incentives (e.g., giving extra credit to students) for study participation that go way beyond what would be considered a reasonable amount for compensating volunteers for their time. For example, a potential study volunteer is recruited to participate in a study while in the waiting room of a public health clinic. The study involves answering four 30-minute surveys over the next 6 months and providing a blood sample to be tested for multiple health indicators. The researcher offers compensation of $250 per each 30-minute survey and $500 to provide the blood specimen. Given that this individual may be in a lower socioeconomic stratum, offering such high levels of financial incentives would constitute coercion because the individual may not truly want to participate but believes he or she cannot pass up this amount of money.

Pressure, on the other hand, is less obvious but infinitely more coercive. Consider as an example a study that recruits people who are on parole from prison. There is a substantial risk that, as a result of their current situation, they may become convinced, rightly or wrongly, that their future depends on cooperating with authorities. If the recruitment efforts in any way come across as implying that participation will ensure that they are not violating their parole, coercion exists. Studies that recruit children (defined as individuals under the age of 18) in school settings (such as the Youth Risk Behavioral Surveillance System conducted by the Centers for Disease Control and Prevention) may also have an element of coercion in that students may enroll to please teachers or to "fit in" with the students already enrolled.

As described previously, the Tuskegee syphilis study used **deception** and misled African American male subjects about the true purpose of the research. Before the new rules and regulations governing research, there were other deception studies conducted, but these were social psychology studies rather than medical, but they still garnered considerable attention because of the results. One in particular, the Milgram Shock Experiment, is described in **BOX 3.3**. After reading about this study and the Tuskegee study, you most likely have gleaned that deception in the research context occurs when investigators provide false or incomplete information to participants for the purpose of misleading research subjects. In general, the use of deception in research is neither ethical nor acceptable. Human subject regulations require that recruitment materials, informed consent documents, oral statements, or any other communication with potential volunteers must disclose the true nature and purpose of the study, its goals, and the exact procedures that are expected to occur relative to study participation. All study protocols, including advertisements for recruitment, must be reviewed and approved by the local IRB. Further, scripted oral messages used in the recruitment process must also be approved by the IRB. As a rule, any

information conveyed and all advertisements and messages should avoid making promises pertaining to the benefits of study participation, be up front and honest about any potential risks, and not emphasize financial or nonfinancial incentives.

Now that you understand what deception is and have read about two famous and horrific deceptive studies, you may be surprised to hear that researchers may still want to use deception in some instances. Of course, researchers must do so in an ethical manner and with IRB approval. But is it possible to use deception ethically? In certain instances, some IRBs will accept the need for certain types of studies to employ strategies that include deception. However, employment of such strategies *must be justified*. Ordinarily, deception is not acceptable if, in the IRB's judgment, the participant may have declined to participate had he or she been informed of the true purpose of the research.

One such instance for the justification of deception may be to investigate what is called the **placebo effect**. The placebo effect has been defined as the positive physiological or psychological changes associated with the use of inert medications, sham procedures, or therapeutic symbols within a healthcare encounter (Guess, Kleinman, Kusek, & Engel, 2002). The use of

BOX 3.3 The Milgram Shock Experiment

One of the most famous and controversial studies in psychology is the Milgram Shock Experiment. The investigator was Stanley Milgram, a psychologist at Yale University, who became interested in how seemingly normal German citizens were influenced into committing atrocious and violent acts during World War II. Throughout his research, Milgram discovered that a large portion of Nazis justified their actions as "following orders." In 1963, Milgram developed a study that investigated how obedience and authority influences an individual's ability to harm others. The study consisted of 40 male individuals who were assigned to be "teachers" and a group of confederates (actors pretending to be study volunteers and acting in secret) who were assigned as "learners." A vital position in this study was the "experimenter," an actor dressed in a white lab coat and assigned to give instructions to participants. The teacher and learner were taken into a room, and the learner was strapped into a chair. The teacher was then taken into an adjacent room where he could hear but not see the learner. The experimenter would explain that the learner was going to be given a learning task: He had to memorize a list of word pairings. The teacher was instructed to test the learner by naming one of the words in the pairing and asking the learner to recall its pairing. If the learner answered incorrectly, the teacher was instructed by the experimenter to administer an electric shock, increasing the voltage after each incorrect answer. The learner, of course, was never shocked, but the teacher believed that he was because the learner would make noises and bang on the wall pretending to get shocked. The learner would mainly give incorrect answers, making sure that the teacher would have to increase the shock level. If the teacher refused to administer a shock, the experimenter would give a series of orders instructing him to continue. More than 65% of individuals continued to the highest shock level of 450 volts, which, if real, would most likely have resulted in death. This study revealed that individuals are extremely likely to follow orders given by an authority figure, even when those orders include harming another individual. Although the results of this study were significant, ethical controversy arose surrounding Milgram's use of deception. Participants were unaware that the learners were confederates and were not actually being shocked. Although participants learned of the deception at the end of the study, the risk of psychological harm was high. When including deception in an experimental study, it is important for the rewards to outweigh the risks.

Modified from McLeod, S. A. (2017, Feb 05). The Milgram shock experiment. Retrieved from https://www.simplypsychology.org/milgram.html

deception is a common feature of research investigating the placebo effect, particularly when the focus is on pharmacological substances or certain drugs. In some studies, deception is somewhat mild in that participants can be told that they will receive *either* the drug or a placebo, but they will not be told which one they have received. However, in other studies, the deception can be more severe. For example, in a study involving 13 women with irritable bowel syndrome (IBS), investigators told the women that four drugs in relation to IBS were being tested. In reality, the participants were administered two different forms of only one drug, along with two placebos. Hence, the participants were deceived by being informed that they would receive drugs that, in fact, were placebo interventions (Vase, Robinson, Verne, & Price, 2003). In the event that a study includes the use of deception, the investigator must provide the following to the IRB for study approval:

- Confirmation that the study design meets all of the criteria for a waiver of consent
- Justification for the deception
- Description of the manner of deception and how the deception will take place
- An explanation as to why deception is necessary to this protocol
- A description of whether the deception results in any increased risk to participants
- An indication of whether the deception may affect a subject's willingness to participate in research
- A description of the poststudy debriefing that includes offering the participant the option to withdraw his or her data from the study
- If an exception to the requirement for a debriefing is requested, the study must be reviewed by the full board of the IRB
- A description of any previous use of deception in similar research and a summary of any actual harms or reactions from participants to the use of deception
- A description of alternatives to deception that were considered and an explanation as to why these alternatives were rejected

Further, since around 2010, social media has seen a meteoric rise as a tool for researchers to recruit study participants. We highlight a few ethical issues that have been raised by these methods. It is important to consider such points as where the recruitment ads will be posted (i.e., which website or social media app such as Facebook), what hours of the day or week the ads appear, and whether anonymity can truly be said to apply given that people will respond from an IP address (Gelinas et al., 2017). Social media recruitment may be

highly effective and cost-efficient, especially when trying to reach more hidden populations but it may also present issues such as people trying to join a study who may not actually meet the study inclusion criteria. It is always wise to consider that people, potential study subjects, can be deceptive as well and are not truthful if they have financial motives. Possible methods of verifying key inclusion criteria such as gender, sex, age, race, and ethnicity should be implemented. In addition, individuals who participate in these online surveys may expect to see results in the future. This presents a complicated question to the researcher regarding distribution of data results. Would the researcher be willing to post the results on the social media site from where the pool of participants was drawn? If not, this again may become a significant ethical issue with regard to study methods.

A final recruitment issue involves low levels of literacy. Despite being a global superpower, the United States is home to more than 30 million people who cannot read. Millions more read at exceptionally low levels of understanding. This sad observation is not only an issue for our economy and national security but also is a challenge for public health research. By necessity and for justice, public health research must be devoted to the obligation to reduce health disparities. Unfortunately, people who lack literacy are also the most likely victims of health disparities; this creates an overrepresentation of low-literacy people who are thus important potential volunteers for public health research studies. So, how does this relate to recruitment? The answer involves the concept of **written informed consent**.

As you will learn in the next section of this chapter, written informed consent is the hallmark of a principle known as **autonomy**. The cornerstone of written informed consent is that potential study volunteers must know exactly what the study will ask them to do, why they have been selected, their rights as volunteers, and their rights to withdraw from the study at any time. These are, in fact, somewhat complicated points to convey effectively when the potential participant does not read at all or reads below the grade level at which the informed consent document has been prepared. Even though many internal review boards require consent forms to be prepared at no higher than an eighth-grade reading level, this may still be too high for millions of Americans.

To rectify the problem of gaining informed consent from people who may have low literacy, guidance from the OHRP suggests the following:

Informed consent is a process, not just a form. Information must be presented to enable persons to voluntarily decide whether or not to participate as a research subject. It is a fundamental mechanism to ensure respect for persons through provision of thoughtful consent for a voluntary act. The procedures used in obtaining informed consent should be designed to educate the subject population in terms that they can understand. Therefore, informed consent language and its documentation (especially explanation of the study's purpose, duration, experimental procedures, alternatives, risks, and benefits) must be written in "lay language" (i.e., understandable to the people being asked to participate). The written presentation of information is used to document the basis for consent and for the subjects' future reference. The consent document should be revised when deficiencies are noted or when additional information will improve the consent process. (Office for Human Research Protections, 2003)

The critical sentence in this guidance is this:

The procedures used in obtaining informed consent should be designed to educate the subject population in terms that they can understand.

This sentence makes it clear that gaining informed consent is very much a process, one that involves educating (i.e., teaching) people about the study and its requirements and in terms they understand. If people do not understand a given term in its written form, is it possible they may also *not* understand it in spoken form? We suggest that the answer is "Yes" and thus believe educating potential study volunteers must be a process that effectively involves feedback loops between the research staff obtaining informed consent and the potential volunteer. A feedback loop occurs when (in this case) the research staff determines how little (or how much) of what has just been "taught" was truly understood and then adjusts the language, pace, and method of "teaching" accordingly. Although this may sound like a reasonable solution to dealing with literacy issues relative to gaining informed consent, in actual practice, it may be difficult and thus not always a standard practice to train staff members in the art of teaching via feedback loops. The result then becomes one of some low-literacy volunteers simply trusting the staff member, nodding their heads to signify agreement, and signing what then becomes written informed consent. The problem is, of course, that the word *informed* does not apply.

This dilemma is one that must be squarely addressed by the supervising researcher (referred to as the **principal investigator**). In the event you are someday a principal investigator, we urge you to work diligently to have all your staff learn the basic principles of effectively teaching people who are of limited literacy in the research procedures. We also urge you to consider a somewhat different but equally important version of this issue of low literacy: the level of English proficiency in a population of non-English speakers or people who speak or read English as a second language. In the event that potential volunteers are literate in a language other than English, OHRP recommends that the written informed consent document should be prepared in the person's native language.

Where informed consent is documented in accordance with §46.117(b)(1), the written consent document should embody, in language understandable to the subject, all the elements necessary for legally effective informed consent. Subjects who do not speak English should be presented with a consent document written in a language understandable to them. OPRR strongly encourages the use of this procedure whenever possible. (Office for Human Research Protections, 1995)

Thus, as a principal investigator, you may someday face a choice between having two or more versions of a written informed consent document available or excluding people from study participation if they cannot read or speak English. We strongly advocate the former solution because the latter may exclude an important segment of your intended target population from the benefits of your research study (bear in mind that findings from a research study can be generalized to populations and subpopulations that were included in the study). Thus, for instance, if you exclude non–English-speaking Latinas from a study then your research findings have absolutely no value for this population in terms of translating that research into widespread public health practice.

▶ What Is Autonomy, Justice, and Beneficence?

In 1979, the *Belmont Report* was published and subsequently served as the primary document guiding the conduct of research with volunteers. The report described three principles, each being equally vital in designing protocols and policies that protect study volunteers from harm (with harm defined as physical, mental, or social ill effects from study participation).

Autonomy: The quality or state of being self-governing: especially the right of self-government. (*Merriam-Webster Dictionary*)

The first principle is **respect for autonomy** and equates with people being provided with full disclosure. This means that potential volunteers must be made fully aware of all possible risks and benefits that may possibly be associated with study participation. The cornerstone of this principle has become known as *written informed consent* (as previously described in this chapter). Obtaining informed consent from each study volunteer provides a high degree of assurance that respect for autonomy has been met, at least in the study's enrollment stage. At this juncture, we—and our public health mascots Snow and Hamilton—hasten to remind you that obtaining consent is a process, one that involves a verbal exchange between the researcher and the potential volunteer (see **FIGURE 3.1**). This process should never be rushed, and it must be conducted based on the learning and developmental needs of the potential volunteer. For instance, although some volunteers may be fully literate, they may nonetheless simply not take ample time to read a consent form. Thus, again, the researcher has an obligation to conduct a paragraph-by-paragraph oral review of the entire document.

The language used in the informed consent form must be "plain and clear," and all possible risks and benefits must have been described. Even more important, the document makes it clear that the

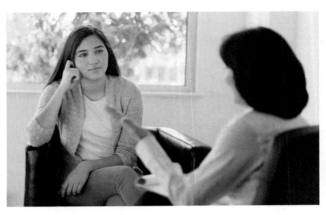

FIGURE 3.2 The Informed Consent Process.
© Tetra Images/Getty Images

volunteer may end his or her participation at any time. This freedom to withdraw without penalty must be made explicit by the researcher *during the consent process* (see **FIGURE 3.2**). As a researcher, you must understand that the consent form language binds you to a type of contract with the study volunteers, which means you must uphold the promises and pledges made within this document.

One common pledge made by researchers often reads something like this: "Your participation in this study may help others like you." For this reason, your entire study is subject to scrutiny by an accredited IRB. The board will determine whether the proposed study procedures are sufficient to reach the study objectives. More vital, the IRB will determine whether the study objectives (if met) make a sufficient contribution to the knowledge base and thus have true value for "others like you."

Justice: The maintenance or administration of what is just: especially by the impartial adjustment of conflicting claims or the assessment of merited reward or punishments. (*Merriam-Webster Dictionary*)

The second principle of the *Belmont Report* is known as **justice**. Departing somewhat from the dictionary definition, this principle involves the simple point that research participants and the larger population to which the findings would apply must be parallel. Consider, for instance, the existence of a new drug designed to treat hepatitis C. The extreme cost of this drug keeps it out of reach for most people in developing nations. What if it had been tested in nations such as Liberia, Mali, Guinea, and Afghanistan? The practice of using people as research participants when these people are unlikely to benefit from the eventual outcome of the study is considered unethical. The intention

ONE DOES NOT *SIMPLY*

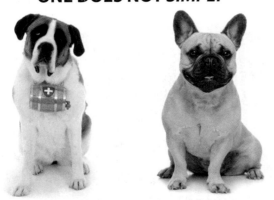

GET INFORMED CONSENT

FIGURE 3.1 Public Health Mascots Snow and Hamilton Weigh in on Informed Consent.
© Eric Isselee/Shutterstock; © Svetography/Shutterstock

BOX 3.4 Example of a Randomized Controlled Trial Possibly Violating the Principle of Justice

Throughout 2004, a multicity trial of the antiretroviral drug tenofovir was conducted in six cities: Phnom Penh, Cambodia; Yaoundé, Cameroon; Accra, Ghana; Lilongwe, Malawi; Ibadan, Nigeria; and Bangkok, Thailand. Although tenofovir has been widely used to treat HIV infections, for these trials it was to be tested for efficacy in preventing the transmission of HIV by giving it before subjects could be infected. This use of the drug was called *preexposure prophylaxis* (PrEP). Some of the key controversies surrounding the trial within these specific settings included the safety of this medication, the assumptions regarding whether tenofovir would be in pill form, the adverse effects especially if taken by an individual without HIV, the possibility of drug resistance, the impact of co-infections with common diseases in the area such as malaria, the care and support of those within the trial, community engagement, and access to PrEP after the trial, the most controversial issue. In addition, one of the biggest ethical concerns of using these locations for the large-scale trial was whether or not low-income individuals within these cities would ever actually be the target population of an expensive, cutting-edge HIV drug. The argument remains that if the target population was essentially, the high-risk populations living in the United States, why was the drug trial carried out within international cities? Ultimately, three location sites shut down the trial based on heavy ethical controversy. This issue of justice would indicate that an ethical study would include one that was conducted within the United States among the targeted populations where PrEP would realistically be available and accessible to the target population (Peterson & Folayan, 2019).

---

here is that the poor or disadvantaged cannot be exploited. **BOX 3.4** provides an example from the published, peer-reviewed literature.

In the same vein, the principle of justice also implies that people should not be excluded from study participation when the study may provide benefits to that population. A great example applies to testing programs designed to avert sexually transmitted diseases (STDs), with populations of persons older than age 17. Although it is convenient to recruit only persons 18 and older (as they can give consent), the epidemiology of STDs suggests that a substantial portion of the annual cases occur in persons younger than 18. Thus, leaving out the younger teens from STD prevention studies is also violating the principle of justice and thus is considered unethical.

One of the best examples (i.e., the most glaring of violations) relative to how justice may not be met involves studies using prisoners, especially those with life sentences (see **FIGURE 3.3**). Prisoners are categorized as members of **vulnerable populations** (e.g., pregnant women, human fetuses and neonates, children, cognitively impaired persons, prisoners, students and employees, and educationally disadvantaged individuals) because of the many unique conditions associated with confinement that compromise their ability to exercise free choice. The word *prisoner* is defined in section 45 of the Code of Federal Regulations (CFR). 46.303(c) as:

any individual involuntarily confined or detained in a penal institution. The term is intended to encompass individuals sentenced

to such an institution under a criminal or civil statute, individuals detained in other facilities by virtue of statutes or commitment procedures which provide alternatives to criminal prosecution or incarceration in a penal institution, and individuals detained pending arraignment, trial, or sentencing.

Thus, consider a study designed to test the safety of a new preventive approach of providing males who are not HIV infected with a drug that is used to treat HIV-infected individuals and is known as **preexposure prophylaxis (PrEP)**. PrEP is designed to prevent people from acquiring HIV. As a daily pill, adherence to PrEP is currently problematic, meaning that many people using this preventive approach fail to take the pills every day and thus are not gaining the

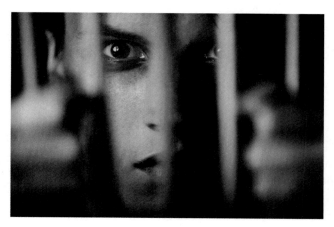

FIGURE 3.3 Male Prisoner Sentenced to Life.
© Arman Zhenikeyev/Corbis/Getty Images Plus/Getty Images

full level of protection. Thus, an innovative solution has been to use an implant method. Much like the use of subdermal (i.e., under the skin) implants that have slow-release hormones used to prevent conception in fertile women, the proposed implants of PrEP are also subdermal and last the same length of time as contraceptive implants (i.e., 90 days). Of course, gaining approval from the U.S. Food and Drug Administration for this new method of delivering PrEP to the body requires research trials, one of which is a safety trial. The study involves implanting PrEP subdermally in males (a primary target population for PrEP—see "Think About It!" toward the end of this chapter). If you were a member of the IRB that was asked to review such a research study, what would your concerns be? Possible concerns include:

- What are the possible side effects?
- If it is not safe, what harm will occur?
- What about inflammation at the site of the implant?
- Will the implants be medically supervised by qualified physicians?
- Can study volunteers have the implants removed on request?

Although each of these concerns is valid, none are as important as the one that should first come to mind: For those serving life sentences, this method of HIV prevention will never be available to them. Thus, the study population has no chance of benefiting from the scientific advances made by the study, so the first reaction any IRB member should have is something like, "This is unethical because it clearly violates the principle of justice as defined in the *Belmont Report*."

Before we take you to the next and final key principle of the *Belmont Report*, we want to quickly offer you a question related to the subject of research with prison populations. As we noted in the previous paragraph, each bulleted concern is entirely valid. Yet each is also amenable to resolution by applying the principle of autonomy. This is because each bulleted item in that list relates to risk; thus, each risk can be clearly defined and explained to people before they decide to participate in the study. However, the key point here is that they must be "free" to make the decision to not participate. **BOX 3.5** provides guidance from the Office for Human Research Protections that gives you an in-depth look at the safeguards in place relative to ensuring that the principle of autonomy is met in prison-based research studies.

Beneficence: The quality or state of doing or producing good. (*Merriam-Webster Dictionary*)

We now present the final principle, **beneficence**, last because it is the most complex. Ultimately,

---

BOX 3.5   A Summary of Added Regulations for Research with Prison Populations

The following guidance is taken from the website for the Office of Research Protections.

HHS regulations at 45 CFR part 46, subpart C provide additional protections pertaining to biomedical and behavioral research involving prisoners as subjects. The regulations are applicable to all biomedical and behavioral research conducted or supported by HHS. See 45 CFR 46.301. It is important to note that the regulations provide that "biomedical or behavioral research conducted or supported by HHS shall not involve prisoners as subjects" unless the research is specifically authorized within the subpart. See 45 CFR 46.306(b).

In the preamble to the final subpart C rule, the drafters noted: "In fact, most testimony before the Commission opposed the use of prisoners in any form of medical research not intended to benefit the individual prisoner." 43 Fed. Reg. 53652, 53653 (November 16, 1978). HHS did determine that some limited research would be permissible but not "until additional and more stringent review procedures are conducted."

B. Subpart C applies where any subject is or becomes a prisoner.

The provisions of subpart C apply to any research conducted or supported by HHS in which prisoners are subjects. This includes situations where a human subject becomes a prisoner after the research has commenced. As the Purpose section of the regulation notes: "Inasmuch as prisoners may be under constraints because of their incarceration which could affect their ability to make a truly voluntary and uncoerced decision whether or not to participate as subjects in research, it is the purpose of this subpart to provide additional safeguards for the protection of prisoners involved in activities to which this subpart is applicable." 45 CFR 46.302. These concerns apply whether the research involves individuals who are prisoners at the time of enrollment in the research or who become prisoners after they become enrolled in the research. In the latter situation, it is unlikely that review of the research and the consent document contemplated the constraints imposed by incarceration.

(continues)

BOX 3.5   A Summary of Added Regulations for Research with Prison Populations   *(continued)*

C. What does the definition of prisoner encompass?

"Prisoner" is defined by HHS regulations at 45 CFR part 46.303(c) as "any individual involuntarily confined or detained in a penal institution. The term is intended to encompass individuals sentenced to such an institution under a criminal or civil statute, individuals detained in other facilities by virtue of statutes or commitment procedures which provide alternatives to criminal prosecution or incarceration in a penal institution, and individuals detained pending arraignment, trial, or sentencing."

D. Special Composition of IRB

In addition to satisfying the requirements of 45 CFR 46.116 and 46.117, when an IRB reviews a protocol involving prisoners as subjects that is conducted or supported by HHS, the composition of the IRB must satisfy the following requirements of HHS regulations at 45 CFR 46.304(a) and (b):

- A majority of the IRB (exclusive of prisoner members) shall have no association with the prison(s) involved, apart from their membership on the IRB.
- At least one member of the IRB must be a prisoner, or a prisoner representative with appropriate background and experience to serve in that capacity, except that where a particular research project is reviewed by more than one IRB, only one IRB need satisfy this requirement.

In the absence of choosing someone who is a prisoner or has been a prisoner, the IRB should choose a prisoner representative who has a close working knowledge, understanding and appreciation of prison conditions from the perspective of the prisoner. In addition, the IRB must notify OHRP of any change in the IRB roster occasioned by the addition of a prisoner or a prisoner representative, as required by HHS regulations at 45 CFR 46.103(b)(3). IRBs should be alert to the impact of roster changes on quorum requirements under HHS regulations at 45 CFR 46.108(b). . . . For research involving prisoners as subjects, the IRB must meet the special composition requirements of 45 CFR 46.304 for all types of review of the protocol, including initial review, continuing review, review of protocol amendments, and review of reports of unanticipated problems involving risks to subjects.

judging the ethics of a proposed research study is similar to judging the guilt or innocence of a person on trial for a crime. The weight of evidence pertaining to guilt must be considered only in relation to the weight of evidence pertaining to innocence. As always, an example may be helpful. Consider a proposed study that has three clear risks: (1) It may cause social harm to participants; (2) if the privacy of study records is somehow compromised, the participants may have legal problems; and (3) participants may learn information about themselves that proves to be psychologically harmful. So far, how do you feel about the ethics of this study? (Before you come to a judgment, we remind you that this "courtroom" has two sides.) The study clearly has two likely benefits: (1) It will establish the efficacy of a drug-dependence counseling program intended for use in street-outreach settings; and (2) if successful, the program being tested has the potential to reduce the rate of deaths from substance use and violence by as much as 50%. Now, has your verdict changed at all? This example illustrates the point that **potential**

risk is only quantifiable in the context of its relationship to likely benefits. **FIGURE 3.4** illustrates this balance.

Indeed, when seeking ethics approval for a study, researchers are asked by the IRB to supply a *benefits-versus-risk* comparison. The following paragraph typifies this type of comparison.

One risk of study participation is the inadvertent disclosure to others that any given volunteer was tested for breast and/or cervical cancer or that any given volunteer tested positive either of these cancers. A second risk involves the inadvertent release of name-identified responses to the baseline or follow-up assessments. Another risk involves personal discomfort in responding to the questions or in interacting with the assigned Lay Health Advisor. The proposed research provides several direct benefits to those who volunteer. First, women will benefit from the social media education program. For those

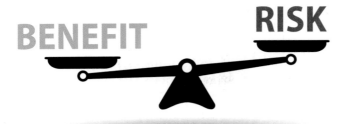

FIGURE 3.4 Weighing the Benefits Versus the Risks of Research.
© Nemanja Cosovic/Shutterstock

randomized to the intervention condition, benefit will occur from interactions with the assigned advisor. Further, all study volunteers will indirectly benefit from the potential future value of the findings relative to the eventual implementation of interventions designed to promote cancer screening for rural Appalachian women.

▶ What Is the Difference Between Exempt, Expedited, and Full-Committee Reviews?

To begin, you have an obligation to select one of three options when asking an IRB for ethics approval. Once you make your selection, you must follow the application instructions provided by the IRB. Once you apply, the IRB may overrule your selection of the option you choose (i.e., exempt, expedited, or full-committee review). As a rule, exempt research is still defined as *human subjects research*, but it is characterized by anonymity and a near complete absence

of risk. It is the category of expedited research that requires more intense consideration and monitoring by an IRB. Guidance from the previously mentioned Office of Human Research Protection has provided a list of seven categories (**TABLE 3.1**). At least one of these categories must apply to the proposed study before it can truly be considered expedited. In cases when the proposed research project is not described by one or more of the categories shown in Table 3.1, the full-committee review most likely applies. This means that a panel of IRB members (as many as 12) will consider the ethical issues, merits, and risk–benefit ratio of the study.

All three forms of review are ultimately equivalent in that they typically result in a letter granting IRB approval for a period of 6 months to 1 year. Before the first approval period expires, the IRB will prompt you (the investigator) to file a continuation review that will be far less demanding than the original application. Continuing reviews of protocols that were initially approved by a full committee are typically handled as expedited reviews. Regardless of whether your research is exempt, expedited, or full-committee review, we urge you to be vigilant in observing one thing: the formulation and construction of the study protocol. Protocols include every possible aspect of the planned research, such as plans for recruitment, retention (if applicable), randomization (if applicable), intervention (if applicable), and compensation for the time that volunteers give to the study. Protocols should include plans for data analysis, and these plans should show that adequate statistical power is available to provide a fair test of all proposed study hypotheses. This last requirement may seem less involved with ethics and more about science. However, as noted previously in this chapter,

TABLE 3.1 Seven Categories That May Qualify a Study for Expedited Review

1. Clinical studies of drugs and medical devices.
2. Collection of blood samples by finger stick, heel stick, ear stick, or venipuncture.
3. Collection of data through noninvasive procedures (not involving general anesthesia or sedation) routinely employed in clinical practice, excluding procedures involving x-rays or microwaves.
4. Research involving materials (data, documents, records, or specimens) that have been collected or will be collected solely for nonresearch purposes.
5. Collection of data from voice, video, digital, or image recordings made for research purposes.
6. Research on individual or group characteristics or behavior (including but not limited to research on perception, cognition, motivation, identity, language, communication, cultural beliefs or practices, and social behavior) or research employing survey, interview, oral history, focus group, program evaluation, human factors evaluation, or quality-assurance methodologies.
7. Continuing review of research previously approved by the convened IRB.

the study must have value to be considered ethical. Volunteers who join a research study do so with good intent (i.e., they want to help), so it is the obligation of the researcher to ensure that this good intent is not misplaced or betrayed in any way.

▶ What Data Security Options Exist to Protect Study Volunteers?

The most important protection that can be provided to study volunteers is not asking them to provide their names or other identifiable information such as Social Security number, date of birth, and so on. Implementing an anonymous study is a distinct possibility if the study perhaps does not involve more than one time point of data collection, and with this occurring immediately after enrollment. In fact, where this scenario is possible, an IRB is likely to also waive the requirement of written informed consent because a signature on such a document creates a name associated with the study records. The informed consent process would still be mandatory; only the signature would be waived as a requirement.

In studies involving any repeated assessments or any form of ongoing data collection (e.g., medical records reviews, prescription records, insurance claims), obtaining the names of volunteers is necessary. This necessity, however, does not need to create substantial risk to volunteers. The associated risks can be mitigated through protocols that replace the names with unique codes and protect the document linking codes to names. In this case, *protection* refers to using a paper record (thus avoiding the inherent risks of storing any record on a server or computer) to link names to the assigned study codes. The paper record must be stored in a locked filing cabinet within a locked office. It should only be accessible to the lead researcher (known as the *principal investigator*) and those on her or his research staff who are certified to collect and view records from study volunteers. This protection is only one of many that must be considered in studies where names and codes are used for ongoing assessments.

A good example of an issue to consider is protecting the confidentiality of volunteers; this includes not disclosing that they are part of the study. Although this may seem a bit odd at first, think about studies that are focused on behaviors such as substance use, sexuality, intimate partner

violence, or illicit behaviors. Studies dealing with potentially sensitive aspects of a person's life may carry such a social or personal stigma that a volunteer might choose to keep his or her participation private. Thus, it is important to design protocols that protect against the risk of inadvertently disclosing that any given volunteer is, in fact, a volunteer. An example of such a protocol follows.

> Confidentiality will be protected by multiple procedures. First, interview response forms will be coded with a number rather than a name identifier—only key study personnel will have access to the links between men's names and their assigned code numbers. Further, the contact information process used to collect multiple forms of future connection efforts with men is structured such that men are asked to provide only the contact information that they believe is safe relative to accidental disclosure. For the information they do provide, men will be asked for "rules" as to how research staff members should and should not proceed when making contact (e.g., "Please do not ask for me by name if you call me—identify yourself first and then I will know who you are").

An additional concern when conducting studies that collect names or other information that can identify someone involves the Health Insurance Portability and Accountability Act (HIPAA). As its name implies, this federal law protects people from being denied insurance based on a negative health condition or even a predisposition to a negative health condition. The essence of the law is simple: People's health information is private, and they cannot be asked to share this with you (the researcher) unless they first sign a waiver of their HIPAA-based protections relative to the specific information you wish to collect. Thus, it is common practice to include language required to obtain a waiver of HIPAA rights as part of the informed consent document.

Perhaps the most crucial safeguard when it comes to protecting the privacy of study volunteers is to be well informed about electronic data security risks. These risks range from the obvious to those that are far from obvious. An obvious risk, for instance, is that data should never be placed on a thumb drive or similar small portable device that stores electronic information and can be easily lost or stolen. Moreover, data files should never be emailed or stored in cloud-based storage at least without first encrypting the file and inputting password protection. To help

TABLE 3.2 Ten Guiding Principles for Data Collection, Storage, Sharing, and Use to Ensure Security and Confidentiality

1. Public health data should be acquired, used, disclosed, and stored for legitimate public health purposes.
2. Programs should collect the minimum amount of personally identifiable information necessary to conduct public health activities.
3. Programs should have strong policies to protect the privacy and security of personally identifiable data.
4. Data collection and use policies should reflect respect for the rights of individuals and community groups and minimize undue burden.
5. Programs should have policies and procedures to ensure the quality of any data they collect or use.
6. Programs have the obligation to use and disseminate summary data to relevant stakeholders in a timely manner.
7. Programs should share data for legitimate public health purposes and may establish data-use agreements to facilitate sharing data in a timely manner.
8. Public health data should be maintained in a secure environment and transmitted through secure methods.
9. Minimize the number of persons and entities granted access to identifiable data.
10. Program officials should be active, responsible stewards of public health data.

Ten Guiding Principles for Data Collection, Storage, Sharing, and Use to Ensure Security and Confidentiality. Retrieved from https://www.cdc.gov/nchhstp/programintegration/tenguidingprinciples.htm

researchers implement protective strategies, the Centers for Disease Control and Prevention (CDC) has published the 10 guidelines shown in **TABLE 3.2**.

A somewhat less obvious risk to data security involves servers. Even the most sophisticated servers are vulnerable to cybertheft. Any such theft of data collected from study volunteers is, of course, a violation of the trust placed in you as the principal investigator by the volunteers when they agreed to enroll. This risk makes it important for you to be a wise consumer when it comes to choosing the correct hardware and software for data collection and storage in your study. Here, more than ever, the maxim of *caveat emptor* applies (meaning it is the buyers' responsibility to thoroughly understand a product before purchasing it). Thus, we urge you to do your homework!

For instance, at a minimum we suggest that any server or system that you use for storing digital data should be protected by advanced firewalls. Further, they should be scanned on a regular basis (at least weekly) to detect any vulnerabilities in the security of the system (with corrections being made immediately). The system should also be checked regularly regarding failover points. A server should have optimal guards to protect participants' confidentiality. Perhaps of greatest importance, safeguards should be in place to deny systems access to anyone other than those authorized and approved by agreement with the internal review board responsible for ethical oversight of the study.

Finally, perhaps the least obvious risk to data security involves the informal exchange or sharing of information about a given volunteer among members

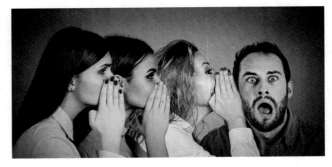

FIGURE 3.5 Gossiping in the Research Context.
© Pathdoc/Shutterstock

of the research staff or between research staff and nonresearch staff members (i.e., others employed in study settings such as clinics, community-based organizations, and schools or colleges). Although the prospect of cybertheft of a study volunteer's personal information is remote, the odds of informal sharing of this information in the research setting is far from remote (see **FIGURE 3.5**). Consequently, as a standing ethic, the principal investigator must be vigilant of this possibility and, therefore, engage in training and monitoring to ensure compliance with the ethic that discussing information obtained from study volunteers is strictly forbidden and may result in being terminated from the staff.

▸ How Do I Prepare an IRB Application?

As with any worthwhile academic endeavor, all research studies begin with an exceedingly long planning phase. This is especially true with IRB applications.

It all begins with first becoming certified to conduct research with human subjects. The certification process functions at a national level through a system known as the Collaborative Institutional Training Initiative (CITI). **FIGURE 3.6** shows the interface you will find on the CITI website. You must, however, enter the CITI website through the university or organization in which you are serving as a research investigator. The CITI training involves reading modules and taking a quiz after each module. We can assure you that the process, although somewhat time consuming, is manageable. Thus, there is no time like the present to do this. After all, it is the first step in preparing an IRB application because your CITI certification number (and certificate) are center stage in this application process.

The next "big step" in applying for IRB approval is to create the **study protocol**. Although the term *protocol* sounds a bit daunting, the process for drafting this document is simply a collection of the study activities laid out in an easy-to-follow and sequential manner. The protocol must focus on exactly what is expected of study volunteers. Points covered should include the following:

- Inclusion and exclusion criteria for the study (i.e., what requirements must be met to be eligible for the study and of those that are eligible, what might exclude some of them?)

- The number of people who will be enrolled in the study
- How the study is important (this includes a literature review showing that the study fills a gap in the research literature—see Chapter 2)
- How potential volunteers will be recruited and from which locations (note that Internet sites are considered a location)
- How written informed consent will be obtained
- How the data will be collected (this section may be extensive as it must describe points such as how and where any face-to-face interviews will be conducted, whether self-administered questionnaires will be used and, if so, what format will be used for this process—e.g., electronic tablet, mobile device, phone calls, or texts)
- How much time will be required of study volunteers and how many, if any, follow-up assessments will occur
- Details on any intervention or prevention program
- Whether volunteers will derive more benefit from the study given the level of risk involved (again, from earlier in the chapter you will recognize this as the principle of beneficence)

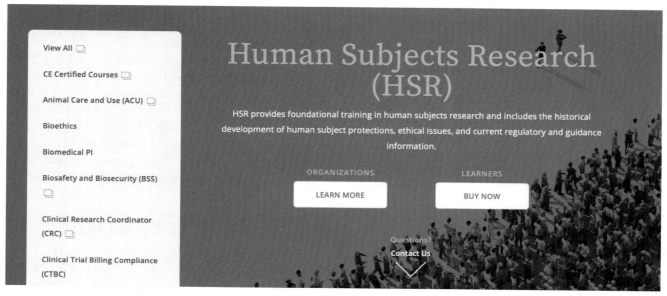

FIGURE 3.6 Screenshot of the Collaborative Institutional Training Initiative for Human Subjects Research Training.
CITI Program. Retrieved from https://about.citiprogram.org/en/series/human-subjects-research-hsr/

■ Whether volunteers will receive compensation for their time (this must be spelled out to precisely state the type and amount of compensation)

Although different universities and organizations have varying requirements for a protocol, none of these requirements should entail any extra writing on your part. This is because the protocol is also the guide for conducting the actual study, training staff, developing assessments, and so on. In other words, you must have a protocol to have a study.

The next "big step" in obtaining IRB approval also varies greatly, depending on your institutional affiliation. This step entails spelling out—in great detail—the exact risks that could occur as a result of study participation (again, this harkens back to the principle of beneficence). **BOX 3.6** provides you a sample of the level of detail typically required in this section of an IRB application.

As you will see from carefully reading Box 3.6, risk does not always mean risk to life or health and may not necessarily be viewed by you as counting as a risk. For instance, calling it a "risk" to have other people find out that you joined this study may seem like a stretch; however, consider a person who has no job security (i.e., the boss can terminate the person's employment easily) and fears that having a negative health condition such as hypertension may prompt such action from that employer. The point here is that even unlikely risks must still be identified and spelled out in this section of the IRB application.

The final big step is to carefully follow the submission instructions published by your institution and then wait for the local IRB analyst to assign a category. At this point, the IRB will review the study protocols, informed consent forms, and other documents. In many instances, you will be asked to change parts of the application or clarify certain procedures. To help you be prepared for one or more rounds with the reviewers at the IRB, think of the application process as iterative rather than as a single event. In fact, you should consider the initial application as nothing more than a method of opening a dialogue with the IRB, one that will continue throughout the life cycle of your study. This is the case because all IRB approvals require periodic (as determined by the IRB) reports and updates regarding progress. More important and implied by IRB approval is that you have an ongoing obligation to communicate with the IRB even after approval is granted. These obligations include the following:

■ Making modifications to the study protocol
■ Adding new personnel to the study
■ Adding items to the assessment schedule
■ Enrolling more volunteers than originally planned
■ Retaining signed consent forms and other required study documents in your files
■ Compromising data security or privacy in any form
■ Avoiding any event that may be considered adverse, meaning that discomfort (physical or mental), harm (of any kind), or actual injury has occurred to one or more study volunteers.

BOX 3.6 Example of a "Potential Risks" Section of an IRB Application

Several potential risks could be associated with any study activity. One important risk is the possibility that volunteers may experience personal discomfort in responding to the questions posed in the web-based assessment. Also, volunteers randomized to the intervention condition may experience personal discomfort in learning about their own high blood pressure and more about the causes and solution to this problem. Accidental disclosure of participation in this study may also be problematic for those volunteers who have kept their visit to the clinic (where they were recruited) secretive. Also, volunteers randomized to the control group may not receive adequate information, motivation, or behavioral-skills training to promote prevention practices related to high blood pressure. As a result, these people may be more vulnerable to subsequent hypertension and its chronic effects on the kidneys, arteries, heart, and so on. Further, being asked for contact information to facilitate their return for planned follow-up sessions may pose discomfort to some volunteers. Failure to safeguard this contact process could cause social discomfort to study participants. Finally, note that any breaches in confidentiality of records could cause psychosocial discomfort to study volunteers. Risks beyond psychosocial discomfort are not anticipated, thus the seriousness of anticipated risk could be considered low to moderate (e.g., physical, legal, and other risks are not anticipated). Remember that volunteers assigned to either condition also receive full standard of care, thus these volunteers are at no more physical risk of hypertension than those who decide not to participate in the study.

As we hope you have garnered from reading this section, IRB approval is simply the beginning of what will become a lasting relationship between you and IRB members. It is vital that you stay engaged with the IRB until the day comes when you submit a form to close out the study.

Think About It!
A Case Study of HIV Prevention

As noted in this chapter, a drug treatment known as *preexposure prophylaxis* is widely used to prevent HIV infection. This is an important prevention strategy, but it may also be one that raises questions about ethics. In this case, it is less about ethics in research than about ethics in practice. You may be surprised to learn that despite widespread protections of research in public health, few such protections exist for actual practice. As an example, consider the following paragraph.

> CDC estimates that one of every two Black men who have sex with men (BMSM) will acquire HIV in his lifetime. This unprecedented estimate places BMSM in the U.S., at a level of HIV risk exceeding that found in many of highly impacted sub-Saharan nations. Consequently, evidence-based interventions applied to promote the use of PrEP for this population are important. However, it is noteworthy, that the most recently published study on condom effectiveness against HIV acquisition among MSM provided a 70% effectiveness rate for persons using condoms consistently (Smith, Herbst, Zhang, &

Rose, 2015). The study, however, did not correct for condom errors among those using condoms consistently, thereby creating bias that underestimates condom effectiveness (Crosby, 2013; Crosby, Charnigo, Weathers, Caliendo, & Shrier, 2012; Graham, Crosby, Sanders, & Yarber, 2006). Assuming 70% as a conservative estimate of effectiveness, correct condom use is nonetheless as effective (or better) than estimates of PrEP efficacy obtained in the original study of MSM (the unadjusted estimate of effectiveness was 44% (Grant, Lama, Anderson, McMahan, Liu, et al., 2010).

Having read the preceding paragraph above, please think about the ethics of prescribing PrEP (which is typically almost completely covered by health insurance) without also providing a corresponding and equally assertive level of clinical guidance. Teaching BMSM how to consistently select and use condoms can help make this equally valid HIV-prevention strategy a practical reality. Consider also that high-quality condoms and lubricants are expensive and not covered by health insurance.

Take Home Points

- The foundation of research with study volunteers is based on carefully planned protocols that provide multiple protections against potential harm, regardless of how likely the risks are to occur and lead to harm.
- The *Belmont Report* is the historical and legal foundation for safeguarding study volunteers. The principles of autonomy, justice, and beneficence are paramount.
- Research can be classified as exempt, expedited, or requiring a full-committee review. The selected category determines the breadth and extent of the application sent to an internal review board.
- Participant literacy levels and not speaking English as a primary language are tremendously important issues to consider when recruiting and enrolling study volunteers.
- Prison-housed populations present a special set of concerns relative to the *Belmont Report*'s principles of justice and autonomy.
- Applying for IRB approval is a time-consuming but vitally important aspect of planning a research study. Once approved, communication between the investigator and the IRB must be open and ongoing.
- The informed consent process is the cornerstone of ethical research practices. This must always be an open and clear exchange between a member of the research team and the potential study volunteer.
- Protecting the privacy of study volunteers is an ongoing obligation of the principal investigator, one involving a set of safeguards during the study and a second involving the security of collected and stored data.

Key Terms

Autonomy
Beneficence
Coercion
Confidentiality
Deception
Institutional review board (IRB)
Justice

Placebo effect
Potential risk
Preexposure prophylaxis (PrEP)
Principal investigator
Privacy
Respect for autonomy
Security

Study protocol
United States Office for Human
   Research Protections (OHRP)
Vulnerable populations
Written informed consent

For Practice and Discussion

1. The Tuskegee study is an extreme example of unethical conduct seen in human subject research. Many other cases of unethical practice have been seen in research studies; although they may not have been quite as unethical, they still posed risks to participants. Using the search engine of Google Scholar, find a public health study that you suspect might have unethical conduct as defined by the standards of the *Belmont Report*. This will seem difficult at first, but consider the notion that every published study is not entirely without ethical fault. The idea is both frightening and true. Because of the considerable efforts in enforcing ethical research practice, however, these shortcomings are less common and less extreme. Once you find an article, cite the article and describe ethical shortfalls and how you would correct the issue. Make sure to explain your reasoning.

2. Using the same article you found for Question 1, determine what level of IRB approval is needed for your corrected version of the study. After doing so, form groups of three to four students and share your case with one another. Feel free to use the textbook or online resources to support your stance.

3. In the authors' experience, students commonly confuse the concepts of beneficence and justice. They are distinct pillars in the *Belmont Report*, and it is critical to understand how they shape ethical human subject research. Working with a classmate, use the following exercise to better your understanding of beneficence and justice.

   Both of you are to create three artificial scenarios that depict at least one example of beneficence and one example of justice. However, be sure not to use the terms *justice* or *beneficence* in your written scenarios. Trade scenarios with your partner and label your partner's examples as either "B" or "J." Discuss the intended answers with one another and make corrections where necessary.

References

Centers for Disease Control and Prevention (CDC). (2014). *Ten guiding principles for data collection, storage, sharing, and use to ensure security and confidentiality.* Washington, DC: CDC and NCHHSTP Program Collaboration and Service Integration. Retrieved from https://www.cdc.gov/nchhstp/programintegration/tenguidingprinciples.htm

Crosby, R. A. (2013). State of condom use in HIV prevention science and practice. *Current HIV/AIDS Reports, 10*(1), 59–64.

Crosby, R. A., Charnigo, R. A., Weathers, C., Caliendo, A. M., & Shrier, L. A. (2012). Condom effectiveness against non-viral sexually transmitted infections: A prospective study using electronic daily diaries. *Sexually Transmitted Infections, 88*(7), 484–489.

Gelinas, L., Pierce, R., Winkler, S., Cohen, I., G. I, Lynch, H. F., & Bierer, B. E. (2017). Using social media as a recruitment tool: ethical issues and recommendations. *American Journal of Bioethics, 17*(3), 3–10.

Graham, C. A., Crosby, R. A., Sanders, S. A., & Yarber, W. L. (2006). Assessment of condom use in men and women. *Annual Review of Sex Research, 16*(1), 2–52.

Grant, R. M., Lama, J. R., Anderson, P. L., McMahan, V., Liu, A. Y., Vargas L., . . . iPrEx Study Team. (2010). Pre-exposure chemoprophylaxis for HIV prevention in men who have sex with men. *New England Journal of Medicine, 363*(27), 2587–2599.

Guess, H. A., Kleinman, A., Kusek, J. W., & Engel, L. W. (Eds.). (2002). *The science of the placebo: Toward an interdisciplinary research agenda.* London, UK: BMJ Books.

Humphreys, L. (2017). The breastplate of righteousness. *Tearoom Trade,* 131–148.

McLeod, S. A. (2017, February 5). The Milgram shock experiment. Simply Psychology. Retrieved from https://www.simplypsychology.org/milgram.html

Meyerson, B. E., Martich, F. A., & Naehr, G. P. (2008). *Ready to go: The history and contributions of U.S. public health advisors.* Research Triangle Park, NC: American Social Health Association.

Office for Human Research Protections. (1995, November 9). *Informed consent of subjects who do not speak English.* Washington, DC: U.S. Department of Health and Human Services. Retrieved from Office for Human Research Protections.

Office for Human Research Protections. (2003, May 23). *Prisoner involvement in research*. Washington, DC: U.S. Department of Health and Human Services. Retrieved from https://www .hhs.gov/ohrp/regulations-and-policy/guidance/prisoner -research-ohrp-guidance-2003/index.html

Peterson, K., & Folayan, M. O. (2019, January). Ethics and HIV prevention research: An analysis of the early tenofovir PrEP trial in Nigeria. *Bioethics, 33*(1), 35–42.

Qualtrics.com. (2018, July 13). Security statement. Retrieved from https://www.qualtrics.com/security-statement/

Smith, D. K., Herbst, J. H., Zhang, X., & Rose, C. E. (2015, March). Condom effectiveness for HIV prevention by consistency of use among men who have sex with men in the United States. *Journal of Acquired Immune Deficiency Syndromes, 68*(3), 337–344.

Vase, L., Robinson, M. E., Verne, G. N., & Price, D. D. (2003). The contributions of suggestion, desire, and expectation to placebo effects in irritable bowel syndrome patients: An empirical investigation. *Pain, 105*(1–2), 17–25.

For Further Reading

Bernheim, R. G., Childress, J. F., Melnick, A., & Bonnie, R. J. (2013). *Essentials of public health ethics*. Burlington, MA: Jones & Bartlett.

Crosby, R. A., Salazar, L. F., & DiClemente, R. J. (2015). Ethical issues in health promotion research. In L. F. Salazar, R. A. Crosby, & R. J. DiClemente (Eds.), *Research methods in health promotion* (2nd ed.). San Francisco, CA: Jossey-Bass Wiley.

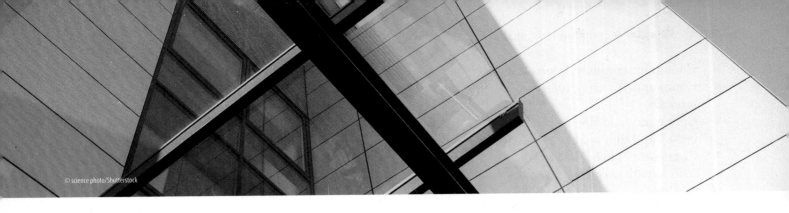

CHAPTER 4

Community-Based Participatory Research

▶ Overview

Before you begin learning about research methods, we must impart one last bit of wisdom stemming from the recent history of public health research and practice, a time when a great many public health efforts were implemented at the community level. Known by many names (all with subtle distinctions in meaning), research at the community level is best summarized by the term **community-based research**. This term implies a partnership with the community (via community members or leaders). Although the exact nature of this partnership can take many forms, the intent remains the same: to ensure program success and sustainability where a working relationship is formed between academic investigators and key leaders of the community where the research effort takes place. However, good intentions do not always translate into good outcomes. Historically, public health research has been criticized for not adequately or appropriately involving community participants, resulting in a negative perception of research. Researchers who come into the community from the outside (i.e., they are not part of the community) with a lack of connection and origin within the community can foster negative issues such as distrust, lack of cultural sensitivity, lack of cultural competence, and incompatibility with local politics, any of which can result in major problems to the research study. These unaddressed issues can typically mitigate the value of the proposed research. In fact, common problems experienced by communities involved in public health research have included the following:

- Irrelevance to the community
- Poor methodology that wastes resources
- Research data and findings that are not given back

- Communities feeling "overresearched"
- Communities feeling coerced to participate in research
- Communities feeling researched on rather than feeling as if they are partners in the process
- Communities being lied to
- Insensitivity to community concerns or issues
- Minimal or nonexistent benefits to communities

As the mission of public health seeks to ensure the health of whole communities while recognizing that the health of individuals is tied to their lives in the community, community-based research ideally should be instrumental in achieving this mission. Unfortunately, as previously stated, this is not always the case. To ensure that the well-being of communities is first and foremost, a public health working group was formed and developed a list of ethical principles to guide public health professionals and institutions in conducting research and practice geared toward populations and focused on prevention (Thomas, Sage, Dillenberg, & Guillory, 2002). These principles are listed in **TABLE 4.1**.

In viewing these principles, community involvement, collaboration, and empowerment are clearly at the heart of these principles. Thus, with some of the previous ethical misgivings, a stark contrast was needed where an honest and true researcher–community partnership could be formed that would transcend these mitigating factors. Thus, a better rendition of community-based research was conceived in alignment with the ethical principles and is known as **community-based participatory research (CBPR)**. CBPR improves on standard community-based research to involve the formation of a true and open partnership between researchers and community members to achieve overall success of a project and satisfaction among community members. As such, CBPR offers broad assurances that the research study will reflect the health needs of the community, have true community oversight, and be compatible with prevailing cultural values. CBPR adheres to the 12 ethical principles of public health research and practice with its emphasis on collaborating with the community as *full and equal partners* in all phases of the research process. Rather than researchers getting funding on their own in isolation and then contacting the community to participate in all of the planned activities, the *participatory* aspect of CBPR means the research agenda is thought out, developed, and carried out by this partnership. CBPR is especially suitable for research that involves vulnerable populations

TABLE 4.1 Principles of the Ethical Practice of Public Health

1. The underlying causes of disease should be the focal point of public health—this prevention orientation is vital.
2. Public health efforts directed at the community level should always be constructed in ways that are consistent with the rights of community members.
3. Community members must have a strong voice in public health policy, priorities, and programs.
4. A key aspect of public health involves advocacy for marginalized community members to obtain the essential needs for achieving and maintaining good health.
5. An important public health obligation involves seeking accurate information regarding how to best implement programs and policies that promote good health.
6. Community involvement in all decisions pertaining to public health programs and policy is a cornerstone of ethical practice.
7. Given the responsibility of protecting people's health, public health professionals must act on new health-related information in a timely manner.
8. All public health programs and policies should use strategies and methods that embrace the values and beliefs of the community.
9. Enhancing the physical and social contexts that shape health behavior is a core function of public health programs and policies.
10. Public health professionals are entrusted with the obligation of guarding the confidentiality of any information with the potential for harm to a community or to specified members of that community.
11. Institutions employing public health professionals have the obligation to constantly ensure the competence of the workforce.
12. Gaining and maintaining the trust of the public is a paramount obligation of public health professionals as they engage in collaborative work to promote good health.

who experience extreme inequities that result in health disparities and that shows great potential for reducing those disparities.

This chapter will provide you with a basic understanding of CBPR and its advantages so that you will be knowledgeable about how to undertake a CBPR approach. Although we do not advocate this approach for all public health research, we suggest that you consider taking this approach when the research takes the form of finding solutions to a specific public health issue within a defined community that experiences inequities and health disparities.

How Does CBPR Result in Better Sustainability?

In addition to adhering to the principles of public health, **sustainability** is another major advantage of CBPR. Unique to public health research, this term applies to intervention research—that is, research that designs and tests public health interventions. The term implies that the program being designed and tested will become integrated into the community and become an ongoing part of the public health structure. Consider a community that has experienced extremely high rates of gun violence. As a public health response, a program known as *Cure Violence* (http://cureviolence.org/) was designed to view violence as preventable and used methods and strategies associated with disease control but it also involved collaborations among multiple levels of community partners, stakeholders, and researchers. The model is depicted in **FIGURE 4.1** and has three main components as shown: interrupt transmission, reduce highest risk, and change community norms.

Cure Violence has been implemented in various states across the United States, and evaluations suggest that it does indeed significantly reduce gun shootings and injuries and save lives. However, after the evaluation research ends, what comes next? Clearly, it would be a disservice to simply declare success, end the program, and walk away. Instead, the public health imperative goes all the way back to the initial design stages of the program. Programs designed by people in the community, with community members being a central aspect of the implementation process, have an inherent ability to stand alone after the research phase ends. In this example, it may be that the program is administered by local health departments and criminal justice offices and involves local police officers, outreach workers, and public health educators, among others engaging in activities that focus on the three components. For example, to interrupt transmission and prevent retaliation once a shooting happens, trained workers immediately work in the community and at the hospital to cool down emotions and prevent retaliations—working with victims, friends and family of victims, and anyone else connected with an event.

By incorporating all program elements into a coordinated community response, Cure Violence can continue to save lives long after researchers have moved on to other public health challenges. Cure Violence is but one example of a successful CBPR approach that holds great potential for long-lasting sustainability.

Do All CBPR Objectives Need to Be Met?

As in life itself, research studies rarely achieve perfection. Thus, despite its great advantages, the principles and practices of CBPR may not always become practical realities. For instance, consider the idea that a main tenet of CBPR is that community needs must drive the research agenda. Although this principle is well intended, it may not always align with the mission of the funding agency sponsoring the research.

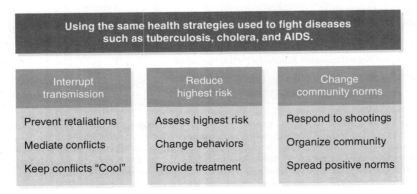

FIGURE 4.1 The Cure Violence Theoretical Model.
Reproduced from Cure Violence Global.

For example, perhaps a community identifies mental health or opioid addiction as the main health issue it wants ameliorated, but the funding agency targets cancer. A basic reality of rigorous research is that it is labor intensive and therefore costly, so funding is vital. Without it, conducting research activities would be nearly unfeasible. Agencies that fund research typically have a preset agenda that drives the allocation of funds. Usually, an agency will announce a funding opportunity by describing possible goals of the research, as shown in **FIGURE 4.2**.

Let's imagine that you feel qualified to respond to the funding announcement in Figure 4.2. Further, you want to apply as many of the CBPR principles as possible to your pending research project. Given the objectives stated in the announcement, however, a community advisory board would clearly have little authority to alter the study aims to fully meet its

Department of Health and Human Services

Part 1. Overview Information

Participating Organization(s)

National Institutes of Health (NIH)

Components of Participating Organizations

National Institute of Allergy and Infectious Diseases (NIAID)

Funding Opportunity Title

Childhood Asthma in Urban Settings Clinical Research Network- Leadership Center (UM1 Clinical Trial Required)

Activity Code

UM1 Research Project with Complex Structure Cooperative Agreement

Announcement Type

New

Related Notices

July 26, 2019- Changes to NIH Requirements Regarding Proposed Human Fetal Tissue Research. See Notice NOT-OD-19-128

August 23, 2019- Clarifying Competing Application Instructions and Notice of Publication of Frequently Asked Questions (FAQs) Regarding Proposed Human Fetal Tissue Research. See Notice NOT-OD-19-137

Funding Opportunity Announcement (FOA) Number

RFA-AI-19-074

Companion Funding Opportunity

RFA-AI-19-073, U01 Research Project – Cooperative Agreement

Number of Applications

Only one application per institution is allowed, as defined in Section III. 3. Additional Information on Eligibility.

Catalog of Federal Domestic Assistance (CFDA) Number(s)

93.855

Funding Opportunity Purpose

The purpose of this Funding Opportunity Announcement (FOA) is to solicit applications for the NIAID Childhood Asthma in Urban Settings Clinical Research Network Leadership Center (CAUSE-LC). The CAUSE-LC will provide the overall scientific strategy and organizational structure to the CAUSE Clinical Research Network and will interact closely with the CAUSE Clinical Research Centers (CAUSE -CRCs) to support the conduct of multi-site clinical studies and trials with the ultimate goal of developing effective interventions or asthma prevention approaches applicable to children residing in low-income urban settings.

FIGURE 4.2 Funding Opportunity Announcement from the National Institutes of Health.

National Institutes of Health. https://grants.nih.gov/grants/guide/rfa-files/RFA-AI-19-074.html. Accessed 2/12/2020.

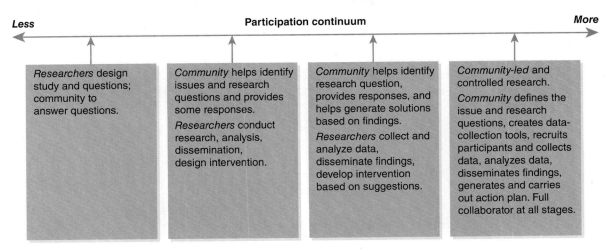

FIGURE 4.3 Continuum of Researcher—Community-Led Participation.

local needs. Consequently (and as a general guideline in this chapter), it may not be possible to follow all of the CBPR principles in any one study that respond to this funding announcement. Indeed, throughout this chapter, we suggest that you view CBPR as one end on a continuum, with the opposing end being a complete absence of community involvement but with varying degrees in the middle as depicted in **FIGURE 4.3**. Depending on these many factors, you as researcher could be on any point of this continuum.

As you can see in Figure 4.3, CBPR is a type of ideal: It exists at the extreme end and thus, as you can easily imagine, endless gradients exist that embrace some but not all of its principles. We suggest that this is a reality of some forms of research and that you do not need to have your study located at the extreme right of this continuum to embrace community engagement and collaboration. This chapter describes the principles of CBPR and advocates adherence to as many principles as feasible to ensure effective and sustainable results while also maintaining the ethical principles to which public health is bound.

▶ What Are the Nine Principles of CBPR?

Although seemingly laborious, learning the nine principles of CBPR is actually quite easy. As you will learn, they are aligned nicely with the principles of public health because each principle revolves around the central ethic of locating project ownership in the hands of a **community advisory board (CAB)** rather than in the hands of the public researcher or public health practitioner. A CAB is key to ensuring that the principles are upheld and it is composed of community members who share a common identity, history, symbols and

language, and culture (Israel, Checkoway, Schulz, & Zimmerman, 1994). For example, gender minority activists and HIV-affected individuals could serve on a CAB for an AIDS clinical trials group interested in recruiting gender-minority participants from the community. Representatives from the African American community (e.g., young women, faith leaders) could serve on a CAB that is linked to a community-based study testing a comprehensive maternal prevention program for high-risk minority pregnant women (Strauss et al., 2001). Think of the CAB as equivalent to a board of trustees for a business corporation. In the case of research rather than business, CAB members may not share common goals, so they must be willing to compromise with one another. Compromise, in turn, implies that constructive discussion and debate be embraced as normal operating procedures. As the convener, your role in this group is to facilitate consensus building through a **nominal group process**. This means that each member offers a solution to a given problem; redundant solutions are then collapsed, thereby narrowing the number of options. **FIGURE 4.4** is an illustration of this process. Next, group members vote by ranking each solution in order of preference—for example, first choice, second choice, and third choice. Discussion ensues until further solutions are eliminated, revoting occurs, and the process repeats until consensus is reached on the one remaining solution. This process should lead to a consensus regarding the research aim and the approach and result in an effective and collaborative project.

TABLE 4.2 delineates the nine key CBPR principles. The first one shown—recognizes community as a unit of identity—is increasingly important to understand. This principle acknowledges that every community is different but each has a sense of connection and identification with others to varying degrees, shared norms

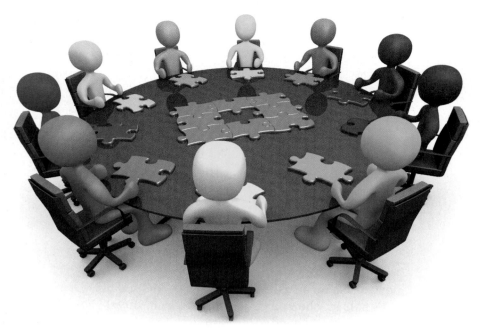

FIGURE 4.4 Community Advisory Board Meeting.
© Konstantinos Kokkinis/Shutterstock

and values, common language and customs, similar goals and interests, and we hope a desire to meet shared needs. The community as a unit of identity can stem from the community's geographic area layered with the community's common sense of identity (e.g., racial or ethnic group, religion, or sexual orientation). CBPR partnerships seek to work with existing communities of identity to enhance a sense of community through the collaborative process. This principle orients the all-too-often vague term of *community* into a more tangible concept: a community of identity.

TABLE 4.2 Nine Key Principles of Community-Based Participatory Research
1. Recognizes community as a unit of identity.
2. Builds on strengths and resources within the community.
3. Facilitates collaborative partnerships in all phases of the research.
4. Integrates knowledge and action for the mutual benefit of all partners.
5. Promotes a co-learning and empowering process that attends to social inequalities.
6. Involves a cyclical and iterative process.
7. Addresses health from both positive perspectives (e.g., wellness) and ecological perspectives.
8. Disseminates findings and knowledge gained by all partners.
9. Involves a long-term commitment by all partners.

The second principle—builds on strengths and resources within the community—is somewhat nuanced. To build on community strengths, the CAB must first identify its assets. Fortunately, this process is achieved by an informal assessment that can be conducted by CAB members. Strengths can take many forms. For instance, a community may be characterized as being "closely linked" relative to communication of health-related information and services. This is a strength that can be used to catalyze most any health-promotion program delivered to that community.

The third principle—facilitates collaborative partnerships in all phases of research—is also somewhat nuanced. CAB members are only the epicenter of the project, and each member must actively forge collaborative relations with outside partners such as non-governmental agencies, organizations, policy makers, governmental offices, and so on. This notion of making connections is central to expanding the CAB's reach and power to include progressively greater numbers of available community assets.

The fourth principle—integrates knowledge and action for the mutual benefit of all partners—asserts that the results of community-based research should not simply be an academic enterprise that adds to the knowledge base of community health but should also be used as a platform to promote local efforts directed at action-oriented community change. Consider, for instance, that a survey of a community of persons who inject drugs provides overwhelming evidence that syringe-exchange programs should be staffed

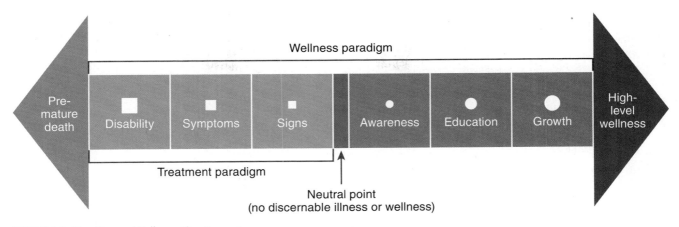

FIGURE 4.5 The Illness–Wellness Continuum.

by trusted members of their community rather than "outsiders" who may be perceived as having a connection to law enforcement. Going the next step and actually helping the community achieve the desired change then becomes an imperative form of action.

The fourth principle—promotes a co-learning and empowering process that attends to social inequalities—means **community empowerment** in service of addressing disparities in health and power. It may be one of the most vital principles, yet one that poses great challenges in the context of a research study. This principle suggests that researchers and community members learn from each other and that it is *the process and results* that ultimately result in community empowerment. Researchers should recognize that no one individual or group can empower someone else or an entire community and that there is inherent inequality among community members and them. The goal of CBPR is to attempt to address these factors by completely sharing all information, making decision-making power equitable, sharing resources, and fully supporting community members.

Turning now to the sixth principle—involves a cyclical and iterative process—the cycle that is alluded to here begins with the CAB and the maintenance of its membership. The CAB actually takes on a rhythm of progressive "wins"—that is, community assessment is the first challenge, followed by problem definition, the development of research methodology, data collection, data analysis, and **dissemination** of findings. This process can be exhaustive, so it is important to view the completion of each step as milestone worthy of congratulations and celebration.

The seventh principle—addresses health from both positive perspectives and ecological perspectives—will require you (as the researcher) to engage the CAB in a bit of education about health and wellness from an ecological perspective. To begin, you can teach CAB members about wellness by using a diagram such as that shown in **FIGURE 4.5**. Be sure to take your time and help them see the value of "moving the community to the right" on this continuum.

Moving now to the eighth principle—disseminates findings and knowledge gained to all partners—the goal is to always treat any study findings like great food. Share these findings with all of your CAB members and ask each member to share the findings with their community contacts (see Principle 3). Chapter 15 provides in-depth information as to how study findings can be most effectively and widely disseminated.

The final principle—long-term commitment by all partners—requires constant efforts to maintain the CAB as well as the community relationships that were formed as a result of the work conducted by you and the CAB. Your goal is to have these multiple and productive relationships continue even in the absence of funding.

▶ How Do CBPR Principles Differ from Those of Traditional Research?

As previously alluded to in this chapter, the notion of a simple dichotomy between CBPR and traditional research is largely academic; in reality, most public health research exists between the two extremes. This dichotomy is nonetheless useful because it provides a learning opportunity relative to your options when you begin to think about a research study that involves a community. **TABLE 4.3** displays multiple examples of **decision points** in research that can be placed along the continuum from "purely a CBPR approach" to "purely a traditional research approach." A decision point

TABLE 4.3 Decision Points Related to a Continuum of CBPR Versus Traditional Research

Decision Points	CBPR Perspective	Traditional Perspective
Should a CAB be formed?	The CAB is an equal partner.	The CAB only gives advice.
How do I find collaborators?	The CAB is well suited.	My own connections will suffice.
How do I learn about the needs of the target audience?	CAB members will conduct this research.	Paid research staff will conduct this research.
Who are the opinion leaders?	CAB members know the leaders.	Key informant interviews will reveal the leaders.
What are the language needs of the community?	Local CAB members will inform you of these needs.	Conduct qualitative research.
How can retention be optimized?	CAB members will have an understanding of this.	Trial and error in retention will inform the retention protocol.

represents opportunities to realistically adopt a given aspect of the CBPR approach to conducting research.

In addition to the decidedly different approaches to resolving decision points, a key difference between these two contrasting styles of research is that traditional research typically moves at a much faster pace, much like the hare from Aesop's fable of the tortoise and the hare (see FIGURE 4.6). This is because CAB meetings and the process of consensus building are not involved. So, this would seem to be a huge advantage, but we caution you not to be overly attracted to meeting or beating timelines, because how quickly you conduct your research has little bearing on its lasting value. Instead, consider whether the research can be substantially improved by the time spent in organizing and maintaining a CAB. We would argue that it definitely can be improved and ultimately you will still get to the finish line—and perhaps even before the other approach would.

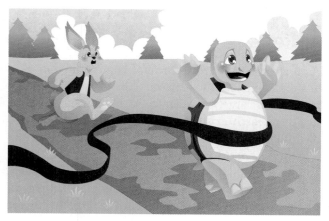

FIGURE 4.6 The Hare and Tortoise.
© Artisticco/Shutterstock

One other key difference that warrants discussion here involves a concept known as **external validity**. Simply stated, when a study is conducted under normal community circumstances, it will have far greater applicability or **generalizability** than one conducted under even somewhat artificial conditions (hence, the term *external validity* means that study findings can be easily generalized to practical, everyday public health applications). By entering and leaving the community as a researcher, your odds of having ample external validity are limited. In contrast, by acting as a mere catalyst to engage key community members in the process of conducting research, your odds of achieving high levels of external validity substantially escalate. This point should be considered in the broader context of public health research, a context that dictates a simple edict: that research only has value when the findings have direct implications for practice. Stated differently, the goal of public health research exceeds the mere completion of a study to include implications for public health.

At this point in the chapter, we do not advocate that all public health research designed to promote community health be conducted using a strict CBPR approach. We do, however, want you to get a feeling for what a **blended approach** looks like in the form of the study abstract. A blended approach is precisely what we have been advocating, one that uses any and all aspects of CBPR that will improve the value of the final research findings. **BOX 4.1** provides an example of a research study that was conducted using an optimal number of CBPR principles.

The research described in Box 4.1 depicts the CBPR principle of an academic–community partnership. Community members were actively engaged in

BOX 4.1	Example of Study Findings and Implications from a CBPR Approach

A suicide-prevention study was conducted among members of the White Mountain Apache tribe. In this population, those under 25 years of age have a suicide rate approximately 10 times that of same-age young people in the United States. The tribe formed an alliance with Johns Hopkins University and engaged in community-based participatory research. The research investigated risk factors for suicide, options for prevention and treatment, and young people's use of mental health services. The project occurred in three phases:

1. A formative phase was designed to enhance existing surveillance related to suicide, to test data-collection methods, and to design assessment tools.
2. A 2-year study of youth who had attempted suicide was then conducted.
3. An intervention program was designed in conjunction with community stakeholders.

Results of the intervention program yielded promising findings relative to the prevention of future suicide attempts in this vulnerable community (Barlow, Craig, Aday, et al., 2005).

conducting the research rather than simply acting in an advisory capacity to their university-based partners. As you can easily imagine, this feature alone was invaluable given that the formative phases (i.e., phases 1 and 2) were highly reliant on the use of one-on-one interviews with tribal youth; these young people may have been far less likely to fully disclose their feeling and experiences to university professors. Clearly, however, not all of the nine principles shown in Table 4.2 are reflected in this application of CBPR. Yet, the suicide-prevention program developed using the collaborative methodology did indeed provide highly encouraging findings.

One final point merits your attention before we leave this section. Public health comprises research disciplines inclusive of epidemiology, food science, environmental health, biostatistics, and health promotion. It is only this final discipline—health promotion—that lends itself to the use of CBPR. One way to think about this point is that health promotion is the response to ongoing activities such as public health surveillance. When that response requires any type of action or behavior change on the part of the affected community, a community-based approach using as many of the nine CBPR principles as possible is necessary.

▶ What Is Coalition Building?

Although your research may or may not include a CAB, a related type of organization you should consider joining or teaming up with is a **coalition** (see **FIGURE 4.7**). Coalitions are composed of various organizations dedicated to filling specific needs in the community. Unlike a CAB, a coalition does not guide the research process; instead, it may sponsor and support the research you have to offer its members.

Given that in the United States, as well as globally, health inequities lead to avoidable differences in health outcomes deemed **health disparities**, which are devastating to the marginalized people who are mostly affected and reflect the ongoing inequities in access to healthcare to obtain treatment for or to prevent disease (National Academies of Sciences, Engineering, and Medicine, 2017). Although Healthy People 2020 has goals to "achieve health equity, eliminate disparities, and improve the health of all groups" (Healthy People .gov, 2019); despite these efforts, limited progress has been made in reducing health disparities specifically for the poor and uninsured and for racial and ethnic minority groups (Agency for Healthcare Research and Quality, 2016). However, this is where community coalitions can make a significant difference. Indeed, coalitions composed of organizations dedicated to filling specific needs of a community can provide a course of action and support for addressing complex social determinants and can work to attenuate inequities and racism via targeted local action (Domlyn & Coleman, 2019). Think of the relationship between communities and coalitions as symbiotic, meaning the relationships are mutually beneficial and play an

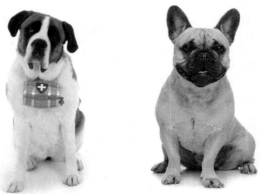

OURS IS THE HUMANE SOCIETY

WHAT'S YOUR COALITION?

FIGURE 4.7 Public Health Mascots Snow and Hamilton Champion for Coalition-Building.

important role in achieving community-level change. Most communities have preexisting coalitions related to various facets of public health. These groups of dedicated public health practitioners and community members welcome community-based participatory research and may even become advocates who can help you access study volunteers and local data useful to your study, as well as help you find gatekeepers who lend credibility to you and your research.

In the absence of a preexisting community coalition that matches your research mission, one last option is to create a new coalition. Far from being an easy task, this process has a well-worn path in public health. For instance, Butterfoss and Kegler (2009) initially provided a framework for establishing and maintaining an effective community health coalition. They delineated possibilities for composition of the coalition and carefully described how to optimally work with the coalition to achieve public health goals, including research projects designed to meet the expressed needs of the coalition.

A key aspect of coalition building is strategically identifying leaders of agencies, groups, and organizations that can substantively add to the collective ability of the coalition to create community-level change. By definition, a coalition is designed with a single goal in mind—for example, detoxification of a local water supply, responding to a local outbreak of hepatitis A, and ensuring the health and safety of people recently made homeless by a natural disaster. An example of a large-scale community coalition whose sole purpose was to combat the obesity epidemic in rural Tennessee is described in **BOX 4.2**. Because coalition members hold central positions in the community, they are well positioned to act as catalysts of change.

BOX 4.2 Example of a Community Coalition to Combat Obesity in Rural Tennessee

The purpose of this initiative was to engage communities in the process of reducing the prevalence of obesity over the long term using the policy, systems, and environment (PSE) model. The PSE model is an ecological approach that seeks to go beyond implementing individual-level programs to include a focus on the systems that create the structures in which people live. The three approaches work in combination with each other, with the whole greater than the sum of its parts. For example, an environmental change such as building walkable sidewalks in a community may be furthered by a local policy (e.g., a tax on sugar-sweetened beverages) or other system-level change. The PSE process theoretically results in more effective and sustainable results than any one approach applied in isolation. An effective PSE approach should seek to reach populations and uncover strategies that are effective and sustainable by effectively integrating approaches into existing infrastructures. This would include involving advocates and decision and policy makers.

The public health community strongly embraces the PSE approach because this model stresses the importance of direct education and recognizes the need to alter the contexts that influence individual health behaviors. Public health efforts have long recognized that to change individual behaviors, a concomitant change must be made to the environment in which the behavior occurs. Four rural counties in Tennessee adopted the PSE approach to address the obesity epidemic in their communities. The community-based participatory initiative, Community Coalitions for Change (C3), was embraced by 67,400 community members and 67 organizations. Community-based participatory practice (CBPP) was the guiding force in conducting C3 activities. This approach used community engagement and empowerment to improve outcomes. It involved building relationships between programs and community members and focused on developing mutual trust and equality; program participants and community members were viewed as important contributors to the entire process. Relationships were developed and maintained throughout the process from identifying critical issues of concern cited by the community to disseminating results.

All four counties participating in C3 activities were rural and had a long agricultural history and a county-based cooperative-extension infrastructure. Across all four counties, the median annual income is $34,563; an average of 27 percent of households live below the federal poverty level, and an average 20 percent of the population reports being food insecure. Three of the four counties are predominately non-Hispanic White, and all have strong faith-based communities. CBPP has been effective in rural communities where healthcare resources are often limited and was effective in this initiative. To address rural obesity rates, coalition members identified key values that included collective community engagement and action. In response, C3 established 25 community gardens and supported 10 existing gardens, resulting in 8,300 community members who received garden produce. Sites began with an average number of 11 physical activity resources, which increased by the third year to an average of 13 resources as a result of C3 activities. Overall, 61 percent (248 of 405) of survey respondents participating in direct education programs reported being more physically active as a result of participating in the programs, 59 percent (117 of 199) reported eating more fruit, and 66 percent (131 of 199) reported eating more vegetables. The results of this initiative support the use of the PSE model coupled with CBPP as an effective ecological approach to reducing obesity in rural areas with few resources (Wallace, Franck, & Sweet, 2019).

Think About It!

Given all you have learned about CBPR and its principles and public health ethical principles, you now feel qualified and confident to enter into CBPR. Let's consider that your public health interest is in preventing HIV among populations that are most at risk. You have studied the research and discovered that Black or African Americans account for a higher proportion of new HIV diagnoses and people living with HIV compared with other races and ethnicities. In 2017, Blacks or African Americans accounted for 13% of the U.S. population but 43% of new HIV diagnoses in the United States and dependent areas. Seventy-three percent of adult and adolescent Blacks or African Americans who received an HIV diagnosis were men. The highest risk transmission is from male-to-male sexual contact where 60% of Blacks or African Americans who received an HIV diagnosis were gay or bisexual men (Centers for Disease Control and Prevention, 2017). You are interested in forming a community–academic partnership that will conduct formative research to inform a HIV-preventive intervention for African American sexual minority male adolescents.

You are able to join a local coalition whose members include university researchers; mental health professionals; local health department representatives; medical treatment providers; and advocates of the lesbian, gay, bisexual, transgender, and queer communities. This partnership worked together to decide what would be assessed, the plan for assessments and research, who would be involved in the implementation, and what resources would be needed to develop a program and sustain it. Part of this process resulted in the consensus that HIV would be the most pressing issue faced by the community, and there was strong support for targeting young African American gay adolescents for prevention. The first phase of the research would involve focus groups within the targeted population so that the results could inform programming efforts. Through the focus groups, the partnership learned that some of the young men would often have unprotected sex with multiple partners in a single day to earn enough money to buy food. Other research findings highlighted the stigma and discrimination experienced by these young men for "being out." For example, several young men had been kicked out of their homes and were homeless or temporarily crashing at friends' homes. Others reported difficulty in getting employment, and some reported being ostracized by their churches. The intersection of race and sexual orientation resulted in some being homeless and experiencing hunger and living in an environment of poverty. Consequently, many turned to drug use and prostitution, putting themselves at heightened risk for HIV and potential arrest. In representing these findings, what ethical considerations might you have in terms of harms to the community? What are potential benefits to the community in having these findings disseminated? Who should decide when and how to present the data? Who should represent these findings, and how should they be represented and disseminated? Although these are not easy issues, we encourage you to think through how to handle sensitive and potential ethical issues to avoid unintended outcomes. Given the tenets of CBPR, the solution would be for the coalition and its members to discuss these issues together and arrive at a consensus that will mutually benefit everyone involved.

Take Home Points

- Community-based research is an essential part of public health research.
- The 12 ethical principles of public health should guide all community-based research.
- When community members play an organized, consistent, and highly active role in community-based research, it is termed community-based participatory research.
- A primary feature of a CBPR approach (one that cannot be abridged) is the formation and maintenance of a community advisory board.
- As one member of the CAB, the researcher will often be able to provide other members with basic education about public health and public health research.
- Consensus building among CAB members can be facilitated by using a nominal group process.
- Although CBPR has nine key principles, rigid adherence to each one may not always be possible. This does not mean that a CBPR approach should be abandoned entirely.
- A primary advantage of an approach that embraces as many principles of CBPR as possible is that doing so greatly enhances external validity of the study.
- Coalitions coupled with CBPR are key to addressing health disparities in communities that experience extreme inequities.

Key Terms

Blended approach
Coalition
Community advisory board
　(CAB)
Community-based participatory
　research (CBPR)

Community-based research
Community empowerment
Decision points
Dissemination
External validity
Generalizability

Health disparities
Nominal group process
Sustainability

For Practice and Discussion

1. In your own words, define and explain the purpose of community-based participatory research. Why would it be beneficial to involve the community in research addressing public health problems?

2. What are the nine principles of CBPR? Explain why it might not be feasible to follow all nine principles.
   a. Provide an example of a real-world public health scenario in which it would not be possible to follow all nine principles.

3. Explain the key differences between CBPR and traditional research.
   a. What are the benefits of using a blended approach?

4. Dr. Wong is a public health professor submitting a grant proposal to the National Institutes of Health to do a community-based intervention to prevent injection drug use in Chicago, Illinois. He wants to use a CBPR approach for this study and form a CAB.
   a. Because NIH typically funds more traditional research studies, how could Dr. Wong incorporate a CAB into this study? Use the decision points related to the continuum of CBPR and traditional research to guide your response.

References

Agency for Healthcare Research and Quality. (2016). *National Healthcare Quality and Disparities Report*. Retrieved from https://www.ahrq.gov/research/findings/nhqrdr/nhqdr16/index.html

Barlow, A. Craig, M., Aday, N. K., et al. (2005). *Employing community based participatory research (CBPR) methods to prevent youth suicide on the White Mountain Apache reservation*. Presented at the 133rd annual meeting of the American Public Health Association.

Butterfoss, F. D., & Kegler, M. C. (2009). The community coalition action theory. In R. J. DiClemente, R. A. Crosby, & M. C. Kegler (Eds.), *Emerging theories in health promotion practice and research* (2nd ed.). San Francisco, CA: Jossey-Bass.

Centers for Disease Control and Prevention. (2017). *HIV surveillance report*, Vol. 29. Retrieved from http://www.cdc.gov/hiv/library/reports/hiv-surveillance.html

Domlyn, A. M., & Coleman, S. (2019). Prioritizing equity: Exploring conditions impacting community coalition efforts. *Health Equity*, 3(1), 417–422.

HealthyPeople.gov. (2019). Washington, DC: U.S. Department of Health and Human Services, Office of Disease Prevention and Health Promotion [cited November 13, 2019]. Available from: https://www.healthypeople.gov/.

Israel, B. A., Checkoway, B., Schulz, A., & Zimmerman, M. (1994). Health education and community empowerment: Conceptualizing and measuring perceptions of individual, organizational, and community control. *Health Education Quarterly*, 21(2), 149–170.

National Academies of Sciences, Engineering, and Medicine. (2017). *Communities in action: Pathways to health equity*. Washington, DC: National Academies Press.

Strauss, R. P., Sengupta, S., Quinn, S. C., Goeppinger, J., Spaulding, C., Kegeles, S. M., & Millett, G. (2001). The role of community advisory boards: Involving communities in the informed consent process. *American Journal of Public Health*, 91(12), 1938–1943.

Thomas, J. C., Sage, M., Dillenberg, J., & Guillory, V. J. (2002). A code of ethics for public health. *American Journal of Public Health*, 92(7), 1057–1059.

Wallace, H. S., Franck, K. L., Sweet, C. L. (2019). Community coalitions for change and the policy, systems, and environment model: A community-based participatory approach to addressing obesity in rural Tennessee. Preventing Chronic Disease, 16, 180678.

For Further Reading

Minkler, M., & Wallerstein, N. (Eds.). (2011). *Community-based participatory research for health: From process to outcomes.* Hoboken, NJ: John Wiley & Sons.

Olshansky, E., & Zender, R. (2011). *The use of community-based participatory research to understand and work with vulnerable populations.* Burlington, MA: Jones & Bartlett.

Satcher, D. (2005). *Methods in community-based participatory research for health.* Hoboken, NJ: John Wiley & Sons.

Wallerstein, N. B., & Duran, B. (2006). Using community-based participatory research to address health disparities. *Health Promotion Practice, 7*(3), 312–323.

Wallerstein, N., & Duran, B. (2010). Community-based participatory research contributions to intervention research: The intersection of science and practice to improve health equity. *American Journal of Public Health, 100*(S1), S40–S46.

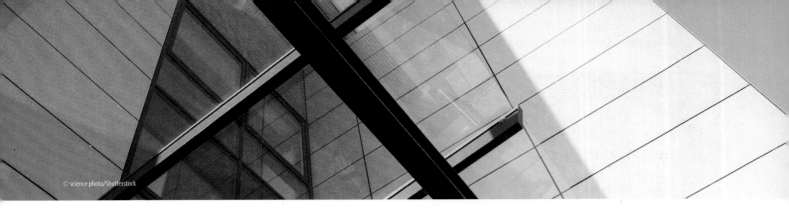

CHAPTER 5

Qualitative Research Methods for Public Health

with Anne Marie Schipani-McLaughlin

LEARNING OBJECTIVES

1. Describe the basic philosophies underlying a qualitative research paradigm.
2. Compare and contrast qualitative research with quantitative research.
3. Articulate three qualitative modes of inquiry.
4. Identify the different types of qualitative data-collection methods.
5. Outline a basic approach to qualitative data analyses.

▶ Overview

When you think of research and data analysis, you probably think of number crunching and statistics: quantitative research. However, **qualitative research**, which is defined as research focused on understanding the *meaning* of phenomena rather than documenting the *quantity*, is an equal and essential part of public health research. Qualitative research complements quantitative research by providing more context and additional understanding of public health problems. As you have seen throughout this text, the main goal of scientific inquiry is to generate knowledge. In public health, we use knowledge to understand health problems such as the incidence and prevalence of diseases, risk factors for diseases, and risk behaviors that can contribute to negative health outcomes, theories, and the effectiveness of public health programs. Qualitative

research is an integral part of this process but uses different methodologies. The goal of this chapter is to provide you with a brief description of the philosophy underlying qualitative research, an overview of the methodologies widely used, qualitative data-collection methods, and a concise tutorial on analyzing qualitative data.

▶ What Are the Underlying Philosophies of Qualitative Research?

Positivism

One general goal of science and its accompanying tool research is to gain a better understanding of our world and how it works. As such, philosophy—which

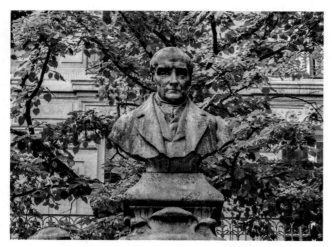

FIGURE 5.1 Statue of Auguste Comte.
© Nadiia_foto/Shutterstock

is derived from the Greek term *philo*, meaning love, and the term *sophias*, meaning wisdom—is integral to science. However, different philosophical perspectives dominate and shape how research is conducted and interpreted. One of these philosophies is known as **positivism**, the view that scientific inquiry should be confined to the study of relations existing between facts that are directly observable. Positivism originates from 19th-century French philosopher Auguste Comte (**FIGURE 5.1**) and refers to the idea that knowledge is limited to what can logically be deduced from theory, operationally measured, and empirically replicated (Glesne, 2011). Positivism has largely shaped current quantitative research methods and is the underlying philosophy for much public health research in addition to the hard sciences.

Interpretivism

In contrast to positivism, **interpretivism** views reality as individual perceptions and makes meaning of their reality in different ways. Thus, reality is socially constructed. This philosophy suggests that research should focus on studying individuals' lives, the context of their lives, and their meaning attached to their experiences. Thus, an interpretivist approach is supported through the use of qualitative modes of inquiry. Just as positivism and interpretivism differ, their modes of inquiry also differ. Quantitative and qualitative modes of inquiry differ in their assumptions of the generation of facts, their purposes, their approaches, and the role of the researcher. These differences are highlighted in **TABLE 5.1**.

▶ What Are the Differences Between Qualitative and Quantitative Research?

More often than not, students are taught that research starts with a quantifiable instrument such as a survey. This survey is often given to a large group of people during data collection, and the data then collected

TABLE 5.1 A Comparison of Quantitative and Qualitative Methods

	Quantitative	Qualitative
Nature of Data	Numerical data	Conversational data via words, observations, or photos
Philosophies	Grounded in positivism	Grounded in interpretivism
Approaches	Uses a deductive approach	Uses an inductive approach
Purpose	Tests hypotheses Provides support of theories Surveils health problems and outcomes	Develops explanatory theories Provides contextual understanding Insight into health barriers and public health programs
Data-Collection Methods	Quantifiable instruments, including surveys or structured quantitative interviews	In-depth and open-ended interviews, focus groups, observations, ethnographies, and case studies
Sample Size	Studies have large sample sizes to ensure statistical power.	Studies have small sample sizes but collect a large amount of data from participants.

through these surveys are analyzed through statistics. This method is considered a form of quantitative research. As shown, Table 5.1 provides a comparison of quantitative and qualitative research attributes. As indicated, quantitative research relies on numerical data to answer the research question. Although quantitative research often starts with theory and examines hypotheses to test this theory, which is also referred to as a *deductive approach* (Glesne, 2011; Patton, 2002), qualitative research relies on data collected through in-depth and open-ended interviews, focus groups, and direct observations. The goal is to *develop* explanatory theories rather than *test* theories and hypotheses, as is done in quantitative research. Qualitative research is used to gain an in-depth understanding of people's behavior, attitudes, perceptions, and experiences that influence and contribute to their decision making and engagement in health-related behaviors. Unlike quantitative research, qualitative research focuses on meanings rather than statistical inferences and estimates.

Another significant difference between quantitative and qualitative research is the difference in sample sizes for each type of research. Quantitative research studies have large sample sizes because, to draw conclusions based on study hypotheses, the study must have statistical power, which is only possible with a large enough sample of study participants. Alternatively, qualitative studies rely on small sample sizes but collect a large amount of data among study participants. Because of this, qualitative researchers study data with detail and depth, exploring themes without predetermined hypotheses or specified theories. In general, the data drive theory development

and provide a level of understanding (e.g., the meaning of binge drinking to a college student rather than the number of college students who binge drink) that cannot be captured by quantitative research.

One overarching goal of public health research is to understand and interpret the social world in which health conditions exist, so it makes sense that qualitative research involves interacting with and speaking to individuals about their experiences. In public health, qualitative research is used to reveal an added layer of context to specific public health problems. For example, let's say we are conducting a quantitative study with residents of a low-income neighborhood about their food and nutritional intake. The findings of this study showed that many residents consume mainly high-fat, low-nutrient foods and experience high rates of obesity. What this research does not uncover are the reasons why people consume these foods. Without performing a qualitative study, we may not gain the contextualized understanding of their dietary choices. For example, the low-income residents may live in a food desert, an area where it is difficult to buy affordable and nutritious foods. In addition, perhaps many residents do not have the time—because they work two jobs to provide for their families—or transportation to travel to a grocery store that offers high-quality and affordable whole foods. These contextual details may not be as evident through quantitative survey results. Qualitative data enrich our understanding of public health problems so that more effective solutions can be determined. **BOX 5.1** highlights a qualitative study that demonstrates the value of this approach in terms of examining and understanding HIV risk among a high-risk population.

BOX 5.1 Qualitative Study of Women Experiencing Abuse and Risk of HIV

In a recent study of African American women living in high-risk areas for HIV infection, a qualitative approach was used to create and validate a theoretical framework that specified the interrelations among those experiencing intimate partner violence or gender-based violence (GBV), psychological, psychosocial, and sociocultural factors; power among heterosexual partners; and HIV risk. The objective was to further our understanding of women's experiences of abuse and how the abuse may lead to less control over condom negotiation and contribute to risky behaviors. Rich themes emerged from this qualitative investigation. For instance, stereotypical gender roles, concurrency (i.e., the male partner having multiple sex partners), and social support from family and friends were described as being influential factors that increased the women's risk of HIV. Several quotes typify these themes. For example:

- "He says that a woman's place is in the home. And that he should be the one that worked, and I [should] stay home and wait on the kids and wait on him."
- "We didn't use a condom all this time, so why start now? [If I asked him to wear a condom] he'd probably get mad and probably say, 'Oh you must cheating on me.'"

(continues)

- "He would cheat and I would forgive. One time he told me he cheated on me with 10 girls. And that should be the point where you [are] supposed to walk out. But I didn't walk out because I felt like he had the problem, not me."
- "Oh my mom, yes she knows, she told me if I don't feel like the relationship's going to work, just get out of it. Because I don't need another bruise again because she knew what I went through with my first husband. She was like you don't need to go through all that again. If he's not going to do right by you, then get out of the relationship."

These qualitative findings led the researchers to conclude that HIV-prevention programs need to address societal, cultural, and relational influences that play a role in men perpetrating GBV while also addressing risk and protective factors for women to engage in safer sex (Wendlandt, Salazar, Mijares, & Pitts, 2016).

▶ What Are Three Widely Used Qualitative Approaches?

Grounded Theory

The first widely used qualitative strategy in public health is **grounded theory**, a general methodology that has been described as a marriage between positivism and interpretivism. Simply put, grounded theory is best used for *understanding* phenomena with the main focus being theory development. The elegance of this approach lies in its strategic method of linking data to the creation and elaboration of a theory. Thus, grounded theory can be used to understand actions and processes. Actions studied could include descriptions of both individuals and groups. Processes could involve the social and psychological processes that underlie whatever problem or issue is under investigation. In the context of public health, the problem could be complex health behaviors

(e.g., smoking), problems (e.g., use of opioids), or conditions (e.g., heart disease). At a basic level, grounded theory focuses on what people are doing, why they are doing it, and what it means to them. The end result should be a theory that ties all of this together and could then be used to guide intervention programs.

To use grounded theory as your approach, you must gather and analyze data in a systematic way. Hence, grounded theory possesses some features of positivism. The approach involves an iterative process referred to as **constant comparative analysis**, which uses the data to first generate a theory; subsequent data are then compared with the initial theory. An assumption is made that the initial theory will be preliminary and subject to changes and modifications as new data are collected and analyzed. A vital part of this process is the use of multiple perspectives (i.e., multiple researchers, multiple types of data) In **BOX 5.2**, we provide an example of how grounded theory was used to inform public health practice for

BOX 5.2 Example of a Grounded Theory Approach to Smoking Cessation

A study of 37 former smokers in Australia provides an example of how a grounded theory approach informed a theory of helping people who are in the process of quitting smoking. The purpose of the qualitative inquiry was to develop "an understanding of the varied contribution of smoking cessation assistance (either pharmacotherapy or professionally mediated behavioral support) to the process of quitting." The data showed discernable patterns from the former smokers relative to times when assistance with quitting was valued and necessary compared to times when assistance was not important or needed in any way. Three patterns were described: (1) quitting without any assistance, (2) quitting without initial assistance followed by assistance and concluding without assistance, and (3) quitting without initial assistance followed by assistance. The theory emerging from these patterns suggests that smoking cessation may best be facilitated by assistance as needed or requested rather than strictly a process requiring complete assistance or complete absence of assistance. As the authors concluded, "Program developers, health promotion practitioners, and social marketers might consider targeting particular audience 'segments' with tailored messages about quitting and use of assistance (Smith, Carter, Dunlop, et al., 2017)."

smoking-cessation programs. In this example, a theory was generated that once applied can be used to guide more effective smoking-cessation efforts.

Ethnography

The second widely used qualitative strategy is **ethnography**. The term is derived from the Greek term *ethnos* (meaning a people, a race, or a cultural group) and the term *graphic* (meaning descriptive). Ethnography is a social scientific description of a people and their cultural beliefs, values, and traditions. As a qualitative research strategy, ethnography focuses on providing a detailed and accurate description of values, behaviors, practices, and beliefs of a given group of people from *their point of view*. Ethnography entails studying people and observing their behavior but goes beyond the gathering of observations and facts to learn *what they mean*. Ethnography requires the researcher to immerse her- or himself, make observations, and then understand the meaning attached from an insider's perspective. An insider's perspective is referred to as the **emic perspective**, meaning "insider participant," whereas an outsider's perspective is referred to as the **etic perspective**, meaning "outsider researcher." Although the emic perspective serves as a valuable lens for synthesizing and interpreting ethnographic findings, a caveat is that it may cause bias on the part of the participant. An example of a researcher taking the emic perspective

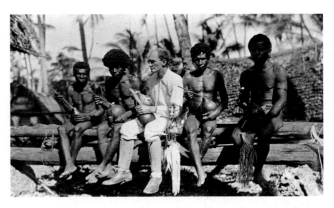

FIGURE 5.2 Bronisław Malinowski, Anthropologist Studying Native Culture in the Trobriand Islands.
© History and Art Collection/Alamy Stock Photo

is provided in **FIGURE 5.2**. World famous anthropologist Bronislaw Malinowski is shown participating fully in the culture and immersing himself with the native indigenous people of the Trobriand Islands to best observe and record the practices that are occurring.

To conduct ethnography, researchers should use multiple data-collection methods such as naturalistic observation, interviews with key informants, gathering of artifacts, and examination of archival data. In this way, they can capture a full description of those aspects of culture that shape people's experiences, behavior, beliefs, and emotions. **BOX 5.3** illustrates an ethnographic study of illicit drug users

---

BOX 5.3 An Example of Ethnography Used to Understand Drug Users' Feelings Toward Opioid Maintenance Treatment

An ethnographic study conducted by researchers Gronnestad and Sagvaag (2016) in Norway was conducted to answer the question, "How do individuals who frequent illicit drug scenes experience opioid maintenance treatment?" The ethnography involved the first researcher spending time in an open illicit drug scene over 1 year. Gronnestad stated that "it was challenging to become accepted and avoid association with the authorities and the power and control they possess," a common issue when conducting research in marginalized communities and when investigating illicit activities. To gain access to the drug users, he first sought out areas in the community where persons using illicit substances would congregate along with service providers. The service providers were highly regarded in the drug community and functioned as gate openers to the drug users.

Data collected were based on field notes and interviews from people with experiences from opioid maintenance treatment (OMT) programs and the open drug scene. They were asked to tell their stories, their experiences with drugs and treatment, how it was to be a man or woman in the drug scene, and their hopes for the future. Interviews were audiotaped and transcribed verbatim. Field notes were written down immediately after the observation describing what happens on the drug scene, how many people, what they do, and what they talk about and also describing the nearest surroundings reaction to the activity on this spot. Four themes emerged as relevant for the participants' experiences with OMT: (1) the loss of hope, (2) being trapped in OMT, (3) insufficient substitution treatment, and (4) stigmatization of identity. The participants found the OMT to be overruling and degrading mainly because OMT does not remove painful emotions; thus, drug users supplemented OMT with illegal substances, violated OMT regulations, and ran the risk of being excluded from the program.

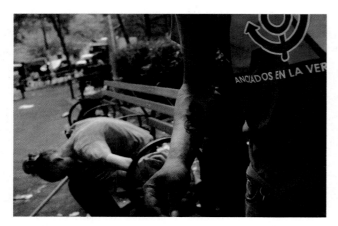

FIGURE 5.3 Individuals Struggling with Heroin Addiction in a Public Park.
© Spencer Platt/Getty Images News/Getty Images

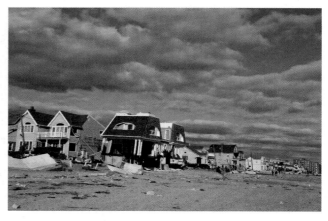

FIGURE 5.4 The Aftermath of Hurricane Sandy, Rockaway Beach, New York.
© Leonard Zhukovsky/Shutterstock

(opioid users) to gain insight into how individuals who frequent open illicit drug scenes experience opioid maintenance treatment (OMT) and investigate how this appears to affect their recovery processes (see **FIGURE 5.3**).

Case Study

The third widely used approach is known as a **case study**. Case studies have been defined as the "polar opposite of survey research" (Scriven, 1991) because they set out to investigate specific topics or single events at a microscopic level. Here, the word *case* is used to denote particular "examples or instances from a class or group of events, issues, or programs, and how people interact with components of this phenomenon" (Moore, Lapan, & Quartaroli, 2012, pp. 243–244). A case could also be a specific event such as a hurricane, flood, recently passed laws affecting immigration, or the implications of healthcare reform on people's use of medical services. People directly affected by the event (the case) are referred to as **stakeholders**. Thus, as you can imagine, case studies interview stakeholders to determine their interactions, decisions, and actions relative to the event under study. For instance, consider the devastating effects of lead poisoning that occurred in the case of Flint, Michigan, in the United States. From an epidemiology perspective, this human-made disaster can be described and quantified relative to its harmful effects on stakeholders using standard epidemiological techniques. From a qualitative perspective; however, case study techniques could answer questions such as:

- How did local healthcare facilities work together to respond to the resulting medical needs of stakeholders?

- How did stakeholders protect themselves from consuming the lead-contaminated water over long periods of time?
- How did the crisis effect the mental health of stakeholders?

Thus, the case study approach can be viewed as a deeper dive into what might otherwise be a fairly standard epidemiological investigation.

Case studies can be applied to a highly restricted—a *bounded*—question pertaining to one aspect that is part of a single event; this is a **single case study**. A **multiple case study** would involve study of a specific question as it applies to several similar cases such as outbreaks of food poisoning from the *Salmonella* microorganism. In the example of *Salmonella*, if the cases are investigated across geographically distinct areas (i.e., states), the design is known as a **comparative case study**.

A single case study was conducted in New York City following the devastation of Hurricane Sandy (see **FIGURE 5.4**) and is described in **BOX 5.4**. The goal of the study was to document the effects of the hurricane on capabilities of local healthcare clinics.

▶ What Are the Methods Used for Data Collection in Qualitative Research?

Interviews

Within qualitative research, **interviews** are one of the most widely used forms of data collection and differ significantly from survey interviews where researchers ask participants questions with close-ended responses

BOX 5.4 An Example of a Case Study to Determine the Impact of Hurricane Sandy

Hurricane Sandy was the largest Atlantic hurricane on record, killing 233 people in its path and landfall. A category 3 at its peak, Sandy was the deadliest and most destructive of the 2012 Atlantic hurricane season with more than $70 billion in damages. Consequently, Sandy posed a relentless number of public health issues, many of which had direct implications relative to the provision of healthcare. To investigate these issues, a 2016 multiple case study of 46 healthcare clinics on the Rockaway Peninsula was conducted. The case study determined how this natural disaster impacted the healthcare facilities. Interviews were conducted with clinic personnel, physicians, and administrators who were familiar with Sandy-related operational challenges. For instance, all but two of the 46 clinics had to close or relocate. Every clinic experienced loss of electricity, Internet access, and landlines. Only nine clinics had an emergency plan in place before Sandy and less than 50% of the clinics developed a posthurricane plan. Perhaps of greatest interest, only 20% of the clinics engaged in problem solving with other clinics, thus suggesting a lack of coordination between stakeholders. The case study concluded that greater attention should be paid to the task of emergency preparedness, as well as emergency responses following a hurricane (Jood, Bocour, Kumar, & Gucla, 2016)

(e.g., strongly agree, somewhat agree) in a highly structured format. In general, interviews within a qualitative context can take several different forms that range from unstructured to structured and may involve interviewing an individual, a dyad, or a group (that is, a focus group). **Unstructured interviews** are more informal conversations than formal interviews. When using this data-collection method, no specific questions are asked; topics emerge and flow from the conversation. The interviewer does ask questions related to the general research topic; however, the process is mostly free association on the part of the participant. Unstructured interviews are used frequently in investigations or inquiries in which the investigator is interested in understanding the meaning behind participants' experiences, events, practices, or behaviors. For example, in the United States, the maternal mortality rate (i.e., 26.4 per 100,000 live births) has risen to be the highest among the developed world (Peterson, 2019), whereas the rate has declined significantly for other countries (World Health Organization, 2019). Preeclampsia is a condition involving a dangerous form of high blood pressure and is a leading cause of maternal mortality. In addition, African American women in the United States experience significant disparities in maternal mortality. A researcher would like to study this phenomenon. Any investigator wanting a "conversation" with an African American pregnant woman would want to start it with a discussion of what it is like to be an African American woman in today's society, what her experiences have been relative to the pregnancy, what stressors she may be experiencing, what her expectations are for the pregnancy, what health behaviors she is engaging in to support the pregnancy, and what her attitudes are toward and how much access she has to prenatal care. Because

this is a highly personal and sensitive topic, it might be best to consider matching the interviewer's gender and race with those of the interviewee (for example, female and African American). This matching may facilitate the establishment of rapport (see **FIGURE 5.5**).

The goal of the unstructured interview is to *explore and probe* the interviewee's responses to develop an in-depth understanding of the phenomenon (see **FIGURE 5.6**). Because this interview is an interaction, the interviewer and the interviewee jointly construct meaning. A skilled interviewer allows participants to describe their experiences and explore their thoughts and opinions about the research topic. This process places a major emphasis on the details of the interviewee's life experiences and social behavior. Even though the interview should be viewed as a conversation, the interviewer must focus on listening to the interviewee. Also, the conversation should begin with less sensitive topics and then gradually ease toward more sensitive and complex issues. An important

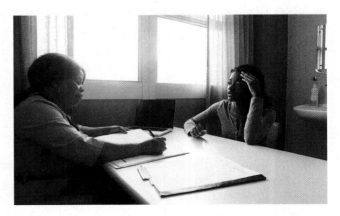

FIGURE 5.5 Unstructured Interview of African American Woman.
© wilpunt/E+/Getty Images

EXPLORING AND PROBING

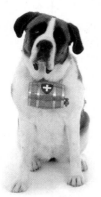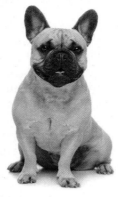

IT'S HOW WE ROLL

FIGURE 5.6 Public Health Mascots Snow and Hamilton Uphold Interviewing Techniques.

© Eric Isselee/Shutterstock; © Svetography/Shutterstock

skill to acquire is being able to be aware of responses that allow for more in-depth probing. **Probing** takes many forms but entails an effort either verbally or nonverbally on the part of the interviewer to elicit more details, to guide the dialogue, or to elaborate on the meaning of something said. For example, the interviewer could ask, "Could you tell me more about that?" Or the interviewer could use the **echo probe** in which he or she paraphrases what the interviewee has just said. The use of phrases such as "I see" and "Yes" are effective, as are nonverbal probes that could include head nodding or simply remaining silent. In any event, the function of the probes is to motivate the participants to communicate more fully and to help them focus on the general topics while keeping the communication flowing.

▶ Semistructured Interview

A more structured type of interview is the **semistructured interview**. This form involves asking a series of questions that are open ended (i.e., free-form questions that are not limited with specific responses) but in a predetermined order. The questions are used to ascertain specific topics related to the research. The interviewer must read the question exactly as it is worded to avoid changing the intention of the question. Although the interviewer is encouraged to use probes, the probes should be as neutral as possible to avoid introducing bias into the process. For example, if the interviewer asks a question and the participant says, "I don't know" or "I'm not sure," one type of neutral probe—a **clarification probe**—could be used—for example, "There are no right or wrong answers, we just want to find out how you feel about this." Although there is more structure to this form of interview, the open-ended questions still allow the participant to elaborate and provide significant details on his or her experiences. Thus, this type of interview is well suited for grounded theory and ethnography when little is known about a certain issue but the research question has a definite direction. An example of a semistructured interview guide that could be used in the study is presented in **BOX 5.5**.

▶ Focus Groups

One frequently used strategy for interviewing people is to conduct the session in a group format. Known as a **focus group**, this format typically involves five to 10 people who have agreed to take part in the

---

BOX 5.5 Semistructured Interview to Assess Food Insecurity Among Young Gay and Bisexual Men of Color

These interviews are being conducted to better understand how access to food and other basic needs may affect young men like yourself. You were asked to complete this interview because you indicated on our survey that you have experienced hunger or had times when you did not have enough food in the last few months. To start with, I want to ask you some questions about your income and work history. If there are any questions you do not feel comfortable answering, just let me know and we will move on.

What is your current living situation?
Do you live at home, on your own, with roommates?
Do you have to contribute to the rent for your home?
About how much is that a month? What other monthly expenses do you have?
To what extent are you able to cover these expenses?
Now, let's talk a little about your work history. What was your first job?
What other jobs have you had? About how much do you make an hour or year?
In general, how consistent has your work history been?
Have there been times when you wanted work but couldn't find it?

Can you tell me more about that?

To what extent does your family help you out financially?

When there are times that you don't have enough money to pay for your basic needs like rent, food, phone, is there someone you can ask for help? Tell me about that.

Thinking specifically about your access to food, about how much would you say you spend on food a month (including eating out and cooking)?

How much do you cook at home or does someone cook for you at home?

How do you decide if you will eat at home or out?

In the past year, have there been times that you were hungry but could not afford to eat?

Can you tell me about that (e.g., how many days, were there family or friends who could help, how did this effect you)?

What kinds of things did you do to try to find food to eat (e.g., food pantry, eat at friends or family, get taken out for dinner)?

How reliable are these strategies?

When using any of these strategies, how do they make you feel?

Have any of these strategies put you in danger or hurt you in any way?

Do you have a place to go for food when you are hungry but cannot buy food? Tell me about this place. What makes it less than easy to go there?

During these times of hunger, were there any strategies that you used that involved your dating or sex partners? (Probe: dating for a dinner out, sex trade.) Can you tell me about these times? (Probes: sexual activity, use of condoms, history with the partner, concerns about STI/HIV.)

Now, thinking about more recently, during the past month have you missed any meals because you did not have enough money to buy food? (Probes: how many days in the last month? How did you cope?)

If you had a choice between spending $5 on food or condoms, what would you pick? Please explain why.

qualitative study, knowing that the interview will occur in a small group (see **FIGURE 5.7**). The first point then is that focus groups cannot be anonymous simply because of the group-based format. However, one great advantage of focus groups is that the responses from one person may stimulate thoughtful discussion from others and thus elicit a host of varied opinions, experiences, and beliefs. In essence, a focus group of seven people, for example, may inspire a greater degree of richness in the data compared with data collected from seven one-to-one in-depth interviews.

Just as one-to-one interviews use a semistructured guide, so do focus groups. The key to making the group-based interview a success involves a skilled facilitator (and sometimes focus groups are conducted with two facilitators). The role of the facilitator is to first establish an environment of trust and respect among group members. This is when rules about protecting the confidentiality of others, for example, must be clearly conveyed. It is also a time when group members should come to understand the importance of listening to others and contributing equally to the conversation (i.e., not dominating the conversation and not being reticent to engage in the conversation). Again, similar to one-to-one interviews, a focus group facilitator will use prompting to draw out information from the group when people are otherwise not forthcoming with providing responses.

Several considerations apply to forming a focus group. A key principle of organizing a focus group is that its composition should be **homogeneous**. This means that participants have similar characteristics that are chosen based on the research question such as gender, age range, socioeconomic status, education level, or race and ethnicity, among others. The size of the selected homogeneous group will depend on the research topic, the age of the participants, and how detailed the session needs to be to meet the needs of the research questions. Further, participants should be chosen on the basis of the research topic. For example, if the research question pertains to teens driving under the influence of alcohol (DUI), the people recruited for the focus group should

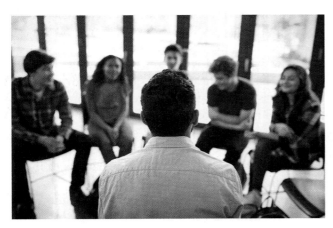

FIGURE 5.7 Focus Group.
© Monkey Business Images/Shutterstock

be teens who have possibly been pulled over for DUI, have been driving under the influence, or have at least been a passenger in a car driven by a teen who was driving under the influence of alcohol.

A final note about focus groups is warranted. It is possible that any given focus group may provide a relatively narrow set of perspectives, opinions, ideas, and so on relative to the questions posed to them during a session. This is fine, but it necessitates the idea of conducting multiple focus groups using the same interview guide. As you move from focus group 1 to focus group 2, you may find a distinctly different set of responses from the second group. This means that you should now move to focus group 3 because it may produce yet another set of responses that differ from the first two focus groups. Once, however, the focus groups begin to substantially overlap in their responses, you have reached what is known as **saturation**. Typically, focus group research (much like one-to-one interviews) should continue until reaching the point of saturation, which requires a minimum of four to six groups.

▶ Observation

Participant observation is a specific type of naturalistic observation in which the researcher has little knowledge of the culture and lives of the people he or she wants to study and immerses him- or herself in a setting. It has been a vital method used in ethnographic research since the late 19th century. This form of data collection entails first gaining access to the setting, whether the setting is public or private, and then spending a significant period of time observing. Researchers can either take part in community activities and assume the life of a local or be less participatory and strictly observe. When embarking on the research, the investigator must decide what role he or she will adopt when making observations. This means he or she must decide on the level of transparency of the research role ranging from covert to overt and his or her level of involvement. Gold (1958) outlined four potential roles moving from the more involved and covert to complete detachment and overt. These roles are depicted in **FIGURE 5.8**.

The first role is that of the **complete participant**, with the researcher allowing the people to see him or her as a participant, not as a researcher. This role is considered covert because the researcher is not explicit in identifying his or her role as a researcher. Because of this, this role may be considered unethical and may present methodological issues because the researcher may affect participants' behavior and

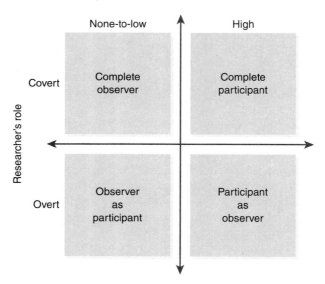

FIGURE 5.8 Potential Roles of Investigators by Level of Involvement.

the setting (i.e., observer effects). Because of these considerations (ethical and scientific), the decision to adopt the role of the complete participant should be well justified. A second role is that of the **participant as observer**. In this role, the investigator is overt by identifying him- or herself as a researcher, thus avoiding some of the ethical issues in the complete participant role. However, some of the methodological issues remain—for instance, observer effects. The third role of **observer as participant** implies that the investigator's main role is that of observer. She or he identifies as a researcher but enters the setting periodically and with limited interaction. In this role, it may be more difficult to gain the perspective of the participants and derive valid interpretation of the observations. Finally, the fourth role, **complete observer**, involves the researcher observing without ever becoming a part of the setting—in other words, watching people without them knowing. This role is more along the lines of an "objective" researcher, with observer effects minimized. Ethical issues are of concern, however, and the researcher loses the emic perspective.

How, what, and when you record your observations depends on the nature of the study, whether or not there is freedom to take notes as the observations are being made. Note-taking is typically is used to record observations. Observations should be broad and descriptive and serve as a guide to identify the key aspects of the setting, people, and behaviors of interest. As the research progresses, the investigator may begin to narrow the focus and record observations but with more detail and elaboration. Creating a list of key words and participants based on your initial observations and then using this list to organize and outline your subsequent observations is recommended. Field notes should be descriptive as well as reflective about what you have seen, heard, experienced, and thought about during an observation session.

▶ How Do You Analyze Qualitative Data?

Organizing the Data

Author A. A. Milne wrote, "Organizing is what you do before you do something, so that when you do it, it is not all mixed up." This sentiment aptly applies to data analysis: You must organize your data before you can begin the process of analyzing your data. You must have a data-management plan that should entail not only a process for documentation but also annotation. Annotating data means providing notes such as interviewer ID, date, participant ID or initials if used, and location or site where collected. This attention to detail will ultimately help with the analyses.

In addition to documenting additional information associated with the data and the research, any interviews or focus groups that were audio or video recorded should be transcribed—and as soon as possible after an interview. The electronic word document containing the transcription of the interview or discussion becomes *the data* that will be stored and analyzed. When conducting a transcript-based analysis, it is critical that the transcripts being coded are **verbatim** transcripts (i.e., word for word). They should include any pauses, additional comments, half sentences, and so on. A verbatim transcript helps provide context about how participants think and feel about the issues being researched. After the first draft of the transcript has been completed, it is important to review it alongside the recording to ensure its accuracy. We highly recommend that you use a database to assist with organizing and managing all of the data, annotations, transcriptions, and other information.

Codebook Development

In a qualitative data analysis, the **codebook** is a critical component and organizes the data at a basic level. Developing the codebook can be viewed as an iterative process. Generally, a **code** is a descriptive word or short phrase that is used as a label and attached to units of data (such as a word, a sentence, or a paragraph) and that represents a **concept** observed by the analyst. In this context, *concept* refers to an idea or notion that is suggestive of the data. For example, college students talking about their experiences in

their freshman year of college related to not knowing anyone, problems with making new friends, and loneliness could be suggestive of the concept of "freshman year isolation" and become the code "Isolation." Developing the codebook is essentially the beginning of data analysis, and it is essential that you and your team develop a codebook that is structured and clear.

Coding Process

Coding the data is a relatively simple task. As you read through the data, you systematically code with respect to the core concepts in your codebook. You can underline or highlight units of data that apply to a particular code. Many qualitative software packages are available to facilitate the entire data-analysis process if desired. After the first round of coding is completed, **intercoder reliability** analysis of the coded transcripts needs to be calculated. Intercoder reliability analysis entails comparing the application of the codes in each transcript. To calculate intercoder reliability, the two most widely used measures for assessing it are **percent agreement** and **Cohen's kappa**. Percent agreement measures the number of times that two coders agreed or disagreed in the coding of a text segment. One simply calculates the number of times raters agree on a rating and then divides by the total number of ratings. This measure can vary between 0 and 100 percent. Cohen's kappa takes into account agreement in coding that can occur from chance and is a more stringent measure than percent agreement. Kappa can be calculated by subtracting the estimated level of chance agreement from the observed level of agreement and then dividing by the maximum possible nonchance agreement. A *kappa statistic* that is ≥ 0.75 is considered an acceptable target.

Interpretation

Interpreting data requires going beyond codes to generate **themes**. A theme emerges from the data during the analysis process and represents the underlying meaning attached to all of the data associated with a particular code. Whereas codes represent direct observation of concepts, themes represent more nuanced levels. For example, *isolation* could be assigned as a code, but *isolation as a risk factor for suicide ideation* would be a theme. When undertaking interpretation, there is no one right way of doing it. It is a lengthy process that should reveal several main themes.

One final note on interpretation. Interpretation is about finding meaning among your codes and themes, but more important, connecting them to your

TABLE 5.2 Four Basic Principles for Writing Qualitative Results	
Principle	**Description**
Be balanced and accurate.	Aim for balance and accuracy in reporting findings, not neutrality. Present multiple sides of the particular issue being studied. Elicit the knowledge, understandings, and insights of the research participants and represent their insights in context.
Ensure no harm to participants.	Ensure that no harm comes to those interviewed as a result of their participation and as a result of the publication, presentation, or dissemination of their views of experiences. Even when the published work does not give names, information could reveal the identity of some participants.
Give public voice to findings by sharing participants' own words.	Present participants' insights in their own words. Try to include quotes or even brief phrases (in participants' original language, along with any helpful translation).
Describe the context of your interactions and disclose your role.	Readers must have adequate information on when and how you gathered information, the nature of your relationship with those studied, and knowledge of your standpoint and motivation in carrying out the study. Also, state all sources of funding for the work.

Modified from Ulin, P. R., Robinson, E. T., & Tolley, E. E. (2005). Qualitative Methods in Public Health: A Field Guide for Applied Research (1st ed.). San Francisco, CA: Jossey-Bass.

research questions or theory and figuring out, "What do our findings mean to the problem at hand, to public health, to society? How can our findings be used to create change?" These questions are meant to guide you in examining the larger context in which the study and your findings should be placed.

Write-Up of Results

Writing up your results involves describing the central or core themes and how they fit together and then using direct quotes from the data to *illustrate* and *support* your insights. The challenge is to create an engaging narrative that explains the phenomena under study. Consider using tables and figures to support your interpretation. An important point to keep in mind is that the write-up of your results is a public communication of the meaning underlying what other people have shared with you. Four guiding principles when

writing your results are presented in **TABLE 5.2** and should be useful as you begin writing up your results.

When beginning the process of writing up the results, using the research questions as a guide to organize themes is recommended. Themes can be presented sequentially followed by a description and one or more illustrative quotes selected from a range of participants. Also, use pseudonyms rather than real names to protect identities. Following the quotes, we also include an interpretation and provide context. **BOX 5.6** provides an example of a write-up from one of our qualitative research studies.

Finally, after your results have been written, in addition to the usual points made in the discussion section of a journal article for qualitative research, effort should be made to acknowledge bias. Some researchers suggest reporting how one's preconceptions, beliefs, values, assumptions, and position may have come into play during the research process.

BOX 5.6 Example of a Theme Write-Up

Influence of Alcohol on Informed Consent

Alcohol facilitates the initiation of sex. The theme of alcohol as a facilitator for sex emerged in three focus groups. Participants indicated that alcohol makes women more "loose," that women are more willing to have sex when they are drinking. Participants also expressed that they become more aggressive in pursuing and initiating sex when they are drinking: "If I've been drinking, yeah, a girl's just gotta stop me cause, like, I'm gonna be more willing to talk her into it, more willing to take off her clothes. . . . So she's really just gotta say, cause if she says 'no,' I'll still stop. . . . I mean, if she's hesitant, and I'm sober, I'm more likely to stop [but if] she's hesitant and I'm drunk, I'm not likely to stop."

Think About It!

Increasingly, social media shapes our world and thus the public health landscape. For instance, Twitter is estimated to be used by more than 100 million people each day, with a daily volume of some 340 million tweets. Given its existence since 2006, Twitter appears to be a form of communication that will be around for decades to come. The question for aspiring public health professionals like you is, how do we harness the power of Twitter to better understand and alter health behavior? So, why are we introducing a section about Twitter in this chapter that pertains to qualitative research?

Think about tweets that you or someone you know have sent and were considered "sensitive and important." Few topics fit this category as closely as sexual abuse and sexual violence. Indeed, as part of the #MeToo movement (see **FIGURE 5.9**), which began in 2017 by activist Tarana Burke, uncounted numbers of women have posted their "Me Too" information on Twitter. So think about it: Is there value in the postings (because postings are "words") as qualitative research? We suggest that qualitative research opportunities are nearly infinite and that social media platforms such as Twitter offer a vast and rich supply of possible data. To illustrate this point, please consider the following study by Bogen, Bleweiss, Leach, and Orchowski (2019).

This study qualitatively analyzed data from 897 tweets classified as "disclosing sexual victimization" and 763 tweets classified as participating in an online forum to discuss personal and social reactions to sexual violence. To begin, consider the point that a larger number of tweets were aimed toward a highly personal behavior (i.e., disclosure of sexual violence) rather than less personal behavior of how people can or should work to react in ways that ultimately help other survivors and raise public awareness about the problem of male-perpetrated sexual violence.

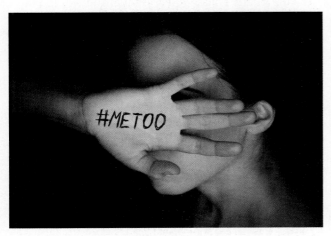

FIGURE 5.9 #MeToo Movement.
© EllieStark/Shutterstock

Of the 897 disclosure tweets, most contained details describing an abuse event. This type of data would not be possible to collect in other forums. Following the category of "describing the abuse event," other categories were qualitatively identified such as (1) who committed the abuse, (2) when it occurred, (3) how it occurred, and even whether the abuser and the incidents were serial in nature. The massive volume of potential data from these 897 tweets is simply beyond the realm of what would be possible in past qualitative research using the more traditional methodologies that you learned about in this chapter. What this means for you as a student and aspiring public health professional (regardless of whether you do work to prevent sexual violence) is that qualitative analyses of social media data represent an entirely new and exciting option for future research endeavors. From a public awareness viewpoint and thus a public health perspective, this type of research can have an immediate and lasting impact on public opinion and thus, by extension, the allocation of financial and even legislative resources to a movement such as #MeToo.

Of the 763 tweets classified as an "online forum" 67% were considered by the research team as being "positive"—meaning that they had content related to advocacy, increasing public awareness, providing emotional support for survivors, and taking social responsibility to address the issues related to sexual violence against women. Although these tweets were distinctly different data than the "sexual victimization disclosure" data, this two-thirds of the 763 tweets provide relevant information regarding women's responses to sexual violence.

Shaping social movements, such as #MeToo, is not necessarily in the realm of public health practice; however, being aware of social movements is at least an initial obligation. Fortunately, that obligation in this case is nicely met through these findings.

As your career blossoms and continues over a lifetime of technology-based innovation and endless public health challenges, we urge you to keep an eye on the things that are happening in real time. The #MeToo movement is indeed powerful and vital, and you can be assured that many other issues (some of which may also involve preventing the perpetration of sexual violence) will be coming along soon. So, think about it, how can qualitative investigations help you and other professionals be better informed as to what people are saying, thinking, and doing?

Take Home Points

- The underlying philosophy of qualitative research is interpretivism, whereas positivism underlies quantitative research.
- Quantitative research is based on numbers and involves hypothesis testing, whereas qualitative research is based on words, observations, images, and behaviors and involves generating meaning and new theories.
- Qualitative research uses grounded theory, ethnography, and case studies as modes of inquiry.
- Interviews, focus groups, and observation are the main forms of data collection in qualitative research.

- Organizing the different types and voluminous amounts of data collected must be achieved by using a data-management system that will facilitate data analysis.
- Transcriptions should be verbatim.
- Codebook development is iterative and entails first identifying concepts and then generating a word or brief phrase that represents the code.
- Coding the data is best conducted by multiple coders, and intercoder reliability must be calculated as an indicator of agreement.
- Interpretation involves identifying themes that convey the deeper, underlying meaning.

Key Terms

Case study	Ethnography	Percent agreement
Clarification probe	Etic perspective	Positivism
Code	Focus groups	Probing
Codebook	Grounded theory	Qualitative research
Cohen's kappa	Homogeneous	Saturation
Comparative case study	Intercoder reliability	Semistructured interview
Complete observer	Interpretivism	Single case study
Complete participant	Interviews	Stakeholders
Concept	Multiple case study	Themes
Constant comparative analysis	Observer as participant	Unstructured interviews
Echo probe	Participant as observer	Verbatim
Emic perspective	Participant observation	

For Practice and Discussion

1. What is qualitative research, and why is it important in the field of public health?
2. Compare and contrast quantitative and qualitative research methods. Discuss the use and application of qualitative research compared with quantitative research in public health.
3. Provide an example of a research question for a qualitative research study on a public health topic. Explain why this research question would be appropriate for a qualitative study.
4. A public health researcher is planning to develop an e-cigarette prevention program for college students in the New York City

area. However, before the researcher begins developing the program, she wants to conduct a qualitative study with college students to understand their experiences and how to tailor the program to fit their needs. Which qualitative data-collection method would you recommend the researcher use for this study and why?

5. How is qualitative data analysis different from quantitative data analysis? Explain the process of analyzing qualitative data in your own words.

References

Bogen, K. W., Bleweiss, K. K., Leach, N. R., & Orchowski, L. M. (2019). #MeToo: Disclosure and reaction to sexual victimization, on Twitter. *Journal of Intrapersonal Violence*, 1–32.

Glesne, C. (2011). *Becoming qualitative researchers: An introduction* (4th ed.). Boston, MA: Pearson Education.

Gold, R. (1958). Roles in sociological field observation. *Social Forces, 36*, 217–213.

Gronnestad, T. E., & Sagvaag, H. (2016). Stuck in limbo: Illicit drug users' experiences with opioid maintenance treatment and the relation to recovery. *International Journal of Qualitative Studies on Health & Well-Being, 11*, 31992.

Jood, R. K., Bocour, A., Kumar, S., & Gucla, H. (2016). Impact on primary care access post-disaster: A case study of Rockaway Peninsula. *Disaster Medicine and Public Health Preparedness,* 10:492–495.

Meyers, M. (2019, May 29). Teachers honored during April LSC meeting. *The Warrior* (Lane Tech College Prep High School, Chicago, IL). Retrieved from https://lanewarrior .com/9018/news/teachers-honored-during-april-lsc -meeting/

Moore, T. S., Lapan, S. D., & Quartaroli, M. T. (2012). Case study research. Pp. 243–270 in S. D. Lapan, M. T. Quartaroli, & F. J Riemer (Eds.), *Qualitative research: An introduction to methods and designs.* San Francisco, CA: Jossey-Bass.

Patton, M. Q. (2002). *Qualitative research and evaluation methods* (3rd ed.). Thousand Oaks, CA: Sage.

Petersen, E. E., Davis, N. L., Goodman, D., Cox, S., Syverson, C., Seed, K., . . . Barfield, W. (2019). Racial/Ethnic Disparities in Pregnancy-Related Deaths—United States, 2007–2016.

MMWR. Morbidity and mortality weekly report, 68(35), 762–765.

Scriven, M. (1991). *Evaluation thesaurus* (4th ed.). Thousand Oaks, CA: Sage.

Smith, A. L., Carter, S. M., Dunlop, S. M., Freeman, B., & Chapman, S. (2017). Revealing the complexity of quitting smoking: A qualitative grounded theory study of the natural history of quitting in Australian ex-smokers. *Tobacco Control, 27*(5), 568–570.

Wendlandt, R., Salazar, L. F., Mijares, A., & Pitts, N. (2016). Gender-based violence and HIV risk among African American women: a qualitative study. *Journal of HIV/AIDS & Social Service, 15*(1), 83–98.

World Health Organization (2019). Trends in maternal mortality 2000 to 2017: estimates by WHO, UNICEF, UNFPA, World Bank Group and the United Nations Population Division. Geneva: Retrieved from: https://www.who.int/reproductivehealth /publications/maternal-mortality-2000-2017/en/

For Further Reading

Glesne, C. (2011). *Becoming qualitative researchers: An introduction* (4th ed.). Boston, MA: Pearson Education, Inc.

Jacobsen, K. H. (2017). Qualitative studies. Pp. 87–93 in *Introduction to health research methods: A practical guide* (2nd ed.). Burlington, MA: Jones & Bartlett.

Ulin, P. R., Robinson, E. T., & Tolley, E. E. (2005). *Qualitative methods in public health: A field guide for applied research.* San Francisco, CA: Jossey-Bass.

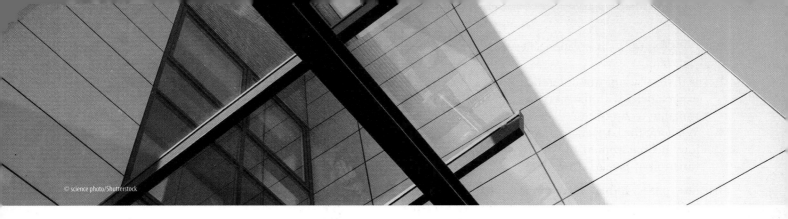

CHAPTER 6

Observational Research Designs

with Anne Marie Schipani-McLaughlin

LEARNING OBJECTIVES

1. Distinguish observational research from other forms of research.
2. Understand the use and applications of different observational research designs used in public health.
3. Understand the principles and advantages of each observational research design.
4. Learn the basic reporting requirements for observational research.

▶ Overview

In Chapter 5, you were briefly introduced to quantitative research and learned about the differences between qualitative and quantitative research. In this chapter, we will focus only on quantitative research. The most common type of quantitative research is best known by the label of **observational research**. As the term implies, this approach to understanding health and its determinants is based on the idea that people can be observed (either at one point in time or over a defined period of observation such as 6 or 12 months or even over the course of 10 years). The word *observed*, however, is loosely used here in this context: We mean measuring people's attitudes, beliefs, and practices via self-report survey questionnaires rather than actually observing their behavior directly as in some qualitative research.

In many ways, observational studies form the backbone of public health research. This is because these types of studies lay the foundation for intervention development, policy change, and even legislation designed to protect health. The range of possible designs in observational research spans from a simple one-time survey to labor-intensive studies of large cohorts that may last for years or even decades. The utility of observational studies lies in their relatively low-cost ability to provide critical data regarding targeted research questions such as:

- Are rural people as likely as their urban same-race and same-ethnicity counterparts to engage in daily aerobic exercise?
- How do men and women differ in their consumption of vegetables?

- Is there a significant difference in life expectancies within a metropolitan area as a function of zip codes?
- What are the barriers to mammography use for low-income women and do barriers differ as a function of race or ethnicity?

Because observational research is quite versatile, it has multiple applications in public health, with many of these applications being somewhat sophisticated in nature. This chapter will provide you with a set of skills to understand and implement five commonly used observational research designs. We begin with the cross-sectional design and proceed to its closest relative, the prospective cohort design. From there, we will lead you into successive independent sample design, then to the classic epidemiologic design, the case-control. We then conclude with the newer case-crossover design. As you learn about each design, keep in mind that choosing the right design for your research question is the single most important decision you will make relative to ensuring rigor in your study and an ability to help shape public health practice.

▶ What Is a Cross-Sectional Design?

By far the most common of all study designs, the **cross-sectional design** derives its name from the idea that it is a "snapshot" in time relative to a given research question. In essence, time is not a factor in these studies because measurements are collected through a survey or questionnaire that assesses variables of interest in the present such as, "Do you have hypertension?" or asks people to recall information from their past such as, "In the past 3 months, on how many occasions have you drunk more than five alcoholic beverages?" Because of the one-time measurement, the cross-sectional design can measure only *differences* between or among people rather than any individual *changes*. Differences can be made in race or ethnicity, gender, age, socioeconomic level, or in exposure to a certain health risk. The cross-sectional study is sometimes conducted anonymously because there is not a need to follow up with participants. Thus, this design works especially well with populations that may be reticent to provide their name as part of the study process. This design is shown in **FIGURE 6.1**.

Cross-sectional designs in public health are used for various reasons. Many cross-sectional studies are conducted to document prevalence of a disease or health-related behaviors or to estimate levels of health-related knowledge, attitudes, and other constructs. The cross-sectional design is also appropriate for use when the research question has an extremely low probability of producing a **spurious finding**—that is, a false finding—that can stem from not being able to establish a temporal order between two variables. For instance, think about the relationship that exists between depression and binge eating. Let's assume that you suspect that depression leads to or causes binge eating. Although your hunch is logical, is it also plausible that the reverse is true? That binge eating could lead to depression? The answer, of course, is yes. So, at this juncture, you now have to ask, "What value does my cross-sectional study have?" The answer

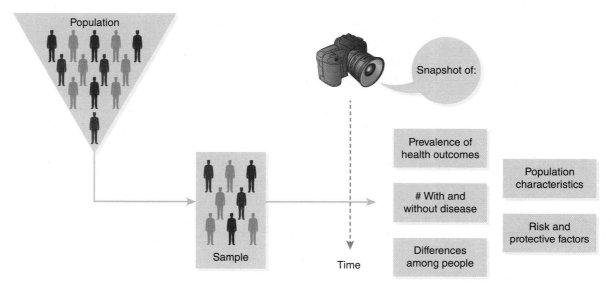

FIGURE 6.1 Cross-Sectional Study Design.

BOX 6.1 Cross-Sectional Study Example

This cross-sectional study compared the risk factors for sexually transmitted infections (STIs) and HIV between young Black cisgender men who have sex with men (YBMSM) and young Black transwomen who have sex with men (YBTWSM). Data for this analysis were drawn from the baseline sample of a randomized controlled trial. Because this study is examining data from *only* the baseline sample, it is considered a cross-sectional observational study. YBMSM (*n* = 577) and YBTWSM (*n* = 32) were recruited from an STI clinic in the United States and completed a computer-assisted self-interview, and their medical records were also abstracted to examine STI and HIV diagnosis information. Independent group *t*-tests and chi-square analyses were used to examine differences in STI risk factors between YBMSM and YBTWSM. Findings showed that more YBTWSM had significantly higher prevalence of chlamydia and gonorrhea compared to YBMSM and that YBTWSM had significantly more risk factors for STIs and HIV compared to YBMSM. YBTWSM had significantly more oral sex partners, engaged in oral sex more frequently than YBMSM, and had a higher likelihood of engaging in sex for money or drugs. In addition, compared to YBMSM, YBTWSM were significantly more likely to have been incarcerated, had a higher likelihood of depending on sex partners for food or money, and were more likely to miss meals because of a lack of money. This study showed that Black transwomen who have sex with men are more likely to experience risk factors associated with STI and HIV transmission compared to cisgender Black men who have sex with men. This novel cross-sectional study revealed that Black transwomen make up a population that is vulnerable to experiencing adverse sexual health outcomes based on sexual history, behaviors, and sociodemographic factors (Crosby, Salazar, Hill, & Mena, 2018).

to this question is that your study still has *some* value. The value here is that cross-sectional designs can always establish a correlation or association between two variables such as depression and binge eating. We caution you, however, that correlation is not indicative of causation. Instead, a correlation merely suggests that a potential cause-and-effect relationship between two variables warrants further investigation using a prospective cohort design. See **BOX 6.1** for an example of a cross-sectional design.

The cross-sectional design has several strengths and weaknesses, which are listed in **TABLE 6.1**. Strengths include the fact that cross-sectional studies are quick and relatively inexpensive because data are collected only once. They also can assess prevalence of health outcomes. There is low or no attrition (i.e., rate in which people drop out). Participation rates are typically high because of low commitment. Results can be used to formulate causal hypotheses that can be tested with more sophisticated designs. Weaknesses include the potential that you may need an extremely large sample size to document prevalence and have statistical power to test hypotheses. Also, you are not able to document rare health outcomes or those of short duration. Results may be affected by selection bias because of accessibility to a targeted population. You cannot establish causation of two variables or incidence of disease, and omission of significant variables can undermine results or result in a third-variable effect (i.e., another unmeasured variable affecting

TABLE 6.1 Strengths and Weaknesses of Cross-Sectional Designs

Strengths	Weaknesses
Inexpensive	Large sample size typically needed
Quick	Cannot establish causation
Document prevalence of health outcomes	Cannot determine incidence
No attrition	Cannot document rare health outcomes
Low commitment of participation	Cannot assess changes over time
Assesses relationships and differences between groups	Does not control for cohort effects

both of the measured variables and causing the two variables to appear correlated with each other). Also, cohort effects are not controlled (such as different ages) and may bias results.

▶ What Is a Longitudinal or Prospective Cohort Study Design?

Sticking with our example of depression and binge eating, assume you want to study a possible cause-and-effect relationship because you are concerned about spurious findings. Cross-sectional designs do not allow us to determine causation, so a better design would be the **longitudinal cohort study**, which is sometimes referred to as a **prospective cohort design**. A prospective cohort design is one in which the same participants are followed over time and interviewed more than once during the time period. Thus, these designs can assess the temporal order of phenomena as well as *changes* in health-related outcomes, behavior, attitudes, and opinions over time. In public health, the purpose of prospective cohort studies typically involves (1) documenting exposure to risk factors and other confounding variables to determine associations with health outcomes over time, (2) determining the predictive ability of certain risk and protective factors as they relate to health-related outcomes over time, or (3) estimating rates of disease or behavior changes during the observation period (e.g., incidence). **FIGURE 6.2** illustrates the prospective cohort study design.

The time period of a longitudinal study could range from months to years. Such a study—sometimes referred to as a *panel study*—begins with a baseline assessment and then proceeds with subsequent follow-up assessments to determine rates of disease, behavior, or other variables of interest in the

cohort during a defined period of observation. So, this upgraded design eliminates the risk of spurious findings. With this advantage, you can now assess the frequency and intensity of depression as the **predictor variable** and binge eating as the **outcome variable**. As the name implies, the predictor variable must occur or manifest before the outcome variable.

Despite its inherent advantages, one major problem with prospective cohort studies is **attrition**. Also referred to as **mortality**, attrition is the loss of participants from the research study and can bias the results. Severe attrition can be dealt with statistically by comparing those who returned for follow-up interviews (or completed follow-up questionnaires) with those who did not, determining critical differences between the two groups and determining whether any bias has occurred.

In addition to attrition, both additional weaknesses and strengths are associated with prospective cohort studies. For example, you do not have to worry about cohort or generation effects. You can study the natural development of multiple health outcomes or disease. You can assess the stability and continuity of several attributes and document trends or patterns over time while establishing a temporal order. Sampling error is minimized, and you are able to assess reasons for any changes or outcomes observed. Weaknesses include the general need for large samples, which means the study will be time consuming and expensive. This design is not especially useful for rare outcomes, and you may have to wait long periods while waiting for outcomes to manifest. Also, assessing individuals multiple times may result in **testing effects**, meaning that participants can be affected by the questions they are being asked on the surveys, which can introduce bias into the study.

Now that you understand the primary advantages and disadvantages of a prospective cohort design, the next step is to learn how to best conduct this type

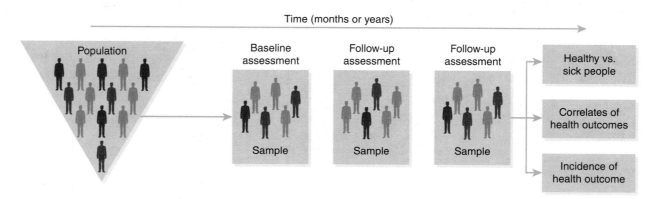

FIGURE 6.2 Prospective Cohort Study Design.

BOX 6.2 Prospective Study Design Example

This prospective study examined the relationship between depression, marijuana use, and sexual risk behavior among truant adolescents. *Truancy* refers to a youth with a history of intentional, unjustified, unauthorized, or illegal absence from school, behavior that presents a serious issue to most school districts in the United States. Data were collected at baseline; 3, 6, 12, and 18 months after intervention from $N = 300$ truant adolescents ages 11–17 who participated in a prospective intervention in the southeastern United States. Overall, results show that truant youth reported high rates of sexual risk behaviors, including engaging in sex without a condom and having sex with two or more partners at each time point. In addition, 48% of male and 42% of female participants had used marijuana and up to 56% of participants reported experiencing symptoms of depression. Longitudinal data analysis revealed that truant female adolescents had higher depression scores. In addition, high depression scores at baseline were predictive of sexual risk behaviors in the future. Study findings suggest that co-occurrence of problem behaviors is typical among truant adolescents, so it is important to incorporate strategies to reduce depression and marijuana in sexual risk-reduction programs for adolescents (Dembo, Krupa, Wareham, Schmeidler, & DiClemente, 2017).

of study. Unlike the simple cross-sectional design (a one-time assessment), the prospective design begins with a sample of people who enroll in the study after agreeing to be contacted periodically for **follow-up assessments**. Typically, a **baseline assessment** is conducted immediately after enrollment; this is when you can assess a large number of predictor variables that may be related to your outcome. Follow-up assessments can then occur at regularly scheduled intervals for as long as needed to fairly test study hypotheses. For instance, a study may have a baseline assessment at enrollment (i.e., month 0), with follow-up assessments every three months thereafter (i.e., end of months 3, 6, 9, and 12). Each follow-up assessment is an opportunity to assess the outcomes of the study. Given that some outcomes may not occur within a 3-month period, it is often the case to have much longer follow-up periods. **BOX 6.2** provides an example of a research study that used the prospective cohort study design.

▶ What Is a Successive Independent Samples Design?

Another design that represents a significant advantage compared with the cross-sectional design is the **successive independent samples design**, also known as a *trend study*. This design is somewhat of a marriage between the cross-sectional design and the prospective cohort design by incorporating a *series* of cross-sectional studies that are conducted over time. However, in contrast to the prospective cohort design, each cross-sectional survey is conducted with a different independent sample, which means that a new sample is drawn for each successive cross-sectional survey. And each sample is assessed only once. This design is used frequently in public health to assess changes in a population characteristic over time, hence the name *trend* study. This design is depicted in **FIGURE 6.3**.

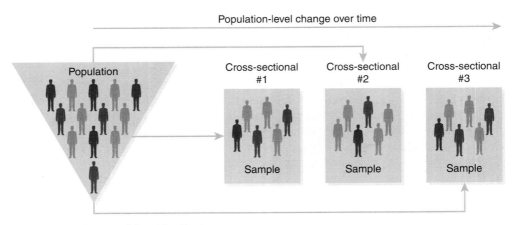

FIGURE 6.3 Successive Cross-Sectional Samples Design.

This type of design is used quite often in epidemiology, which is the discipline studying the incidence, distribution, and control of disease in a population. In fact, federal, state, county, or city health departments may want to document the change in certain health risk behaviors or the prevalence of disease for a *given population over a period of time* to inform new programs and policy or to determine effects of newly implemented policies. The successive cross-sectional design would be the appropriate design to obtain these types of information. In fact, the Centers for Disease Control and Prevention (CDC) conducts and sponsors many studies using the successive independent samples design; a prime example is the National HIV Behavioral Surveillance, which collects independent cross-sectional samples each year from different high-risk populations and assesses the prevalence of engaging in HIV-risky behaviors. A recent example of a successive cross-sectional study is presented in **BOX 6.3**.

Although a vast improvement over regular cross-sectional designs, the successive cross-sectional design still suffers from weaknesses. For example, with this design, you still cannot identify *causes* of documented changes, and each independent sample must be drawn from the same population and be equally representative of that population. However, you can document trends or patterns over time, and typically there is low attrition and refusal rates because each sample is assessed only once. **Internal validity**, or a high degree of confidence in the results because of the level of rigor in the study design and methods, is also higher in successive cross-sectional designs than in cross-sectional designs.

▶ What Is a Case-Control Study Design?

In Chapter 1, we briefly introduced the story of John Snow, the British physician aptly referred to as the father of modern epidemiology (and whose namesake is one of our public health mascots). As you may recall, Snow is famous for his investigation of a cholera epidemic in 1854 in Soho, London. First by conducting interviews and making observations, he formed a hypothesis that suggested contaminated water from a public water pump was the source of the cholera epidemic. He mapped where victims lived and then marked the sites of public water pumps on the map. Snow was able to determine that one particular water pump (the Broad Street pump) lay at the center of a cluster of cholera cases; in fact, every local cholera patient had consumed water from this one pump. Other pumps on his map were shown to be used much less frequently. Accordingly, Snow concluded that this pump (i.e., the water source flowing from it) was the source of the infection and persuaded health officials to remove the pump handle so that its use would be discontinued. His interviews with people who had cholera and with those who did not enabled him to determine differences between the two groups, and these led him to his conclusion. His study formed the basis for the case-control study.

Since Snow's study, the **case-control design** has been used extensively in public health research. The design requires that participants are selected on the basis of whether or not they have the disease or other

---

BOX 6.3   Example of a Successive Cross-Sectional Samples Study

This successive cross-sectional samples study, also referred to as a *trend study*, examined changes in diet quality (i.e., healthy eating patterns) over a 16-year period among U.S. adults with diabetes and trends in socioeconomic disparities specifically related to the diet quality. Data for this study are drawn from eight cycles of the National Health and Nutrition Examination Survey (NHANES) that was administered from 1999 to 2014. Each year, a nationally representative sample in the United States was surveyed. The current study examined NHANES data collected from adults aged 20 or older with type I or II diabetes. Statistical analyses were performed to examine whether diet quality differed based on socioeconomic factors (education and income) and whether differences varied over time.

Diet quality was measured using the Healthy Eating Index (HEI) in which HEI scores range from 0–100 with higher scores indicating better diet quality. Results indicate significantly better diet quality and healthy eating patterns from 1999 to 2014, with increases in HEI scores from 49.4 to 52.4 over 16 years. Findings showed that participants with low income, education, and food security had significantly worse diet quality than those with high incomes, education, and food security. Moreover, despite the large increase in HEI scores among U.S. adults with diabetes from 1999 to 2014, these differences in diet quality between low and high income, education, and food security did not significantly change over the 16 years. This trend study showed that diabetic U.S. adults' overall diet quality has improved over the past 16 years but that consistent health disparities related to diet quality and nutrition persist (Orr, Keyserling, Ammerman, & Berkowitz, 2019).

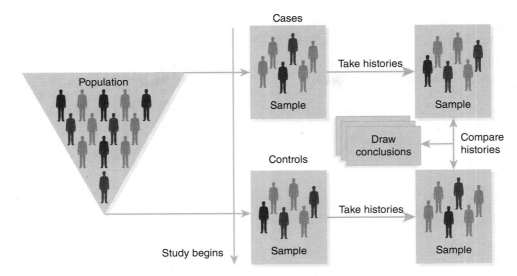

FIGURE 6.4 Case-Control Study Design.

health-related outcome of interest. Those who have the disease or outcome are termed **cases**, and those who do not are termed **controls**. Although assessment occurs once, as is the case in a cross-sectional design, exposure to hypothesized risk factors is assessed retrospectively for both cases and controls. Then comparisons are made to determine the likelihood of the contribution of different risk factors deemed **exposures** to the outcome. For instance, people who have diabetes (cases) could be compared with people without diabetes (controls) in terms of their eating habits (exposure) to determine whether more cases were unhealthy eaters than controls. Thus, the central feature of the case control is the comparison of the cases' and controls' exposure *histories*. The case-control design is depicted in **FIGURE 6.4**.

When conducting a case-control study, because by definition, cases have the disease or outcome, they are typically selected from available cases at some type of medical care clinic or facility. When selecting the controls, it is vitally important that controls' characteristics mirror those of cases as closely as possible. Thus, cases and controls should be nearly the same except for the disease or outcome of interest (see **FIGURE 6.5**). Characteristics to be considered include age, gender, and race or ethnicity in addition to the hypothesized risk factors. The key to choosing controls is that comparability is more important than representativeness.

In terms of risk factors or exposures that should be assessed, researchers should consider many possible determinants to explain the outcome, including physical, biological, social, cultural, and behavioral factors. Interviews or surveys with cases and controls can be used to assess risk factors, or any available preexisting sources can be used such as medical, pharmaceutical, registry, employment, insurance, birth, death, and environmental records.

Case-control designs are considered cost-efficient because a large sample is not necessary as with a prospective cohort design. This efficiency is particularly true when the disease or outcome is rare (i.e., less than 20% of the population). In fact, when the outcome is extremely rare, case-control studies may be the only feasible approach. As an example, consider the CDC's early investigations into the possible methods by which HIV could be transmitted from person to person. This case-control study occurred among 50 gay men with either Kaposi's sarcoma (KS) or Pneumocystis pneumonia (both of which are common opportunistic infections among people living with

EVER WONDER WHETHER

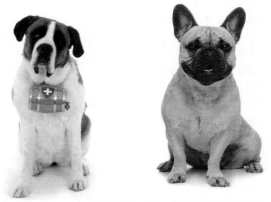

YOU'RE A CASE OR CONTROL?

FIGURE 6.5 Public Health Mascots Snow and Hamilton Deliberate on Their Research Roles.
© Eric Isselee/Shutterstock; © Svetography/Shutterstock

BOX 6.4 Case-Control Study Example

A case-control study conducted in a hospital setting examined the relationship between experiencing intimate partner violence (IPV) during pregnancy and adverse birth outcomes among pregnant women in Ethiopia. This study used an unmatched case-control design and was conducted in four hospitals in a region of Ethiopia. A total of 954 expecting mothers were recruited (318 cases and 636 controls), and data were collected using in-person interviews with participants. Roughly 41% of these women had experienced IPV during pregnancy, and 68% had experienced IPV sometime in their lives. Data were analyzed using logistic regression, and findings showed that women who experienced IPV during pregnancy were three times more likely and women who experienced physical violence were five times more likely to give birth to a child with low birth weight and have a preterm birth compared with those who did not experience IPV. This case-control study provided compelling evidence that experiencing IPV during pregnancy can severely impact childbirth and newborn health, suggesting a need for maternal health programs in Ethiopia to address IPV (Berhanie, Gebregziabher, Berihu, Gerezgiher, & Kidane, 2019).

HIV or AIDS). The controls were 50 gay men who were healthy at the time of study enrollment. Controls were matched to the cases based on three criteria: age, race, and city of residence (Jones & Salazar, 2016). The following shows a partial chronology of this early HIV and AIDS study.

> Early in 1982, CDC conducted a national case-control study that included most living patients with Kaposi Sarcoma, or other opportunistic infections reported in the United States. The 50 cases among gay men were compared with control gay men matched by city of residence, race, and age. The studies, led by Drs. Harold Jaffe and Martha Rogers, found that case patients tended to be much more sexually active than controls and were more likely to have had other sexually transmitted infections. (Curran & Jaffe, 2011)

As you can see from this highlight, the case-control study design was relied on early in the HIV epidemic (again, because the outcome—in this case, HIV infection—was relatively rare).

In addition to these strengths, case-control studies are useful for outbreak investigations or new diseases (such was the case in 1982 with HIV and AIDS) and are well suited for diseases with long latency periods. Also, case-control studies allow for the examination of multiple risk factors to help identify causal factors with the outcome of interest. Weaknesses are that this design cannot account for rare exposures, and it is restricted to only one outcome. Also, because peoples' histories are assessed when determining significant risk factors, recall bias is an issue. Sample bias may also be a problem, especially when creating the groups, especially if controls are not properly matched to cases. Finally, this design cannot determine incidence.

An example of a recent case-control study is presented in **BOX 6.4**.

▶ What Is a Case-Crossover Study Design?

Imagine that you need to know whether a health-related outcome increased immediately after exposure. By *immediate*, we mean that the disease or condition has a relatively abrupt onset period and it is not necessarily long-lasting (i.e., it is a not a chronic disease). Examples include asthma attacks, myocardial infarctions, traffic accidents, and work injuries.

Often in public health, the key to understanding these "immediate onset" diseases or outcomes lies in linking them to intermittent environmental risk factors. This is when the **case-crossover design** is your best choice. A basic requirement of the design is that people in the study serve as both cases and their own controls and must have "crossed" from lower to higher levels of exposure. For instance, the case-crossover design would be an appropriate design to test whether being under the influence of certain drugs while driving (a transient exposure) was associated with being in a traffic crash. In this example, the risk-exposure period (called the **hazard period**) is the time period right before the crash, such as the 16 hours preceding the crash. The exposure (taking of the drug) would be assessed during this defined period of time occurring in tandem with the risk exposure period—this is known as the **case-exposure window**. During this window of time, the person is deemed a case. The **control window** refers to an earlier period such as the 24 hours before the day of the crash or perhaps even the most recent

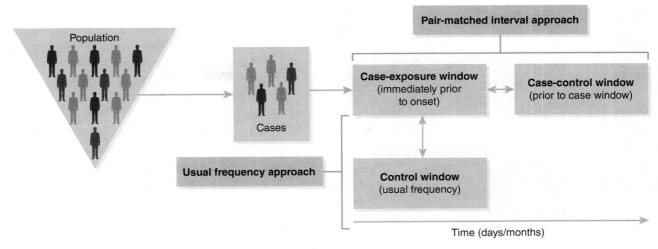

FIGURE 6.6 Case-Crossover Design.

day before the crash when the person drove. In this example, we would record drug use during the case-exposure window and during the control window. The risk exposure during the case window is then compared statistically to risk exposure during the control window. This two-window comparison is known as the **pair-matched interval** approach.

In addition to this comparison, some case-crossover studies conduct a second comparison where risk exposure during the case exposure window is compared with the **expected frequency** of exposure. Expected frequency is based on a subject's reported usual frequency over a specified time period *before* the outcome occurred. This provides a more in-depth understanding of the typical levels of exposure leading up to onset and can be compared with the case window. In our example, this would be the drug use behavior over the course of the previous months leading up to the car crash. This alternative approach is called the **usual frequency approach**. The case-crossover design, using both of these approaches, is depicted in **FIGURE 6.6**. Regardless of which approach is used, the case-crossover design has tremendous utility when it comes to linking environmental hazards with acute health outcomes; see, for example, Jaakkola (2003); Jaakkola, Tuomaala, & Seppänen (1994); Lee & Schwartz (1999); Maclure (1991); Nafstad et al. (1998);

Neas, Schwartz, & Dockery (1999); and Reinikainen, Jaakkola, & Seppänen (1992).

Again, a key requirement of using this design is that the outcome must be something that occurs abruptly rather than slowly develops over a protracted period of time. The onset of a serious asthma attack, for instance, could be investigated as a result of environmental triggers. In this second example, levels of air pollution would be measured during the case-exposure window and also during the control period preceding the attack. Notice here that the crossing over occurred naturally and was not manipulated by the experimental design in any way. Of course, this type of opportunity to observe people while they engage in a natural crossover requires careful attention to building a base of research participants. Other examples include car crashes involving texting while driving, heart attacks involving exposure to extreme temperatures, and negative health outcomes involving exposure to lead. Please notice that the case-crossover design is quite distinct from the other designs discussed in this chapter. The distinction regards the investigation of environmental causes. Clearly, the environment has always been (and always will be) highly influential in determining the health of any given geographic population or populations defined by their "home surroundings."

Think About It!

Vaping and the use of e-cigarettes has become a widespread practice (see **FIGURE 6.7**). Among adolescents, this practice has been shown to produce nicotine dependence within 12 months of onset

(Vogel, Prochaska, Ramo, Andres, & Rubenstein, 2019). Given this information, an essential question is, What are the health effects of vaping or the use of e-cigarettes? Although promoted as

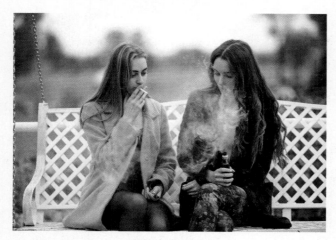

FIGURE 6.7 Teens Smoking and Vaping.
© Aleksandr Yu/Shutterstock

having no serious side effects, this is nonetheless an important empirical question. So, let's consider this an opportunity to apply either a case-crossover design or a prospective cohort design. Both have strengths and weaknesses with regard to this study objective.

Beginning with the prospective cohort option, you can easily imagine a study that begins with a cohort of teens who vape or use e-cigarettes on a daily basis. A requirement to be enrolled in the cohort would be something like "currently vaping or using e-cigarettes." Thus, once you locate prospective study volunteers and enroll them in the study, over time—let's say 12 months—you would need to track the level of vaping or use of e-cigarettes, the substances used in the e-cigarettes, and several health indicators. These indicators might be:

- The onset of asthma or other respiratory illness
- Shortness of breath
- Frequency of colds or upper-respiratory infections
- Elevated blood pressure or heart rate (or both)
- Pain in the chest or lungs

Take Home Points

- Observational research is used to measure people's attitudes, beliefs, and behaviors using self-report surveys.
- Observational research studies range from a one-time survey to large cohort studies that last for years or even decades.
- There are five types of observational research designs: cross-sectional, longitudinal or prospective cohort, successive independent

As the 12-month period of observation unfolds, you may have several issues with the cohort, such as first people enrolled quitting their use of vaping or e-cigarette use or not being able or willing to attend periodic assessments for the indicators (shown in the preceding bulleted list). Given that you could maintain a reasonable percentage of the cohort over 12 months, you would then have the ability to use the assessments to conduct analyses that detected relationships between average number of weekly hours of vaping or e-cigarette use, the substances inhaled, and the onset of symptoms or actual disease conditions.

Now, let's consider how this study would look using a case-crossover design. In this scenario, you might consider enrolling people who use e-cigarettes and reported to an emergency room (ER) with serious health issues such as a heart attack or severe respiratory issues. Once you have enrolled these participants, you would assess their actual e-cigarette use for a specified time period preceding the ER visit, such as 1 week. This would be considered as being in the hazard period or the case-exposure period. You would then assess them retrospectively for their usual frequency of e-cigarette usage during another period of time (the control window) that preceded the ER visit and that would encompass a longer time period such as the 6 months before the hospital visit. Again, you would apply the same assessment protocol during the control window period of time to assess use of e-cigarettes and also the substance in the e-cigarette (i.e., nicotine or THC—the high-inducing compound in marijuana). With this design, you could assess the relative risks of e-cigarette use to an asthma attack, for example, by using the case-exposure period and the control window. This would allow you to determine whether exposure to e-cigarettes was lower during the control window compared with the hazard period. Ultimately, both the prospective cohort study and the case crossover present multiple (and highly challenging) issues to conducting a rigorous study. So, for practice, please think about which one you would use and why that option is better.

samples, case-control designs, and case-crossover designs.
- Establishing a correlation between two variables in cross-sectional studies is possible, but correlation is not indicative of causation.
- A longitudinal or prospective cohort study design refers to an observational study in which individuals are followed over time.

- A successive independent samples design, also called a *trend study*, refers to multiple cross-sectional studies conducted over a period of time.
- Case-control studies are used to make comparisons of different risk factors that contribute to disease outcomes.

- Somewhat similar to case-control studies, case-crossover studies are also used to make comparisons of different risk factors that contribute to disease outcomes but the same sample is used for both the case and control period.

Key Terms

Attrition
Baseline assessment
Case-control design
Cases
Case-crossover design
Case-exposure window
Control window
Controls
Cross-sectional design

Expected frequency
Exposure
Follow-up assessment
Hazard period
Internal validity
Longitudinal cohort study
Mortality
Observational research
Outcome variable

Pair-matched interval
Predictor variable
Prospective cohort design
Spurious finding
Successive independent samples
  design
Testing effects
Usual frequency approach

For Practice and Discussion

1. What is observational research and how is it used in the context of public health? Compare the five different observational research designs described in this study and explain how each is used.
2. A researcher is interested in studying whether smoking is related to physical activity in a sample of college students. Which observational research design would be appropriate to use given this research question, and why?
3. Which observational research design would allow you to assess changes in a health problem over time and why? Explain this design in your own words.
   a. What are the strengths and weaknesses of this design?

4. Develop a research question for an observational research study on a public health topic of your choice.
   a. Explain why your research question is appropriate for an observational study.
   b. Which type of observational research design would you use for your study and why?
   c. What is the predictor, and what is the outcome variable for your study?

References

Berhanie, E., Gebregziabher, D., Berihu, H., Gerezgiher, A., & Kidane, G. (2019). Intimate partner violence during pregnancy and adverse birth outcomes: A case-control study. *Reproductive Health, 16*(1), 1–9. https://doi.org/10.1186/s12978-019-0670-4

Crosby, R. A., Salazar, L. F., Hill, B., & Mena, L. (2018, June). A comparison of HIV-risk behaviors between young Black cisgender men who have sex with men and young Black transgender women who have sex with men. *International Journal of STD & AIDS, 29*(7), 665–672.

Curran, J. W., & Jaffe, H. W. (2011). AIDS: The early years and CDC's response. *Morbidity and Mortality Weekly Report, 60*, 64–69.

Dembo, R., Krupa, J. M., Wareham, J., Schmeidler, J., & DiClemente, R. J. (2017). A multigroup, longitudinal study of truant youths, marijuana use, depression, and STD-associated sexual risk behavior. *Journal of Child and Adolescent Substance Abuse, 26*(3), 192–204. https://doi.org/10.1080/1067828X.2016.1260510

Lee, J. T., & Schwartz, J. (1999). Reanalysis of the effects of air pollution on daily mortality in Seoul, Korea: A case-crossover design. *Environmental Health Perspectives, 107*, 633–636.

Jaakkola, J. J. K. (2003). Case-crossover design in air pollution epidemiology. *European Respiratory Journal, 23*, 81–85.

Jaakkola, J. J. K., Tuomaala, P., & Seppänen, O. (1994). Air recirculation and sick building syndrome: A blinded crossover trial. *American Journal of Public Health, 84*, 422–428.

Jones, J., & Salazar, L. S. (2016). A historical overview of the epidemiology of HIV/AIDS in the United States. Pp. 19–41 in E.R. Wright & N. Carnes (Eds.), *Understanding the HIV/AIDS epidemic in the United States: The role of syndemics in the production of health disparities.* Switzerland: Springer International Publishing.

Maclure, M. (1991). The case-crossover design: A method for studying transient effects on the risk of acute events. *American Journal of Epidemiology, 133,* 144–153.

Nafstad, P., Øie, L., Mehl, R., Gaarder, P. I., Lødrup-Carlsen, K. C., Botten, B., et al. (1998). Residential dampness problems and development of bronchial obstruction in Norwegian children. *American Journal of Respiratory Critical Care Medicine, 157,* 410–414.

Neas, L. M., Schwartz, J., & Dockery, D. (1999). A case-crossover analysis of air pollution and mortality in Philadelphia. *Environmental Health Perspectives, 107,* 629–631.3

Orr, C. J., Keyserling, T. C., Ammerman, A. S., & Berkowitz, S. A. (2019). Diet quality trends among adults with diabetes by socioeconomic status in the U.S.: 1999–2014. *BMC Endocrine Disorders, 19*(1), 54. https://doi.org/10.1186/s12902-019-0382-3

Reinikainen, L. M., Jaakkola, J. J. K., & Seppänen, O. (1992). The effect of air humidification on symptoms and the perception of air quality in office workers: A six period cross-over trial. *Archives of Environmental Health, 47,* 8–15.

Vogel, E. A., Prochaska, J. J., Ramo, D. E., Andres, J., & Rubenstein, M. L. (2019). Adolescents' e-cigarette use: Increases in frequency dependence and nicotine exposure over 12 months. *Journal of Adolescent Health, 64,* 770–775.

For Further Reading

Jacobsen, K. H. (2017). Cross-sectional surveys. Pp. 45–48 in *Introduction to health research methods: A practical guide* (2nd ed.). Burlington, MA: Jones & Bartlett.

Jacobsen, K. H. (2017). Case-control studies. Pp. 49–58 in *Introduction to health research methods: A practical guide* (2nd ed.). Burlington, MA: Jones & Bartlett.

Jacobsen, K. H. (2017). Cohort studies. Pp. 59–70 in *Introduction to health research methods: A practical guide* (2nd ed.). Burlington, MA: Jones & Bartlett.

Mann, C. (2003). Observational research methods. Research design II: cohort, cross-sectional, and case-control studies. *Emergency Medicine Journal, 20*(1), 54–61. https://doi.org/10.1136/emj.20.1.54

Rosenbaum, P. R. (2010). *Design of observational studies.* New York, NY: Springer Verlag.

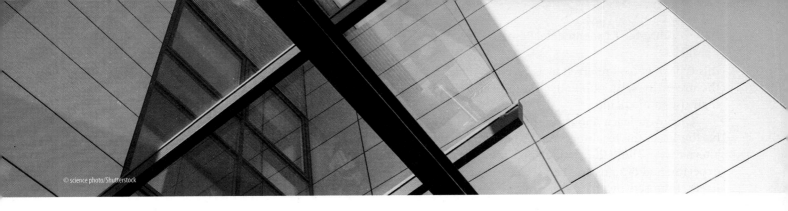

CHAPTER 7

Experimental Research Designs

with Anne Marie Schipani-McLaughlin

LEARNING OBJECTIVES

1. Identify how experimental research designs can be applied to inform public health practice.
2. Distinguish between internal and external validity.
3. Describe the basic threats to the internal validity of experimental designs.
4. Identify the principles and advantages of several experimental research designs.
5. Determine how best to align the research question with the optimal experimental research design.

▶ Overview

In Chapter 6, you learned about the value of observational research to public health. In this chapter, we take you to the next level of complexity: evaluating public health intervention programs designed to protect and promote the health of a population. In many ways, testing interventions represents the culminating point of both qualitative research (Chapter 5) and observational research because these types of studies are used many times to inform public health interventions. Much of the ultimate success in public health relies on rigorous testing of intervention programs developed through our research findings. Experimental designs are most often used to test interventions.

To begin, you may not be aware of this, but many medications available to you over the counter or by prescription were probably first tested with one specific type of experimental design: the randomized controlled trial. For instance, consider the ibuprofen you might take to resolve muscle pain. You might not

realize that the ibuprofen was tested for safety and efficacy with two groups of people—those randomly assigned to either receive the ibuprofen or receive a **placebo** (a neutral substance without any related biological effects). Most likely, the results of this trial showed that people randomly assigned to take ibuprofen fared better in terms of relief compared with those taking the placebo. If the difference in "relief" is greater than would be expected by chance alone, the ibuprofen is considered to be **efficacious** (meaning that it worked as expected). In fact, thanks to public health policy and legislation that regulates drugs, most medical drugs that you have taken were tested in a randomized controlled trial (RCT) and shown to be safe and efficacious.

Unfortunately, the leap from medical RCTs to those used to test public health interventions may be fraught with issues. For instance, ibuprofen is relatively easy to make, and each tablet is standardized in terms of dosage. Public health interventions, on the other hand, may vary from one time to the next. It is this type of issue—referred to as **fidelity**—that makes the use of RCTs in public health quite different from their use in medicine.

Once you learn about the RCT, this chapter will be the basis for teaching you about four important alternatives. Thus, the chapter provides five types of experimental designs you can select from to align the needs imposed by the nature of the research question and the capacities and strengths of each design. Ultimately, we want you to exercise logic and versatility in the selection of the optimal experimental design for your study. As you read this chapter, be mindful that an *intervention program* can also include new public health regulations (e.g., adding requirements to the accreditation of hospitals), public health policy (e.g., environmental tobacco smoke policies in workplaces), and public health law (e.g., taxes on sweetened beverages), in addition to public health educational programs.

▶ What Is Internal Validity and What Are the Common Threats to This Concept?

Before we review the five types of experimental designs, understand two crucial concepts that help us gauge the value of a study: **external validity** and **internal validity**. External validity pertains to whether the results from an experiment can be generalized to other people who did not participate in the study. This is a question best addressed by concepts related to sampling (see Chapter 10); however, when conducting experimental research, external validity is typically less of a priority. Internal validity is concerned with rigor and pertains to the experiment itself: Did it create conditions for a fair test of the intervention program? How confident are we that the results obtained can be attributed to the intervention program and not some other influence? Internal validity specifically refers to the degree of control exerted over potential **confounding variables** to reduce alternative explanations for the effects of various treatments. For most research involving an experimental design in public health, internal validity is prioritized over external validity.

A major threat to internal validity is confounding. *Confounding* occurs in a study when changes observed in the dependent variable could be attributed to variations in **extraneous variables** (Spiegelman & Zhou, 2018). Extraneous variables are those variables that may have an influence on an outcome variable but are not of interest to the research. The degree of control

exerted over potential extraneous variables determines the level of internal validity. By minimizing the potential for an alternative explanation for treatment effects, you will have more confidence that observed effects are the result of the independent variable. Thus, it is critical to understand what the potential confounders could be for your study and control them (see **FIGURE 7.1**).

To assist you with identifying potential confounding variables, **TABLE 7.1** displays nine common threats to the internal validity of an experimental study. Once you understand these threats, you can include steps in your research design to control for them. As shown, each category has a somewhat different effect on internal validity, but each can be mitigated by a somewhat simple set of preemptive design features. Primary among these is the use of a *comparison group*, which is also known as a *control group*. To truly understand the value of a comparison group, consider the threat known as **history**. We illustrate this point by using the recent story of Beyoncé having an emergency cesarean section.

In 2018, the popular performer Beyoncé publicly announced that she had toxemia, one form of a condition known as *preeclampsia*. Preeclampsia is a condition in pregnancy characterized by abrupt hypertension (a sharp rise in blood pressure), albuminuria (leakage of large amounts of the protein albumin into the urine), and edema (swelling) of the hands, feet, and face. Preeclampsia is the most common complication of pregnancy. In the case of Beyoncé, her preeclampsia necessitated having an emergency cesarean section, one that drew a tremendous amount of public attention. Events such as a celebrity having a life-threatening prenatal condition constitute *historical*

GOT YOUR CONFOUNDERS

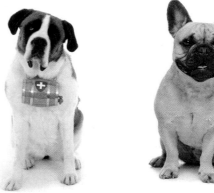

UNDER CONTROL?

FIGURE 7.1 Public Health Mascots Snow and Hamilton Get a Grip on Confounders.

TABLE 7.1 Nine Common Threats to Internal Validity

Threat	Cause	Research Design Affected
Hawthorne effect	Results might be from the time and attention paid to participants.	One-group design and two-group design without attention-placebo group
Diffusion	Results might be from contamination of the control group.	Two-group or multigroup design
History	Results might be from an event that occurred between observations.	One-group design
Maturation	Results might come from participants growing older, wiser, stronger, or more experienced between observations.	One-group design
Testing	Results might be from the number of times responses were measured.	One-group design
Instrumentation	Results might be from a change in the measuring instrument between observations.	One-group design
Statistical regression	Results might be from the selection of participants based on extreme scores; when measured again, scores move back to an average level.	One-group design
Differential selection	Results might be from differences that existed between participants in groups before treatment occurred.	Two-group or multigroup design
Differential attrition (mortality)	Results might be from the differential loss of participants from each group.	Two-group or multigroup design

events and have an unintended effect on other people's behaviors, attitudes, and knowledge.

Consider the following scenario. After conducting extensive qualitative and observational research, you have developed an intervention program designed to promote mammography use by women due or overdue for this lifesaving screening procedure to detect breast cancer in its earliest possible stages. Unfortunately, your intervention is launched in the month immediately before a celebrity endorses mammograms and has an on-air mammogram. So, if all of the women enrolled in your study were assigned to receive your intervention program and scheduled their mammogram appointments, how confident would you be that your program was a great success? The answer here is "Not very confident," and the reason for the lack of confidence is that the uptake in mammogram screening may

have been the result of this historical event. In this scenario, the historical event constitutes what is called the *history effect* and is deemed a threat to internal validity.

Fortunately, a reliable method for controlling history effects exists and is basically the use of a **comparison group**. A comparison group is typically formed immediately after study enrollment and baseline assessment. It is best formed by a simple procedure known as **randomization**. In fact, randomization is the hallmark of a true experimental design and involves a procedure, depending on the form of randomization, in which study participants are assigned to different groups (Rosenberger & Lachin, 2015). For example, there are several different techniques such as simple randomization, block randomization, or stratified randomization, all of which are implemented differently. However, regardless of the specific

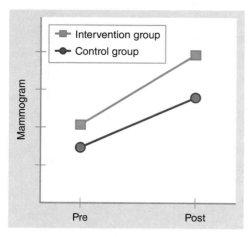

FIGURE 7.2 Example of a Line Graph Depicting Findings from an RCT of an Intervention Designed to Promote Mammography.

randomization technique implemented, each subject must be assigned to his or her respective group by way of the chosen randomization procedure. With a two-group study, this means that some subjects will receive the intervention program (the treatment group) and some will receive an innocuous alternative (a *placebo* in the parlance of a medical RCT). We can assume that if a historical event took place, *all* enrolled participants were likely exposed to it. With this assumption in mind, any differences between groups relative to the study outcome (e.g., scheduling a mammogram) can be attributed to the presence or absence of the intervention program. In this example, we would ideally see an increase in both groups—but a more dramatic increase among those randomly assigned to the intervention group. In graphic form, the findings may look like those shown in **FIGURE 7.2**. Although there are other threats to internal validity in addition to history shown and briefly described in Table 7.1, note that a two-group design eliminates many but not all of them. For example, diffusion, differential selection, and differential attrition are threats for two-group designs.

▶ What Is the Pretest–Posttest Randomized Controlled Design?

As described in the Overview to this chapter, the pretest–posttest randomized controlled trial is widely used in medical research and is considered the gold standard of research designs. The RCT also has an important place in public health research. Specifically, the RCT is useful for testing public health interventions that are intended for application at the individual level. By individual level, we mean intervention

attempts to favorably alter attitudes, beliefs, and practices of people through a strategy applied directly to them such as education, counseling, skill acquisition, or some other form of instilling motivation.

Simply put, the RCT is the most effective and most rigorous design for testing the efficacy of a program or treatment because it allows for causal inference and has the highest level of control possible in a real-world setting. As mentioned previously, the RCT involves random assignment of study participants to groups but it also involves control over extraneous variables, hence the name. Controlling for the effects of extraneous variables can be accomplished either by holding them constant, meaning the investigator would look to recruit participants with similar levels of these extraneous variables; or by randomizing their effects across the different treatment levels. In addition, the RCT entails multiple assessments: assessing groups at baseline (before randomization—i.e., the pretest) and then one or more follow-up time periods (i.e., the posttest or posttests). *Group* in an RCT is also referred to as the *treatment condition* or the **study arm**. Within the context of experimental research, the number of treatment conditions or number of study arms equates with the number of levels of the **independent variable (IV)**. The IV in this scenario is subject to **manipulation** by the researcher and is the public health intervention. Most RCTs have two arms—an intervention condition and a comparison condition—so there would be two levels to the IV in this case. However, three-arm RCTs are not uncommon (see **FIGURE 7.3**). In this case, you would find two intervention conditions (perhaps similar in nature but with one being less costly and labor intensive) and a single comparison condition. The RCT uses both a **between-subjects factor** (this is the comparison of the groups on the outcome measure) and a **within-subjects factor** (this is the movement of time across the various follow-up assessments). All of these features, including the sequence of assessment, intervention, and then follow-up assessment, allow for a temporal order to be established. The goal of an RCT from the perspective of the person designing and testing the intervention is to show that the intervention group demonstrates more favorable effects on the **dependent variable (DV)** (or outcome measure) than the comparison group (or comparison groups) over time.

Implementation of an RCT involves five important steps:

1. Conducting a thorough assessment before randomization
2. Randomizing participants into groups

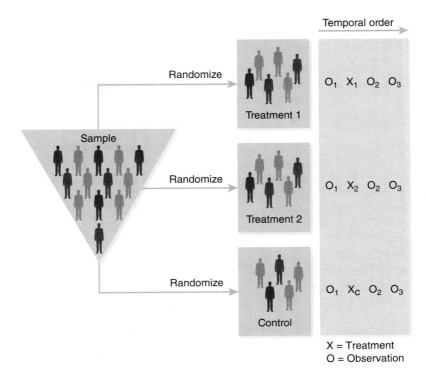

FIGURE 7.3 A Three-Arm Randomized Controlled Design.

3. Exposing the groups to the intervention program or the provisions specified for the comparison condition
4. Assessing participants after completion of the intervention or comparison condition programs and procedures
5. Optionally, continuing to assess participants after the intervention or comparison condition is completed, a process that may continue for months or even years

Before introducing the next study design, note that generally the RCT is a labor-intensive and, therefore, costly option. A primary determinant of the time and expense incurred by an RCT involves the sample size needed to fairly determine whether the intervention group significantly outperforms the comparison group on the predetermined study outcomes. Determining how large the sample size must be for an internally valid trial is beyond the scope of this text, so we urge you to learn more by consulting the highlighted readings in the "For Further Reading" section.

As noted in the previous paragraph, "generally the RCT is a labor-intensive . . . option." At this juncture, however, we wish to leave you with the point that RCTs are sometimes used in studies of college students. It is in these circumstances—if the intervention is not medical in nature—when the RCT is often seen as a more low-scale option that can produce important results. To give you a recent illustration of this point, please take a close look at **BOX 7.1**.

BOX 7.1 Example of a Randomized Controlled Trial Conducted Among College Students

The practice of *mindfulness* has become a method that more and more people use to avoid and manage stress. Given the overwhelming role of stress in the onset of disease and given that stress may be occurring at record levels, this tool can be an important ally to public health practice. Typically, mindfulness is considered to have five dimensions:

1. Observe
2. Describe
3. Act aware
4. Remain nonjudgmental of inner experiences
5. Remain nonreactive to inner experiences

Reliable and valid self-reported measures exist to assess the degree to which these five dimensions of mindfulness are occurring for a person. Thus, it is conceivable (and important) to know whether an intervention program may

(continues)

BOX 7.1 Example of a Randomized Controlled Trial Conducted Among College Students *(continued)*

have a positive impact on mindfulness over time. Keeping pace with the world, it is further conceivable that a mobile app could be used to deliver this intervention. Finally, given a general surplus of daily stress among *most* college students, it is easy to imagine that a trial of such an app might occur with this population. Indeed, this box is devoted to summarizing the results of a recent RCT designed to assess the effects of a mindfulness app (we thought you would like this one).

Students attending a large, state-owned university in the southwestern United States were recruited for the study via social media. Contrary to what we stated previously about large sample sizes being needed to detect changes in dependent variables, the study had adequate statistical power with only 88 study volunteers. The discrepancy in small sample size and statistical power may be attributed to the nature of the dependent variable, which was self-reported behavior as opposed to the more common medical RCTs that assess dependent variables that occur on a less-than-common basis (e.g., incidence of disease) and are typically biologically or medically confirmed.

The 88 volunteers were assessed at three points in time (baseline, 8 weeks after randomization, and 12 weeks after randomization) on the following dependent variables: (1) a measure of perceived stress, (2) five subscale measures of mindfulness (see the preceding list), and (3) a measure of self-compassion. Immediately following the baseline assessment, volunteers were then randomized to receive and use the mobile app for the next 12 weeks or to be on the waitlist control, meaning they were offered the app after the 12-week assessment period ended.

The findings from this relatively inexpensive and low-resource RCT were quite remarkable. To begin, however, we are obligated to explain that statistically significant differences (either demographically or pertaining to the dependent measures) between the two randomly assigned groups were not found at baseline, meaning a "level playing field" existed before the intervention began. Now for the findings. First, at the 8-week assessment, significant between-group differences favoring the intervention condition were found for all dependent variables. At this juncture, our only point we wish to express to you is that this sweep of all the measures is a rare and stunning occurrence. At 12 weeks, the majority of these favorable changes persisted, thus providing further evidence supporting the utility of this mobile app to promote mindfulness (so it was a happy ending).

To help you practice what you have been learning in this chapter (specifically *this section* of the chapter), you can now perhaps see where the larger and more expensive RCT could be valuable. If, for instance, students somaticizing their stress to the point of disease (or at least symptomology of disease) were to use the mobile app for an entire school year, is it conceivable—in light of the study of 88—that their physical issues may partially or fully abate during that time. We hope your answer to this was "Yes," and we hope also that you realize that this more extensive study measuring disease outcomes would more closely resemble a resource-intensive RCT that you first learned about in this section of the chapter.

Modified from Hubert J, Green J, Glissman C, Lackey L, Puzic M, & Lee C. (2019). Efficacy of the mindfulness mediation mobile App "Clam" to reduce stress among college students: a randomized controlled trial. *Journal of Medical Internet Research, 7,* e14273.

▶ What Is the Posttest-Only Control Group Design and When Is It a Good Choice?

The posttest-only control group design is considered the weakest of experimental designs and is considered a between-subjects design. Unlike the RCT, it does not involve a within-subjects factor. Stated differently, groups are formed by random assignment and then presented with either the treatment or some type of control. Posttests are then given to determine if a difference between or among groups or arms exists. However, because this design lacks a pretest assessment, the element of change before and after the intervention *within groups* is not one that can be considered as part of this design. Thus, groups are compared on the DVs using data assessed following the intervention and at one or more follow-up periods. This design is presented in **FIGURE 7.4**.

At this juncture, a key question you may have in mind is, "Why would a study design not have a pretest?" The answer involves the threat to internal validity known as *testing* (see Table 7.1). To illustrate this threat and thus the possible advantage of not having a pretest, think about a study that uses daily dietary choices such as the DV. Consider that this outcome is assessed based on records kept through daily food diaries. If you have ever kept a daily food diary, you may be familiar with the idea that doing so tends to somewhat alter what you eat. In other

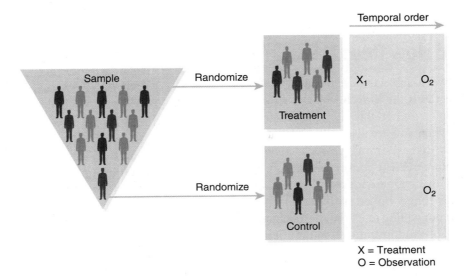

FIGURE 7.4 Posttest-Only Control Group Design.

words, your diet may change as a function of keeping a food diary. This is a classic example of a testing effect. Thus, to avoid having this testing effect confound your study, you would measure daily dietary choices on a one-time basis and then ideally at the end of study following the intervention. Note that other than the lack of pretest, the posttest-only design has all of the features found in the RCT, and its major strength is having a control group. Beyond the advantage of avoiding the threat of testing effects, the posttest-only control group design does not offer any other special feature that makes it a superior choice. It should only be used when

testing effects are likely to occur. Other weaknesses are that, without a pretest, it is also difficult to determine definitively if any differences observed at the end of the study are the result of an actual change stemming from the treatment. Also, differential selection and attrition are issues with this design. Randomization should theoretically control for differential selection; however, without a pretest, we cannot be assured that randomization worked and truly created an equivalency between groups. An example of a study that used the posttest-only control group design is described in **BOX 7.2**.

BOX 7.2 Example of a Three-Arm, Posttest-Only Experiment

This posttest-only design study tests the effect of information about behavioral and psychological symptoms of dementia (BPSD) on stigmatizing attitudes toward people with dementia and what factors, if any, influence these effects. Participants aged 18 to 83 years (*n* = 200) were recruited as part of a convenience sample from a college campus, community centers, and social centers in Hong Kong. After providing informed consent, participants were randomized to one of three conditions: control (*n* = 68), cognitive symptoms (*n* = 65), and BPSD (*n* = 67). The cognitive symptoms group viewed vignettes describing fictitious older adults with memory impairment; the BPSD group viewed the same vignettes that were expanded to include descriptions of BPSD, and the control group did not view any vignettes. All participants then completed self-administered questionnaires consisting of measures on stigma and demographics. Analysis of variance was conducted to examine whether exposure to information about cognitive and behavior symptom effects on stigma scores as the dependent variable. Findings showed that there was no significant experimental effect on stigma. In addition, having a relative with dementia or positive prognostic belief did not affect individuals' stigma level. Age and education were the only factors that were significantly associated with stigma. Individuals with little or only primary education reported greater stigma than those with college educations. Furthermore, participants ages 18 to 29 showed a higher level of stigma than participants aged 30 to 59. This study showed that information about BPSD may not influence stigma toward dementia. This posttest-only design allowed for an immediate assessment of stigmatizing attitudes after participants were presented with information regarding cognitive, behavioral, and psychological symptoms of people with dementia (Thrasher, Anshari, Lambert-Jessup, Islam, Mead, Popova, … Lindblom, 2018).

▶ What Is the Matched-Pairs Design and How Does It Work?

Another type of between-subjects design that is useful in public health research is the **matched-pairs group design**, which is depicted in FIGURE 7.5. This design is most advantageous when you are aware of a particular subject characteristic that is strongly associated with any intended study outcome. The concern about subject characteristics is that an attribute such as opioid use, for example, may be so strongly linked with the outcome measure that you are not willing to let the role of chance (which is the nature of randomization) determine the relative composition of people's opioid use in the randomized groups. Randomization does not ensure equal distribution of this attribute, so its use could result in a significant amount of bias to the study. Thus, to ensure that the characteristic is distributed equally, subjects can be matched on the characteristic (in this case, their current frequency of opioid use) *before* randomization. By matching, we mean that pairs of people are first formed based on the attribute. Then, taking each pair at a time, each subject within the pair is randomly assigned to the intervention or comparison conditions. The main advantage of this design is a significant reduction in the potential confounding effect of the attribute that is closely linked with outcome variable because each group will be equally balanced in terms of the attribute.

Applied to our example of opioid use, consider a two-arm randomized trial. Before randomization into the intervention or comparison condition, subjects would be assessed relative to their frequency of opioid use. Those reporting similar frequencies (i.e., two people reporting daily use) on this matching variable would be paired together. Next, each subject within each pair would be randomly assigned to one of the two conditions.

Regarding threats to internal validity, the matched-pairs design allows for the control of differential selection (see Table 7.1). It essentially creates a balance between groups relative to key variables that otherwise may introduce bias into the study design. This advantage is one that makes the matched-pairs design a superior choice when it is clear that one or more subject characteristics cannot be left to the fate of randomization. A weakness, however, of the matched-pairs design is that it is a time-consuming method and thus may add greatly to the overall cost of conducting the study. Also, it may not be possible to truly match all participants in one group with a suitable partner in the other group. An example of a study that utilized the matched-pairs group design is described in BOX 7.3.

> **BOX 7.3** Example of a Matched-Pairs Study
>
> This matched-pairs study evaluated the feasibility, acceptability, and effectiveness of an implementation strategy aimed at improving physicians' adherence to clinical guidelines for opioid prescriptions in primary care settings. This study tested a blended implementation strategy using a mix of the following approaches: audit and feedback, academic

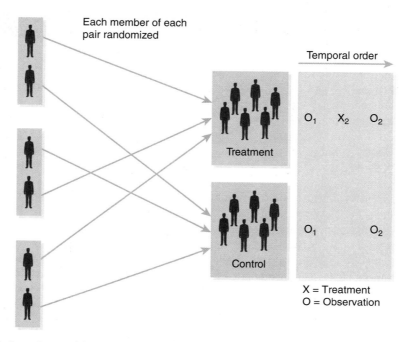

FIGURE 7.5 Matched-Pair Experimental Design.

detailing, and external facilitation. Using a matched-pairs design, the research team randomized four primary care clinics to receive the intervention and four clinics to act as the control condition. The intervention clinics implemented the clinical guidelines around opioid prescription during a 6-month period. Data collection involved a mixed-methods approach—that is, both qualitative (focus groups, structured interviews, and ethnographic field research) and quantitative (surveys) data collection occurred. Data were analyzed, and results indicate that 80% of staffers at the intervention clinics reported that their clinic had a better process for prescribing opioids and were more familiar with the guidelines for opioid prescription. At 6 months postintervention, intervention clinics showed significant improvements in mental health screening, treatment agreements, urine drug tests, and opioid co-prescribing and, at 12-months postintervention, the daily dose of morphine-equivalent drugs was significantly reduced compared with control clinics. This matched-pairs implementation study demonstrated the feasibility, acceptability, and effectiveness of the implementation strategy to improve physicians' adherence to clinical guidelines for prescribing opioids in primary care settings. Findings of this study have the potential to improve clinical guidelines within the healthcare system and alleviate the prevalence of opioid addiction (Quanbeck, Brown, Zgierska, Jacobson, Robinson, Johnson, … Alagoz, 2018).

▶ What Is the Within-Subjects or Repeated-Measures Design and When Should It Be Used?

The within-subjects or repeated-measures design (see **FIGURE 7.6**) is our next design in this chapter and one that is quite different from the first three. The difference is that a comparison or control group is not used, so randomization is not part of the design. Because this design has only one group and does not have random assignment, it *cannot* be considered a *true* experimental design. This one-group design is referred to as a *within-subjects* or *repeated-measures design* and because its lack of a control group, the study is vulnerable to multiple threats to internal validity (see Table 7.1). The reason this sacrifice may be well worth making, however, involves time, costs, and even ethical considerations. Ethical considerations would involve withholding a public health program from some individuals or groups on the basis of randomization (Rosen, Manor, Engelhard, & Zucker, 2006). Because there is only one group used, between-group differences are not considered. Instead, this within-subjects design involves each subject acting as his or her own control. Having subjects act as their own controls reduces **error variance** (in statistics, the portion of the variance in a set of scores resulting from extraneous variables such as individual differences and measurement) and increases the power of the study to detect effects in the DV. Translation of this design into practice occurs by having all subjects exposed to all levels of the IV. Thus, if the investigator wanted to test an intervention for its efficacy with this design and wanted to use both a treatment and a comparison condition, this design entails exposing all subjects to both conditions.

For example, imagine a smoking-cessation program is tested with this type of design. The investigator could first administer the pretest or baseline assessment and then have subjects go through the first condition (a self-guided, web-based program) and then expose them to the other condition, a nicotine-replacement patch. The self-help phase would be condition 1, and the nicotine replacement would be condition 2. Subjects would be assessed three times: before condition 1, after condition 1 but before condition 2, and then after condition 2. Thus, you can see how this design captures change over time on a person-by-person basis. That change is detected only through the repeated assessments of the same people,

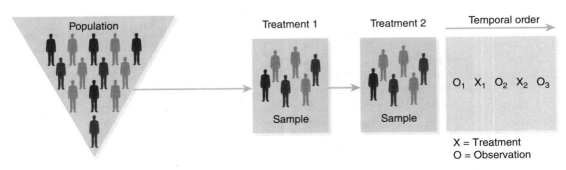

FIGURE 7.6 Within-Subjects or Repeated-Measures Design.

timed in conjunction with the intervention conditions and giving rise to the name *within-subjects* or *repeated-measures* design. In a sense, the *within* here means that people are serving as their own comparison standard; if we see significant change within a given subject over time, that change can be attributed to the intervention conditions.

Although the within-subjects design is economical and avoids the issue of providing a placebo comparison condition, the within-subjects design suffers from what are called **carryover effects**, which occur when exposure to the first treatment affects the subjects' performance (either enhancing it or reducing it) during subsequent treatments. For example, one type of carryover effect is called **learning** (enhancement of performance after the second treatment but resulting from the first treatment). Other types of carryover effects include **fatigue** (deterioration in performance from being tired from the first treatment), **habituation** (repeated exposure to stimulus leads to reduced responsiveness), **sensitization** (stronger responses to stimuli stemming from initial exposure to a different stimulus), and **adaptation** (adaptive changes to a stimulus lead to a change in outcome). An example of a study that appropriately used the within-subjects design is described in **BOX 7.4**.

To control for some negative carryover effects, a specific form of the within-subjects design has been developed called the **crossover trial** (Sedgwick, 2014). The crossover trial uses **counterbalancing** to balance the carryover effects. First, it creates groups and then randomizes each group to receive each level of the independent variable but varies the order in which each group receives each level. Similar to the classic repeated-measures within-groups design, the same group of subjects is exposed to all levels of the independent variable, but the order in which groups are exposed is varied. Thus, for every possible order combination, a group is formed. For example, using the same example of the smoking-cessation study with a crossover trial, researchers would randomly assign half the subjects to receive the nicotine patch first, followed by a "washout period" and then the self-guided web-based program, while the other half receives the self-guided web-based program first followed by a washout period and then the nicotine patch second. The washout period allows the effects of the first treatment to dissipate. The crossover occurs when each group of subjects switches from the first treatment condition to the next. By random assignment into the groups in this way, the more simple within-subjects design can be classified as a true experiment.

The crossover trial design is appropriate only for studies where the effects of a treatment are short-lived and reversible (such as in drug efficacy trials). Crossover designs should not be used when the condition of interest is unstable (e.g., asthma) and may improve regardless of intervention. This design improves on the basic within-subjects repeated measures because it allows for group comparisons and each subject acts as its own control and balances carryover effects.

BOX 7.4   Example of a Within-Subjects Study Design

A study identified the characteristics of messages in cigarette pack inserts that aimed to help smokers quit using a within-subjects design through direct-choice experiments, which are used widely in marketing research to determine the independent effects of certain product characteristics on decision-making and the choices people make. The research team recruited 665 adult smokers 18 to 50 years of age in the United States to participate in the direct-choice experiments using a within-subjects design that systematically manipulated cigarette insert characteristics based on image, informational or testimonial text type, cessation resources, call to action, and four message topics on response efficacy (e.g., benefits of cessation for life, financial gain of quitting) and self-efficacy (e.g., dealing with cravings, using social support when quitting). Participants evaluated nine choice sets, each with four inserts and rated inserts based on scales from those that were the most to least helpful for quitting, as well as the most to least motivated to quit. The researchers analyzed data to examine participants' choices based on insert characteristics, controlling for sociodemographic variables and smoking-related variables. The research team also assessed the interactions between insert characteristics and smokers' attributes (i.e., intention to quit, education, self-efficacy). Study findings showed that participants found it most helpful and motivated to quit when the inserts included an image, provided smoking-cessation information, or referenced the benefits of quitting related to well-being and financial gain. Significant interactions between insert characteristics and smokers' attributes indicated that inserts with information about smoking-cessation resources were more helpful and motivating to smokers with low self-efficacy, intentions to quit, or lower education level. Overall, this noteworthy study demonstrated that cigarette pack inserts with images and smoking-cessation information could be a powerful tool to promote smoking cessation (Lindblom, 2018).

▶ What Is the Randomized Stepped-Wedge Design?

Increasingly, public health research involves work that exceeds the individual level of intervention. The stepped-wedge cluster randomized trial is a novel research study design that is increasingly used in the evaluation of service-delivery–type interventions that are positioned at a higher level (Hemming, Haines, Chilton, Girling, & Lilford, 2015). The design involves random and sequential crossovers of **clusters** from control to intervention until all clusters are exposed. A cluster is simply a defined collection of similar units constituting the potential target of a pending intervention effort. For example, consider the task of investigating whether intervening with pharmacists who work in clinics to help them greatly restrict the distribution of oxycontin might reduce the severity of the opioid epidemic. The level of intervention in this case is, let's say, pharmacists operating within clinics located in a defined geographic region (for instance, a number of small counties in one area of a single state). As you might imagine, some training will be necessary relative to helping pharmacists work with providers to be more restrictive in their prescription of oxycontin or other prescription opioids. In case you are unaware, clinic-based pharmacists have expertise in the management of chronic conditions and are uniquely positioned to provide thorough recommendations with regard to a patient's opioid requirements. Also, pharmacists are subject matter experts on current literature and new developments, so they are able to provide continuing education to providers. Therefore, clinic-based pharmacists are uniquely positioned to provide a thorough assessment of a patient's pain-management needs and supplement the limited time providers have with patients. Pharmacists can also serve as advocates for prescribing naloxone and using urine drug screens to collaboratively evaluate a patient's pain-management needs. Thus, an intervention targeted to clinic-based pharmacists could include additional training and emphasis on collaboration with providers on evaluating the chronic pain-treatment plan for the patient and recommendations communicated with the provider before the patients' clinic visit. For this level of intervention, it would be prudent to begin targeting clinic pharmacists one county at a time and thus staggering the start times for the intervention period. Given that the first county where training and intervention occurs is also used for a control period, each selected county would have a control period and a defined period of intervention.

These time frames, however, *will not* be equal across the counties.

Given that this design involves the random assignment of clusters rather than individuals, we have to designate what we are defining as each cluster. Typically, but not always, clusters can be defined by geography. For instance, the small counties in our clinic pharmacists' example may have been naturally occurring clusters, with each containing an approximately equal number of clinic-based pharmacies. The eloquence of identifying clusters lies in gaining the ability to manipulate (via randomization) which clusters will become first recipients, second recipients, and so on in receiving the planned structural-level interventions.

The randomized stepped-wedge design is specifically advocated when pragmatic concerns preclude rolling out the intervention at only one point in time. By staggering intervention start dates, the stepped-wedge design allows for a staged and sequential rollout of the intervention program, thereby corresponding with two key points: (1) the reality that making structural-level change seldom has an instant effect, which means that change may more likely occur in stages and (2) the point that delay periods before the rollouts serve as the ideal control period. It is the second key point that makes this design one of great practicality as well as one that has a strong ethical character (because the intervention is never withheld from any one cluster, only delayed).

Returning to our example, the planned training efforts of the clinic pharmacists—within clusters—will be made practical and possible because training will occur in distinct areas at differing times. This means that the size of the research team responsible for this training still needs to be large enough to handle the volume of one county's entire employed clinic-based pharmacists until the training and other intervention objectives are fully met. Of great advantage in this example, the randomized stepped-wedge design allows every participating clinic pharmacy to be part of the intervention condition. This is a crucial aspect of buy-in for the pharmacies as they are recruited for the study.

The randomized stepped-wedge design is increasingly being applied to service-delivery studies. Inherent in the design is that intervention time periods will not be equivalent across steps because of the aforementioned staggering of rollouts. In the parlance of this design, *rollouts* represent the time when a randomly designated control condition switches over to become an intervention condition. The design refers to the time between rollouts as *step length*.

Randomized	Baseline	Step 1	Step 2	Step 3	Step 4	Step 5	Step 6
Clusters 21-24	O	X, O	O	O	O	O	O
Clusters 9-12	O	O	X, O	O	O	O	O
Clusters 17-20	O	O	O	X, O	O	O	O
Clusters 13-16	O	O	O	O	X, O	O	O
Clusters 5-8	O	O	O	O	O	X, O	O
Clusters 1-4	O	O	O	O	O	O	X, O

Time

O = Observation

X = Intervention

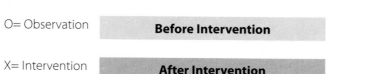

Before Intervention

After Intervention

FIGURE 7.7 Randomized Stepped-Wedge Design.

FIGURE 7.7 displays an example of a randomized stepped-wedge design. Please notice that the clusters are not shown in numerical sequence because they have been randomly assigned to this sequence. The design shown in this figure involves six steps of 1-month duration each. Notice that the number of control periods and the number of intervention periods is never the same for any one cluster. In our example of clinic pharmacies and sales of oxycontin, pharmacy sales records of oxycontin would be tracked throughout each 1-month period of observation. These 1-month time periods correspond with points in time when clusters are scheduled to switch from the control condition to the intervention condition. Ultimately, the goal in this case is to detect immediate and lasting changes in the clusters 21–24 clinic pharmacies when they switch from the control to intervention conditions. Next, for clusters 9–12 pharmacies, you hope for changes starting in the step four 1-month period of observation (and lasting throughout the study) followed by changes for the clusters 17–20 pharmacies.

Of course, you can imagine all kinds of public health intervention programs that can and should be tested using a randomized stepped-wedge design. Again, we urge you to reserve this somewhat more complex design for interventions that exist beyond the individual level. Examples include the following:

- Providing community meal programs in places where people lack adequate nutrition to maintain a healthy body weight
- Training street-based outreach workers to conduct intensive testing for hidden cases of HIV and hepatitis C in various communities
- Installing a sweetened-beverage tax in 2-month intervals across five counties within a single greater metropolitan area.

Think About It!

The breadth and scope of the devastating public health effects of climate change are already being experienced throughout the world. These effects include mass starvation, lack of potable water, and emerging diseases. As we write this textbook, it is daunting to us how much you (the student, as opposed to us, two professors who recall the 1970s perfectly) will ultimately have to work to reduce the carbon footprint of the United States. Although many citizens have chosen to simply "trust our leaders" and wait for a solution to climate crisis, we hope that your advanced standing as a college student will preclude such passive action. So, think about what you and others like you might take immediate action to lower your carbon footprints. This kind of creativity is exactly what it takes to inspire future public health practice—the next "pump handle" may, in fact, be a gas nozzle or a thermostat.

You learned previously in this chapter that a randomized controlled trial may initially occur among college students to determine whether it's effective before launching it on a wider scale. Accordingly, we challenge you here to think about (and even design) a small-scale RCT that you could feasibly test with college students. The goal would be to test only one or two small but highly repeatable actions that students could take to independently lower their carbon footprints. Indeed, this is a great learning experience because once you identify the "one or two things," you have to be sure they are measurable and prone to showing change as a result of the intervention action you might also propose. This leads to your larger challenge of creating some kind of nonpolicy (thus, think *behavioral*) intervention program that you could test as a method of leveraging this change. As you go through this exercise mentally, be inspired by Greta Thunberg, the Swedish teenage environmental activist on climate change whose campaigning has gained international recognition (see **FIGURE 7.8**). She first became known for her activism in August 2018 when, at age 15, she began protesting during school hours outside the Swedish parliament to call for stronger action on global warming. The word quickly spread over the world, and other students engaged in similar protests in their own communities. This school climate strike

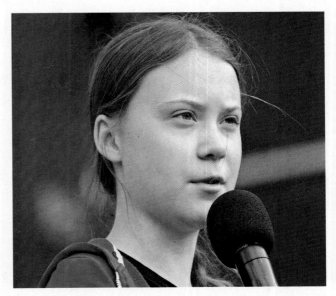

FIGURE 7.8 Environmental Teen Activist and Global Influencer Greta Thunberg.
© Liv Oeian/Shutterstock

movement became "Fridays for Future" (https://www.fridaysforfuture.org/). After Thunberg addressed the 2018 United Nations Climate Change Conference, student strikes took place every week somewhere in the world. In May of 2019, Thunberg was featured on the cover of *Time* magazine, and she sailed across the Atlantic Ocean in a 60-foot racing yacht equipped with solar panels and underwater turbines to address the U.N. Climate Action Summit in New York City in August of 2019, where she made an impassioned and targeted speech.

Take Home Points

- The purpose of experimental research is to determine whether an intervention is efficacious.
- Internal and external validity are pertinent to the value of an experimental study.
- Randomization indicates an experimental research design and involves randomly assigning participants to different study groups.
- The five types of experimental research designs are pretest–posttest randomized controlled trial, posttest-only control group design, matched-pairs design, within-subjects or repeated-measures design including crossover trials, and randomized stepped-wedge design.
- The pretest–posttest randomized controlled trial is considered the gold standard of research designs because it involves randomization, control of extraneous study variables, the use

of two or more study arms, and experimental manipulation.
- The posttest-only control group design is appropriate to use when there is the threat of testing to internal validity.
- Participants are matched based on specific characteristics before randomization in matched-pairs design research studies.
- Within-subjects or repeated-measures design studies do not involve randomization or the use of a control group unless it is augmented as the crossover trial.
- The randomized stepped-wedge design provides a rigorous design to test for efficacy interventions aimed at a higher level (clusters), with all clusters sequentially randomized to receive the intervention following a period of control.

Key Terms

Adaptation	Efficacious	Internal validity
Between-subjects factor	Error variance	Learning
Carryover effects	External validity	Manipulation
Clusters	Extraneous variables	Matched-pairs group design
Comparison group	Fatigue	Placebo
Confounding variables	Fidelity	Randomization
Counterbalancing	Habituation	Sensitization
Crossover trial	History	Study arm
Dependent variable (DV)	Independent variable (IV)	Within-subjects factor

For Practice and Discussion

1. What does it mean for a public health intervention to be efficacious? How are experimental research studies used to test the efficacy of intervention programs?
   a. Why is it important that programs are efficacious in the field of public health?

2. What is the difference between internal and external validity? Why are internal and external validity each important to determining the value of a research study?
   a. What are some strategies researchers use to minimize threats to internal validity in experimental research? How do these strategies help to strengthen a research study?

3. Explain the purpose of randomization. Why is it important within the context of experimental research designs?

4. Find a journal article that uses a randomized controlled trial to evaluate an intervention on a public health topic of your choice.
   a. How many study arms are in the trial? Define the study conditions, explaining the intervention and comparison groups.
   b. What are the independent and dependent variables in the study?
   c. What is the within-subjects factor in the study? What is the between-subjects factor?
   d. Based on the five steps of conducting an RCT as described in this chapter, was this trial conducted with rigor and replicability in mind? Explain why or why not.

References

Hemming, K., Haines, T. P., Chilton, P. J., Girling, A. J., & Lilford, R. J. (2015, February 6). The stepped wedge cluster randomised trial: Rationale, design, analysis, and reporting. *BMJ, 350*: h391.

Hubert, J., Green, J., Glissman, C., Lackey, L., Puzic, M., & Lee, C. (2019). Efficacy of the mindfulness mediation mobile app "Clam" to reduce stress among college students: A randomized controlled trial. *Journal of Medical Internet Research, 7*, e14273.

Quanbeck, A., Brown, R. T., Zgierska, A. E., Jacobson, N., Robinson, J. M., Johnson, R. A., . . . Alagoz, E. (2018). A randomized matched-pairs study of feasibility, acceptability, and effectiveness of systems consultation: A novel implementation strategy for adopting clinical guidelines for Opioid prescribing in primary care. *Implementation Science, 13*(1), 1–13. https://doi.org/10.1186/s13012-018-0713-1

Rosen, L., Manor, O., Engelhard, D., & Zucker, D. (2006). In defense of the randomized controlled trial for health promotion research. *American Journal of Public Health, 96*(7), 1181–1186.

Rosenberger, W. F., & Lachin, J. M. (2015). *Randomization in clinical trials: Theory and practice.* Hoboken, NJ: John Wiley & Sons.

Sedgwick, P. (2014). What is a crossover trial? *BMJ, 348*, g3191.

Spiegelman, D., & Zhou, X. (2018). Evaluating public health interventions: 8. Causal inference for time-invariant interventions. *American Journal of Public Health, 108*(9), 1187–1190.

Thrasher, J. F., Anshari, D., Lambert-Jessup, V., Islam, F., Mead, E., Popova, L., . . . Lindblom, E. N. (2018). Assessing smoking cessation messages with a discrete choice experiment. *Tobacco Regulatory Science, 4*(2), 73–87.

For Further Reading

Friedman, L. M., Furberg, C. D., DeMets, D. L., Reboussin, D. M., & Granger, C. B. (2015). *Fundamentals of clinical trials* (5th ed.). New York, NY: Springer International Publishing.

Jacobsen, K.H. (2017). Experimental studies. Pp. 71–86 in *Introduction to health research methods: A practical guide* (2nd ed.). Burlington, MA: Jones & Bartlett.

Julious, S. A. (2013). *Sample sizes for clinical trials*. New York, NY: Taylor & Francis.

Kirk, R. E. (2012). *Experimental design: Procedures for the behavioral sciences* (4th ed.). Newbury Park, CA: Sage.

Sedgwick, P. (2015). Randomised controlled trials: Understanding power. *BMJ, 350*, h3229.

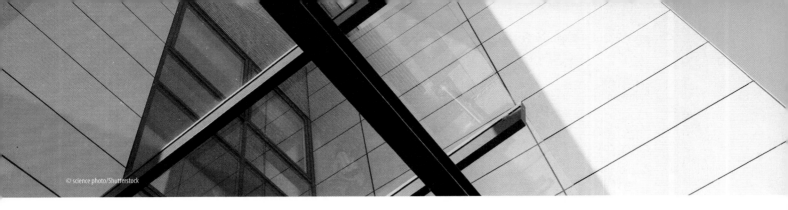

CHAPTER 8

Quasi-Experimental Designs for Public Health

LEARNING OBJECTIVES

1. Distinguish between experimental and quasi-experimental designs.
2. Articulate why quasi-experimental designs are uniquely suited to the needs of public health research and practice.
3. Understand the principles and advantages of several commonly used quasi-experimental designs.
4. Describe the threats to the internal validity of each quasi-experimental design.

▶ Overview

As a public health practitioner, you will have an obligation to ensure that your public health research is firmly grounded in the realities of practice. This means that the research, as much as possible, should be practice based. Indeed, leading scholars in the field of public health have widely advocated the need to make a shift from evidence-based research (such as tightly controlled, randomized, controlled trials) to research that more closely resembles the public health obligation to intervene at the upper levels of the socioecological model such as targeting entire populations (e.g., communities, states, or nations) rather than the one-at-a-time individual level (Green & Glasgow, 2006; Glasgow et al., 2006). In Chapter 7, you learned about the main experimental designs that are typically used to test individual-level public health programs. However, these designs are not as well suited to testing public health interventions that extend beyond the individual level and

may target schools, entire communities, and even the larger society. As a reminder about the nature and mission of public health, remember that the socioecological model is the hallmark of the principles and practices that best protect and promote the health of a population. **FIGURE 8.1** displays the socioecological model and illustrates the point that other types of research designs extending beyond the individual level are indeed a critically valuable part of public health research and, thus by extension, public health practice.

To delve deeper into research capable of testing interventions implemented at the community-level and above, this chapter offers you design options that can easily be added to your professional repertoire of research skills. Known as **quasi-experimental design**, this expanded level of research designs comprises the tools that must be used to determine efficacy of community-level (and higher-level) intervention programs. The prefix *quasi* represents the idea of "approximating" an experimental design.

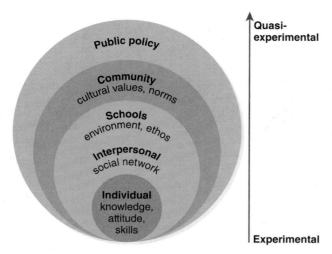

FIGURE 8.1 Socio-Ecological Levels and Corresponding Research Designs.

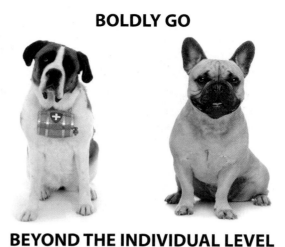

FIGURE 8.2 Public Health Mascots Snow and Hamilton.
© Eric Isselee/Shutterstock; © Svetography/Shutterstock

What this means essentially is that quasi-experimental designs share similar characteristics to experimental designs but differ on one major characteristic: random assignment. Quasi-experimental designs do not involve randomization. One reason for this is that evaluations of public health interventions that target higher levels of the socioecological model such as clinics, communities, schools, and so on would require implementation among large enough samples of these entities to ensure sufficient numbers at that level to randomly assign to conditions. Another reason is that in some instances, random assignment is neither ethical nor practical. Nonetheless, quasi-experimental designs are still considered appropriate and acceptable research designs and are widely used to estimate the causal impact of an intervention on target populations.

As an example, imagine that you have developed a policy-based intervention intended to impact the incidence of type II diabetes among young people residing in an urban area. The program is based on a combination of three key actions: (1) a citywide sweetened-beverage tax, (2) mandatory in-school screenings for elevated levels of blood sugar among high school students, and (3) the construction of easily accessible public recreation facilities for all city residents. Notice here that each program component involves everyone in the city. This means that randomizing people to one condition versus another is simply not plausible. Thus, the standard randomized controlled trial design is one that cannot be used to test your policy-based program. Consider, instead, that you could begin a study designed to test your policy-based intervention by selecting two fairly equivalent cities. You implement the policy-level intervention in one city while the other experiences a 2-year delay before launching.

This 2-year period then becomes a time when you can compare the two cities relative to recent changes in the incidence of adult-onset diabetes among young people. As you can readily understand, this type of design is radically different from the experimental designs previously discussed. This chapter will guide your professional development by describing this type of research design and several other design options needed to conduct rigorous and bold public health intervention research that extends beyond the individual level (see **FIGURE 8.2**).

▶ What Is the Nonequivalent Groups Pretest–Posttest Design?

The **nonequivalent groups pretest–posttest design** is one of two main types of designs that fall under the general category of nonequivalent groups design (NEGD) (see **FIGURE 8.3**) and is a highly practical method of testing community-level interventions. NEGD relies on naturally formed or intact groups that are similar to some degree and can be used as treatment and control groups. Because randomization is not used to create the groups, the groups by definition are not equivalent to each other. Because many of the tools of the public health trade such as social marketing, community organizing, and advocating for policy change all affect entire geographic areas, these areas would constitute the groups. Consequently, you can think of a community as being the recipient or target of an intervention. To control for potential threats to internal validity such as history effects, a comparison community is necessary,

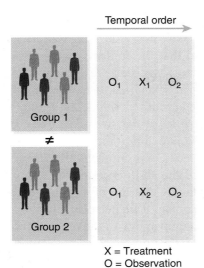

FIGURE 8.3 Nonequivalent Groups Pretest–Posttest Design.

although the comparison community should meet several requirements:

- It must be as demographically similar to the intervention community as possible.
- It must be geographically separate from the intervention community—that is, it cannot be geographically contiguous.
- The appropriate agencies, people, or clinics in the community must agree to regularly scheduled waves of data collection.
- It must be a community with preexisting public health practices and policies that are similar to those of the intervention community.

Once you have carefully selected both an intervention and control community, implementation of the nonequivalent groups, the pretest–posttest design involves a temporal order of steps:

Step 1: Data collection before implementation of the intervention

Step 2: Implementation of the intervention

Step 3: One or more postintervention data collections

Your first step is quite simple: Collect baseline data in each community for a period of months or even a full year. By definition, baseline or pretest measurements provide a starting point within which to gauge any changes following the intervention and also—and this is important—provide a method of adjusting for any differences between the two communities that would otherwise introduce bias into your study findings. Following baseline data collection, you would then implement the different components of your community-level intervention. Once the intervention components have been implemented (and this type of intervention may take years), follow-up data collection would ensue. Thus, with the nonequivalent groups' pretest–posttest design, you are able to assess differences on study outcomes between the two cities following implementation of the intervention. Because of the nonequivalence of groups, however, the NEGD is especially susceptible to the threat of **differential selection**, which means that prior differences among groups may affect the outcome of the study. Even with controlling for any differences observed via the pretest assessment, there still may be differences that were not measured and are essentially unobserved. Under the worst circumstances, this can lead us to conclude that our community-level intervention did not have an effect when it did or that it did have an effect when it did not. An example of a community-based intervention that was evaluated with this quasi-experimental design is presented in **BOX 8.1**.

BOX 8.1 Example of a Community-Level Intervention Study Using a Nonequivalent Control Group Design

This study evaluated the effects of a chronic disease-management program to increase elderly patients' adherence to hypertension medication using a nonequivalent control group design. The community-based intervention includes patient education, recall and remind services, and reducing out-of-pocket payments; in fact, this was implemented in 2012 in Hongcheon County, Korea. This study sample was drawn from the Korean National Health Insurance Big Data set and included a cohort of patients ($N = 5370$) with hypertension aged 65–85 living in Hongcheon County (intervention group, $n = 2685$) or Hoengseong County (control group, $n = 2685$) for 5 years between 2010 and 2014. Because patients were from two different counties, patients from each were matched on key characteristics (i.e., age, sex, type of insurance, and income rank) to ensure groups were as equivalent as possible. Analyses revealed that roughly the same percentage of patients in both the intervention and control groups had medical insurance and that hypertension medication adherence was significantly higher in patients in the intervention group compared with those in the control group. Findings suggest that this community-based intervention may help elderly patients better manage their hypertension and therefore has powerful implications for chronic disease management (Son, Son, Park, Kim, & Kim, 2019).

▶ What Is the Nonequivalent Control Group Posttest-Only Design?

The **nonequivalent groups posttest-only design** is the second main type of design that falls under the general category of NEGD. The nonequivalent groups posttest-only design is similar to the nonequivalent groups pretest–posttest design in that it also involves the use of two groups, one serving as the treatment group and one as the comparison group—or possibly two program groups, each receiving a different version of the program. However, it differs in that there is no pretest data collection. Rather, it consists of collecting data only after the intervention has been implemented; thus, you cannot assess preintervention differences and control for them. The main question is, why would you use this design instead of the pretest–posttest design? This design would be used when, for some reason, you are unable to do a pretest. For example, a principal of a school wanted to evaluate their new sexual health curriculum although *it had already begun*. This design was used where one group of students at one high school received an abstinence-only program while students at another school received a comprehensive sexual risk–reduction program. After 12 weeks, a test measuring sexual debut (i.e., first experience of sexual intercourse) and risky sexual behaviors was administered to see which program was more effective in reducing these behaviors. As previously stated, a major problem with this design is that the two schools might not be the same before the program takes place and may differ in important ways that may influence the outcomes. Thus, differential selection is a threat to internal validity. For instance, if it is found that the students in the abstinence-only program reported a delay in sexual debut and less engagement in sexual risk behavior compared to students in the sexual risk–reduction group, there is no way to determine if they were less likely to engage in those behaviors before the program or whether other factors existed. For example, students at the school who received the abstinence-only program may come from households that are of a higher socioeconomic status and contain a higher percentage of two-parent households compared with the other school. Thus, the students from the former school may differ in their levels of parental monitoring or parental communication about sex, and these differences may have influenced their sexual behavior. For this reason, this design cannot definitively show whether observed changes are the result of the treatment or the differences that existed between the groups before treatment. An example of a study that used the nonequivalent groups posttest-only design is provided in **BOX 8.2**.

In addition to differential selection, the nonequivalent groups posttest-only design has other weaknesses such as **differential attrition** as well as additive and interactive effects, meaning that threats to internal validity can be layered with such factors as **selection history**, which occurs when history affects one group but not the other. For example, in the school example, imagine that a major event occurs at one school (e.g., a rape or shooting) but not at the other school, and this event affects the outcome of the study. The design is depicted in **FIGURE 8.4**.

BOX 8.2 Example of a Nonequivalent Groups Posttest-Only Design

This study used a nonequivalent control group posttest design to examine the effects of using an Xbox Kinect™ along with standard physical therapy on range of movement, early activity levels, and discharge outcomes among children in a pediatrics burn unit (PBU) in South Africa. The use of video games in burn rehabilitation has increased in recent years because it facilitates and encourages patients' range of motion and distracts from pain. This study used a nonequivalent posttest-only control group design and took place over a 14-month period. It was not possible to randomize children admitted to the PBU because children in the PBU stay in the same room, are exposed to the same environment, and undergo the same treatment. Participants included $N = 66$ children aged 5–12 in the PBU. The control group received standard physical therapy, and the intervention group received standard physical therapy plus the Xbox Kinect sessions. During these sessions, children played either Kinect Sports™ or Dance Central 3™ games for 15–30 minutes twice a week. Data collection involved physical assessments of range of movement and interviews using the following quantitative measures: Activities Scale for Kids and a modified enjoyment-rating scale. Analyses revealed that the Xbox Kinect group had significantly greater range of motion, fun, and enjoyment, as well as more positive discharge outcomes between discharge and follow-up compared with the control group. This innovative intervention found that using the Xbox Kinect, along with standard of care among children in PBUs, may lead to a more positive and enjoyable rehabilitation and should be considered in future interventions (Lozano & Potterton, 2018).

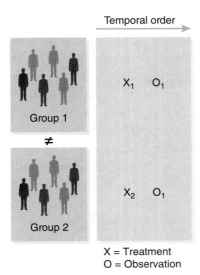

FIGURE 8.4 Nonequivalent Groups Posttest-Only Design.

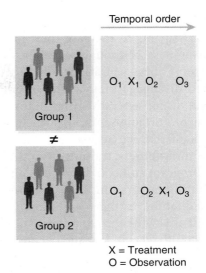

FIGURE 8.5 Nonequivalent Groups Pretest–Posttest Design with Switching Replication.

What Is the Nonequivalent Groups Pretest–Posttest Design with Switching Replication?

Although the nonequivalent groups pretest–posttest design is considered rigorous among the quasi-experimental designs, it can be further improved by adding what is called **switching replication**. This design works by starting out exactly like the traditional nonequivalent groups pretest–posttest design: The pretest measure of your dependent variable (DV) is administered first to both groups, then the non-equivalent intervention group receives the treatment intervention while the nonequivalent control group receives the comparison intervention or receives nothing (i.e., true control); both groups are then assessed again. However, this next step is where the switching replication comes in and deviates from the traditional NEGD design: After the postintervention assessment of the DV, the treatment intervention is then implemented (i.e., "the switching") among the nonequivalent control group and then finally the DV is assessed one last time. The switching replication allows for the control group to receive the treatment intervention; thus, overcoming the ethical issue of withholding needed programs. Yet what is so advantageous is that the switching replication also maintains a degree of internal validity by allowing for comparisons among the treatment intervention and control groups on the DV before the switch. This design is depicted in **FIGURE 8.5**.

As a concrete example, let's say we wanted to introduce a mindfulness-based intervention (MBI) for smoking cessation for minorities. **Mindfulness** is defined as paying attention in a particular way, on purpose, to the current moment and without judgment. Mindfulness, therefore, involves self-regulation to attend to what is being experienced in the current moment, as well as being open and accepting toward one's experience (Shapero, Greenberg, Pedrelli, de Jong, & Desbordes, 2018). A key feature of MBIs is education in formal and informal mindfulness meditation practices to train individuals in both attentional control (i.e., "staying in the present") as well as the nonjudgmental attitudinal aspects of mindfulness. MBIs typically involve formal meditation practices, mindful movement such as yoga (see **FIGURE 8.6**), and a focus on bodily sensations.

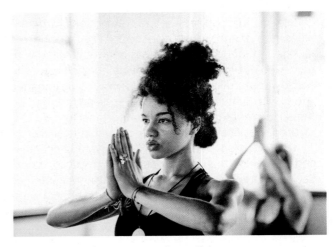

FIGURE 8.6 Yoga as a Form of Mindfulness.
© Thomas Barwick/DigitalVision/Getty Images

An MBI for smoking cessation would involve teaching participants to increase their moment-to-moment awareness of thoughts, feelings, and sensations; observe these sensations nonjudgmentally; and learn to disengage their attention and choose more skillful responses (rather than automatic reactions) to uncomfortable sensations (including cravings) and high-risk situations (e.g., Spears et al., 2019). The mindfulness training would consist of an 8-week program and could include daily practice of formal sitting meditation, body scan meditation, walking meditation, eating meditation, and gentle yoga. To test this MBI for efficacy in smoking cessation, we could recruit low-socioeconomic-status minority participants who are smokers from a county health clinic to serve as the treatment group. For the nonequivalent control group, we could recruit similar participants from another county health clinic. We first measure rates of daily smoking in both groups and then introduce the 8-week MBI intervention to the treatment group patients but hold off on introducing the MBI to the control group participants. After the 8-week MBI, we then measure daily smoking rates in both groups and perhaps then one more assessment 6 months later. If the MBI is effective, we should see a reduction in or complete cessation of smoking among clinic patients (who received the MBI treatment) but not in the clinic participants who have not yet received the MBI. Finally, following the final follow-up assessment, we would introduce the MBI to the other group of participants and then we could also assess their smoking rates

at follow-up. Now and only now should we see the control groups' levels of smoking decrease or cease.

One strength of this design is that it includes a built-in replication. In the example given, we would get evidence for the efficacy of the MBI in two different samples (patients from two different health clinics). Another strength of this design is that it provides more control over history effects. It becomes rather unlikely that some outside event would perfectly coincide with the introduction of the treatment in the first group and with the delayed introduction of the treatment in the second group. For instance, if a change in taxes on cigarettes occurred when we first introduced the treatment to the first group of patients—and this explained their reductions in smoking at follow-up—we would see smoking rates decrease in both groups. Similarly, the switching replication helps to control for **maturation** and **instrumentation**. Both groups would be expected to show the same rates of spontaneous smoking cessation. Also, if the instrument for assessing smoking behaviors happened to change at some point in the study, the change would be consistent across both groups. Of course, **demand characteristics**, **placebo effects**, and **experimenter expectancy** effects can still be problems. But they can be controlled by using some of the methods described in Chapter 5. An example of a nonequivalent group pretest–posttest design with switching replication study is described in **BOX 8.3**.

BOX 8.3 An Example of a Nonequivalent Groups Pretest–Posttest Design with Switching Replication Study

Civic engagement involves individual and collective actions designed to identify and address community issues and needs. Through service and connections with others, civic engagement is thought to bring about mutual gains for both individuals and society. One specific form of civic engagement is volunteering. Many studies have found that volunteering has been associated with lower depression levels, increases in life satisfaction and perceived health, higher levels of well-being, slower declines in self-perceived physical and emotional health, and lower mortality rates. Other forms of civic engagement such as intergenerational programs that pair older adults with school children have also been found to be beneficial in both cognitive and physical well-being. Past research has demonstrated the importance of civic engagement for older adults, yet previous studies have not focused specifically on the potential benefits of civic engagement for older adults with functional limitations.

This pilot study explored the feasibility and effectiveness of an intervention designed to promote civic engagement in this growing and often overlooked population. A convenience sample was recruited from two adult day health centers ($N = 43$). A multicomponent intervention was implemented comprising education, service, and recognition phases. The study employed a nonequivalent switching-replications design. In this design, one site received the intervention, whereas the second site served as the comparison group, in this case receiving services as usual in the adult day program. Services as usual included activity programs that involved arts and crafts, physical activity, or intellectual stimulation such as discussion of current events. No activities were completed specifically for the benefit of serving other individuals or groups such as in the civic-engagement intervention. The second site then received the intervention, and the intervention was withdrawn from first site for comparison purposes. In scientific notation (NR = nonequivalent, not randomized):

NR_{site1}	O_1	X	O_2		O_3
NR_{site2}	O_1		O_2	X	O_3

The switching replication design was selected because it controls history and testing threats to internal validity and allows for testing of the lasting effects of the intervention. In addition, it allows for the intervention to be provided to the comparison group later. Data were collected at baseline before the intervention (O_1), at the point at which the intervention was switched from site 1 to site 2 (O_2), and at the completion of the study (O_3). Using the nonequivalent switching-replications design, researchers compared participants receiving the civic-engagement intervention with participants receiving treatment as usual. Participants receiving the intervention reported higher yet nonsignificant levels of purpose in life, self-esteem, and perceived physical health when compared with those in the control group. However, five weeks following the withdrawal of the intervention, participants reported a significant decrease in self-esteem and perceived physical health. Civic-engagement interventions appear to be beneficial for some older adults with physical and cognitive limitations, such as those enrolled in adult day health programs. Future studies should examine the nature and amount of engagement needed to maximize the benefits of such interventions (Dabelko-Schoeny, Anderson, & Spinks, 2010).

▶ What Is the Switching-Replication-Without-Treatment-Removal Design?

In a basic pretest–posttest design with switching replication, the first group receives a treatment (which is then discontinued) and then the second group receives the same treatment later. In contrast, in a switching-replication-without-treatment-removal design, the treatment can be continued for the first group even when the treatment is added to the second group. Once again, let's assume we first measure smoking rates of one group of clinic patients who are smokers and compare with a second group of different clinic patients who are also smokers. Then we only introduce the MBI smoking-cessation intervention to the first group of clinic patients. After they have been exposed to the MBI for the 8 weeks, we assess smoking rates again in both groups. If the intervention is effective, we should see smoking levels decrease in the treatment patient group but not the control group. Next, we would encourage the treatment group of clinic patients to continue with their newly learned MBI practices. So, we would encourage them to continue to practice meditation, yoga, etc. At the same time, we would implement the MBI among the control group. After 8 weeks of the control-group smokers learning and using mindfulness practices, and with the original treatment group also continuing to practice, we would reassess smoking levels. Now, if the intervention is effective, we should see that the smoking rates have now decreased significantly in the control group but also that smoking rates have continued to decrease in the original treatment group (because they are still practicing mindfulness). This design is depicted in **FIGURE 8.7**. Demonstrating a treatment effect in two groups staggered over time can provide strong evidence for the efficacy of the treatment. In addition to providing evidence for the replicability of the findings, this design can also provide evidence for whether the treatment continues to show effects over longer periods of time.

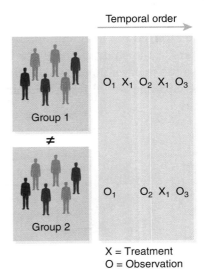

FIGURE 8.7 Nonequivalent Groups Pretest–Posttest Design with Switching Replication.

▶ What Is the Nonrandomized Stepped-Wedge Design?

A key aspect of quasi-experimental designs is the ability to evaluate public health interventions that are targeted to the upper levels of the socioecological model. In addition to the NEGDs, another suitable and practical design for evaluating public health interventions targeted to entire areas or clusters is the **stepped-wedge (SW) design**. The advantage of the SW design is that it enables all targeted clusters or groups to eventually receive an intervention during the study period. Before the study period, each cluster or group serves as its own control, thus maintaining high internal validity. Typically, in the SW design, all units or clusters start out untreated, and then *randomly chosen* units switch to intervention at sequential time points until all receive intervention. As you recall, because randomization is involved in this instance, this type of SW design would be considered a true experimental design. However, as we have already come to understand, randomization is not always feasible or ethical. Thus, the nonrandomized stepped-wedge (NR-SW) design (units switching to intervention are not randomly chosen) is the better design to use when withholding critically needed interventions is unethical or impractical. Because this chapter is focused on quasi-experimental designs, the NR-SW design rather than the randomized SW design will be discussed.

The way the NR-SW design works is that it allows *each* cluster to receive the intervention following the baseline assessment period; however, each cluster receives the intervention at *differing* start times. One cluster typically starts immediately following baseline assessment, and then the next cluster perhaps starts several months afterward, and so on and so on until all clusters have received the intervention. Thus, if there are six clusters in the study, perhaps the first cluster could receive the intervention immediately following baseline, the next one would receive the intervention

1 month later, and so on until all six clusters received the intervention. The NR-SW design is depicted in **FIGURE 8.8**, which shows how this design got its name: By adding clusters over time, you create steps within a wedge.

An example may be helpful to illustrate how this design is implemented. Considerable racial and socioeconomic disparities have been documented in breast cancer diagnosis and treatment. Although numerous evidence-based interventions (EBIs) aimed at reducing breast cancer screening barriers among the underserved exist, there is a lack of uptake of EBIs in community and clinical settings. Researchers in Houston, Texas, considered the idea of using patient navigators to improve the uptake of and adherence to mammography screening tests among underserved women attending health clinics (Highfield et al., 2015). This intervention called the "Peace of Mind" program used a tailored, telephone counseling reminder call to help women overcome barriers to appointment attendance. In this example, a cluster was defined as a federally qualified health center or a charity clinic that served a particular area of Houston. This study included nine clinics in total; three groups of three clinics each were formed to facilitate timing of the intervention. Each clinic group was scheduled to begin the intervention phase of the study at different time points. Group 1 started the intervention at week 13, group 2 started at week 33, and group 3 started at week 48. In this example, the **intervention phase** was defined as the period of time that patient navigators were placing the counseling calls to the women, whereas the **control phase** was the period of time that elapsed between the first month of the research study (when baseline assessments were being completed) and the start date of the intervention phase. Thus, the period of time for the control phase and for the intervention phase is not identical across the three groups.

One great advantage of the NR-SW design is purely pragmatic. Again using the example of patient navigators to increase adherence to mammography, it

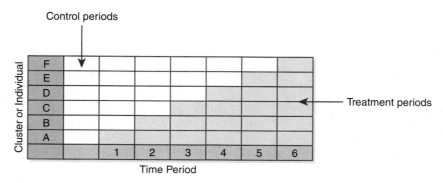

FIGURE 8.8 The Nonrandomized, Stepped-Wedge Design.

This study examined the effects of a workplace health literacy intervention on pain intensity, pain-related absences, and bothersomeness of pain (i.e., reported frequency of pain affecting employees' work) using a quasi-experimental stepped-wedge cluster design. This design involved repeated measurements of study outcomes, which allowed for the clusters to cross over from the control group to the intervention group at specific time points. The research team recruited a single municipality in Denmark with the highest number of nursing homes in the country. The study included nursing home employees and supervisors or managers, representatives from the municipality, and the director general of health and care. The intervention itself included the following two elements: (1) courses for employees and management to develop a curriculum on pain prevention and management along with communication tools and (2) structured conversations between employees and supervisors to develop action plans to reduce and prevent pain. Six nursing homes participated in the study and crossed over from control to intervention at a point determined in an agreement between nursing home managers and the research team. Data were collected through text messages every 4 weeks to assess employees' pain intensity, pain-related absences, and bothersomeness of pain during and after the intervention. Participants included $N = 405$ employees, and data were analyzed using linear mixed models. Results indicate that employees' pain intensity was significantly reduced postintervention, but there were no significant differences in bothersomeness or sickness absence. This study revealed that this workplace health literacy intervention was both feasible and effective in decreasing pain among employees at nursing homes; thus, these interventions could be a useful approach to improve nursing home employees' health and work environment (Larsen, Thygesen, Mortensen, Punnett, & Jørgensen, 2019).

would be logistically complex during a study to provide in-person training to all of the patient navigators working in a large city at the same time. Instead, training one-third of the patient navigators in the city would be much more manageable. Thus, each of three groups would be trained to implement the new practice at staggered points in time during the study. This, of course, means that some clusters are exposed to the intervention condition for much longer periods of time than others. Fortunately, statistical techniques can be applied to account for this unequal exposure. Because the NR-SW design allows *every* participating clinic to be part of the intervention condition while also using the preintervention phase as the control condition, these aspects are the greatest advantage of this design. This is a crucial aspect of buy-in for clinics when being asked to participate in the study because it would be unethical to ask health centers to serve *only* as control sites.

A final note about the NR-SW design is warranted: It is important to stagger rollouts for the intervention phase using a time period that makes sense relative to the outcome variables of the study. Thus, an outcome that may occur rather quickly (e.g., uptake of mammography appointment) would require a shorter lag time between steps than a study using an outcome requiring more time for valid assessment (e.g., reduced incidence of adult-onset diabetes). The design refers to the time between rollouts as the **step length**. Typically, a step length of a few months is used in a NR-SW design; however, this may be extended to periods as long as 1 year. Another example of a study that used the NR-SW design is described in **BOX 8.4**.

What Is the Interrupted Time-Series Design?

The **interrupted time-series design (ITSD)** is considered by many as the strongest quasi-experimental approach for evaluating the *longitudinal* effects of interventions. As its name implies, ITSD involves collecting a series of data points over time before and after the implementation of some kind of intervention. The intervention can be a health-promotion program, the passing of a new health policy, or new legislation such as an imposed tax increase on the sale of cigarettes. A critical aspect of the ITSD is that the outcome variable must be assessed at *multiple data points before and following the intervention*. Thus, a critical question involved in implementing this design is, how many data points are needed? The number of observations needed depends on the type of statistical analysis that will be conducted. For example, if ordinary least-squares regression approach is used, only four observations—two before and two after intervention implementation—may suffice. However, if using **autoregressive integrated moving average** models, a general rule is that 50 observations are needed. Data used in a time-series design can range from individual behavior such as getting a mammogram, using a condom, or exercise to reduce rates of cumulative incidence of diseases such as cancer and type II diabetes. Another critical factor to implementing the ITSD is that knowledge about the specific time in which the program or intervention occurred is required. Although it seems as if knowing the exact date when the intervention was implemented should be obvious and usually is, in some instances—such as the passing of a new policy by a city council that restricts smoking in outdoor public places—the date to be used in the ITSD may not be as straightforward. Do you use the date that the new law was passed? Or should you use the date when signs went up in the city and local law enforcement started enforcing the law? In this latter example, the research team should decide what makes the most sense when choosing the start date.

As an example, an ITSD was used by researchers who were interested in understanding changes in traffic fatalities following the passing of legislature legalizing recreational cannabis sales (RCS) (Lane & Hall, 2019) (see **FIGURE 8.9**). In this study, researchers used an ITSD and examined data from three states that legalized RCS and their respective neighboring states. In this study, the intervention date was the month and year of the new legislation. Data were collected before and after the dates legislation was passed for the following:

1. Colorado (January 2014) plus Kansas, Nebraska, New Mexico, Oklahoma, and Utah;
2. Washington state (June 2014) plus British Columbia and Oregon; and
3. Oregon (October 2015) plus California and Nevada.

To ensure that each state had at least 1 year of monthly traffic fatality data, the study period start date was 2009

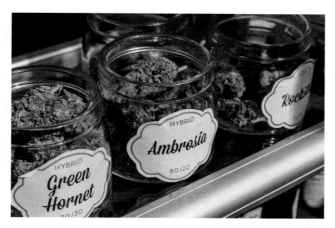

FIGURE 8.9 Recreational Sale of Cannabis or Marijuana.
© Stuart Dee/Stockbyte/Getty Images

and was then extended to 2016 to sufficiently capture before and after RCS implementation. Researchers also implemented a control group by collecting data from U.S. states that had not implemented the legalization of medicinal cannabis, recreational use of cannabis, or RCS during the study period. Data used for analyses included monthly traffic fatalities rates per million residents using mortality data from large, publicly available data sets: the CDC WONDER and RoadSafetyBC. An advantage of collecting a series of observations both before and after the treatment is that a reliable picture regarding the outcome of interest can be gleaned—in this example, monthly traffic fatalities. Thus, the time-series design is sensitive to trends in performance. The results revealed that in the year after RCS implementation, traffic fatalities temporarily increased by an average of one additional traffic fatality per million residents in both the legalizing states of Colorado, Washington, and Oregon and their neighboring jurisdictions (Lane & Hall, 2019). Thus, they concluded that the legislation had a temporary effect in both the states in which it was legalized and neighboring states as well.

Because the ITSD design involves an examination of an intervention's effect using data before and after the intervention period, the overarching aim is to determine whether or not this effect occurred *over and above* any **trend** present in the data. For example, the data collected before the intervention may reveal several trends in the data such as a **maturational trend** (in which observations involve human subjects who are changing their behavior as they age) or a **seasonal trend** (in which observations are influenced by the season in which data are collected). The good news is that any trend found in the data can be identified and then assessed, thus allowing for the identification of any treatment effect. If the pattern of postintervention responses differs significantly from the pattern of preintervention responses, meaning there is some sort of break in the pattern of pre- and postintervention responses, a treatment effect can be determined. Hence, the term *interrupted* in the name of this design. For example, an effect is demonstrated when there is a significant change observed in the level or slope of the postintervention responses compared with the preintervention responses. This type of interruption effect is shown in **FIGURE 8.10**.

The most basic of the ITSDs is the simple interrupted time series, in which there is only one experimental group and no control or comparison group. **BOX 8.5** describes a study that used the simple ITSD. The simple ITSD experiences the same threats to internal validity as the other one-group designs

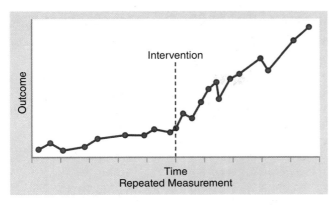

FIGURE 8.10 Demonstrated Intervention Effect with Interrupted Times Series Design.

Design
Simple interrupted time series
O_1 O_2 O_3 O_4 X_1 O_5 O_6 O_7 O_8
Interrupted time series with nonequivalent control group
O_1 O_2 O_3 O_4 X_1 O_5 O_6 O_7 O_8
O_1 O_2 O_3 O_4 O_5 O_6 O_7 O_8

FIGURE 8.11 Interrupted Times Series Designs with and Without Nonequivalent Control Group.

described in this chapter, but the greatest threat to the internal validity of this design is history. History is a major threat because, as stated previously and described in the example involving recreational cannabis sales and traffic fatalities, the length of time involved in collecting data for both the preintervention and postintervention periods (sometimes years for both) increases the likelihood of a historical or related event occurring that might affect the outcome. One historical event that could affect traffic fatalities might be a severe economic downturn such as a major recession. In fact, in the ITSD study described, the researchers excluded data from before 2009 because of the global financial crisis, which had shown a reduction in traffic fatalities during this period (Noland & Zhou. 2017).

Other threats to internal validity affecting the simple ITSD include instrumentation, which is likely if data-collection methods change over time. When data-collection periods span years, depending on the nature of data collected, changes in *how* the data are collected are likely to occur. Maturation may also be an issue if the data points represent assessments with human subjects or other outcomes that would normally change over time. Testing could also pose a threat if archival data (i.e., data collected routinely as part of data-collection systems such as criminal justice data) are not used, although testing would most likely become evident in the preintervention phase. The simple ITSD is diagrammed in **FIGURE 8.11**.

To significantly improve on some of these limitations, if possible, add a nonequivalent control group to the simple ITSD as was done in the study of traffic fatalities. This ITSD with nonequivalent control group design is also diagrammed in Figure 8.11. As shown, a series of observations are collected both before and following the administration of the treatment for the experimental group; during

BOX 8.5 An Example of an Interrupted Time-Series Design

A quasi-experimental study using an interrupted time-series design examined whether voter referenda specific to lesbian, gay, bisexual, and transgender (LGBT) groups has an effect on homophobic bullying among adolescents in California. The research team examined data collected from 14 consecutive waves of the California Healthy Kids Survey (CHKS), the largest statewide cross-sectional survey in the United States to understand homophobic bullying trends before and after the 2008–2009 academic year, which includes the period when Californians passed Proposition 8, which banned same-sex marriage. Participants included ($N = 4,997,557$) high school students in California who participated in the CHKS between 2000 to 2014. An interrupted time-series analysis showed that the passage of Proposition 8 was a turning point for homophobic bullying, which significantly increased and accelerated in the period right before Proposition 8 was passed and gradually declined after its passage. These trends were not observed among students who reported that they experienced bullying unrelated to their sexual orientation. In addition, the presence of a gay–straight alliance at schools was considered a protective contextual factor against homophobic bullying for LGBT youth, and it was also associated with a smaller increase in homophobic bullying before Proposition 8's passage. Study findings provide compelling evidence that public campaigns promoting LGBT-based stigma and homophobic beliefs may increase the risk of bias-based bullying among youth (Hatzenbuehler, Shen, Vandewater, & Russell, 2019).

BOX 8.6 Example of an Interrupted Time-Series Design with Nonequivalent Control Group

Childhood obesity is a public health priority in the United States. The prevalence of childhood obesity has more than doubled from 7 percent in 1980 to nearly 18.5 percent in 2014; currently, more than one in three children are overweight in the United States. Children who are overweight or obese are likely to become overweight or obese adults. A major risk factor for childhood obesity is the overconsumption of calories compared to calories expended. This condition is referred to as *positive energy balance*. The drivers of positive energy balance in children are lack of physical activity and caloric overconsumption often characterized by poor diet quality. The Dietary Guidelines for Americans recommend at least five servings of fruits and vegetables daily, yet these foods are lacking in the majority of American children's diets. In 2011, the National Afterschool Association adopted the Healthy Eating and Physical Activity (HEPA) standards to address snack quality and physical activity in afterschool programs. Public health policy makers and researchers have recognized the potential of afterschool programs as a place to promote nutrition and physical activity policies. Afterschool programs across the nation have adopted the HEPA standards. Although research has indicated promise in the adoption of these policies, less is known about local adoption, implementation, and effectiveness. In this study, we aimed to compare the quality of snacks served at program sites pre- and postadoption and to determine the quality of nonprogram snacks compared to program snacks. An interrupted time-series design was used to collect pre- and postpolicy data. Data were collected at different points in both pre- and postpolicy adoption phases with the interruption being the adoption of the policies during the summer break for afterschool programs. Data were collected at sites during prepolicy for five weeks during April and May 2014. Each site was visited 10–14 times during the afterschool period of 3–6 PM. Postpolicy data collection occurred after the adoption of the policies over 6 weeks during September and October 2014. During the follow-up period, each of the five sites was visited 10 times. Data collected included snack type, brand, and amount consumed using a modified quarter-waste method (a visual estimation of food remaining on a student's plate or tray). Analysis on nutrient content of snacks was completed using Nutrition Data System for Research software. The results showed that adoption of the HEPA standards among policy-adopting sites did not result in significantly better snack quality. Across all sites, program snacks were healthier than nonprogram snacks. Pursuing additional components of the HEPA standards related to implementation may be necessary to significantly improve snack quality. Environmental supports such as limiting the amount of nonprogram snacks available on-site may improve snack quality (Helmick, Esmond, Hedrick, Zoellner, You, & Hill, 2019).

---

this same time period, a series of observations are also collected for a comparison group. This design sometimes often but not always allows the researcher to control for history effects because a historical event would most likely affect both treatment and control groups equally. An example of the ITSD with nonequivalent control group is described in **BOX 8.6**. What may be problematic, however, is when one group experiences a unique set of events (selection history). Note that for a historical event to pose a threat to internal validity, the event must occur at close to the same time as the intervention or treatment was implemented. Other threats to the internal validity are similar to the basic NEGD, with differential selection being the greatest threat and the interaction of selection with threats other than history such as **selection-maturation**, **selection-instrumentation**, and **selection-regression**.

Think About It!

You just received funding to implement and test the efficacy of a community-level intervention to reduce HIV through the administration of preexposure prophylaxis (PrEP), a type of drug that prevents HIV acquisition. This intervention will be implemented and tested in a metropolitan city with some of the highest rates of HIV in the country. You proposed to conduct a randomized controlled trial as your research design because this is the gold standard of research designs and will allow you to have high confidence in your results. You plan to randomize individuals who meet study inclusion criteria and are at high risk of HIV to either the intervention condition, in which they will receive PrEP, or the control condition. The control condition would consist of receiving a placebo drug. However, now that you are ramping up to conduct the study, you are preparing for your first meeting with your community advisory board (CAB) and anticipate pushback on the design from board members. They may want you to switch to a nonrandomized design of some sort so that all participants have equal opportunity to receive the intervention. With this in mind, think about possibly switching your design. Which of the quasi-experimental designs would allow you to test the efficacy of the intervention while maintaining a high level of rigor and satisfying the CAB's ethical concerns? What are some of the practical considerations you need to work out to switch designs? For example, if you are targeting individuals, how would you form groups or clusters where you could use the nonrandomized stepped-wedge design? Perhaps you instead favor the switching replication design. Thus, is it possible for you to form two nonequivalent groups to execute this design?

Take Home Points

- Quasi-experimental research designs are widely used to determine the efficacy of interventions implemented at the community level or higher levels of the socioecological model.
- Randomization does not take place in quasi-experimental research designs.
- Quasi-experimental research designs are appropriate for testing community or policy-based interventions in which randomization is not possible or is not ethical.
- The nonequivalent groups pretest–posttest design designates an intervention and control community and measures differences between groups at baseline and at posttest, or after the intervention is implemented.
- Less rigorous than the nonequivalent groups pretest–posttest design, the nonequivalent groups posttest-only design designates an intervention and control community and measures differences between groups only at follow-up after the intervention is implemented.
- The nonrandomized stepped-wedge design uses clusters such as clinics, communities, and so on that undergo both the intervention and control phases at designated time points throughout the study period.
- The interrupted time-series design involves collecting a sufficient number of data points before and after the implementation of the intervention to determine whether the intervention had a significant effect over and above any trends observed in the data.

Key Terms

Autoregressive integrated moving average
Control phase
Demand characteristics
Differential attrition
Differential selection
Experimenter expectancy
Instrumentation
Interrupted time-series design (ITSD)

Intervention phase
Maturation
Maturation trend
Mindfulness
Nonequivalent groups posttest-only design
Nonequivalent groups pretest–posttest design
Placebo effects
Quasi-experimental design

Seasonal trend
Selection history
Selection-instrumentation
Selection-maturation
Selection-regression
Step length
Stepped-Wedge (SW) Design
Switching replication
Trend

For Practice and Discussion

1. What is a quasi-experimental design? Explain the differences between quasi-experimental research designs and randomized controlled trials.
2. When is it appropriate to use a quasi-experimental research design? Provide an example of a situation in which a quasi-experimental design would be the most appropriate choice for a research study.
3. Find a journal article on a research study that uses a quasi-experimental design to address a public health problem.

a. Which type of quasi-experimental design do the researchers use in the study?

b. What is the purpose of the study? Based on the study purpose, is the type of quasi-experimental design used the most appropriate design for the research study? Explain why or why not in your own words.

4. What are the strengths and weaknesses of the following quasi-experimental designs? Please explain.
   a. Nonrandomized stepped-wedge design
   b. Nonequivalent groups pretest–posttest design
   c. Interrupted time-series design

References

Dabelko-Schoeny, H., Anderson, K. A., & Spinks, K. (2010). Civic engagement for older adults with functional limitations: Piloting an intervention for adult day health participants. *The Gerontologist, 50*(5), 694–701.

Hatzenbuehler, M. L., Shen, Y., Vandewater, E. A., & Russell, S. T. (2019). Proposition 8 and homophobic bullying in California. *Pediatrics, 143*(6), e20182116. https://doi.org/10.1542/peds .2018-2116

Helmick, M., Esmond, A. C., Hedrick, V., Zoellner, J., You, W., & Hill, J. L. (2019, October). The adoption of the Healthy Eating Standards in local afterschool programs does not improve quality of snacks. *Journal of School Health, 89*(10), 809–817.

Highfield, L., Rajan, S. S., Valerio, M. A., Walton, G., Fernandez, M. E., & Bartholomew, L. K. (2015, October 14). A non-randomized controlled stepped wedge trial to evaluate the effectiveness of a multi-level mammography intervention in improving appointment adherence in underserved women. *Implementation Science, 10*(143).

Lane, T. J., & Hall, W. (2019). Traffic fatalities within U.S. states that have legalized recreational cannabis sales and their neighbours. *Addiction, 114*(5), 847–856.

Larsen, A. K., Thygesen, L. C., Mortensen, O. S., Punnett, L., & Jørgensen, M. B. (2019). The effect of strengthening health literacy in nursing homes on employee pain and consequences of pain: A stepped-wedge intervention trial. *Scandinavian Journal of Work, Environment & Health*, 0–10. https://doi .org/10.5271/sjweh.3801

Lozano, E. I., & Potterton, J. L. (2018). The use of Xbox Kinect™ in a paediatric burns unit. *South African Journal of Physiotherapy, 74*(1), 1–7. https://doi.org/10.4102/sajp.v74i1.429

Noland, R. B., & Zhou, Y. (2017). Has the great recession and its aftermath reduced traffic fatalities? *Accident Analysis & Prevention, 98*, 130–138.

Shapero, B. G., Greenberg, J., Pedrelli, P., de Jong, M., & Desbordes, G. (2018, January 24). Mindfulness-based interventions in psychiatry. *Focus* (American Psychiatric Publishing), *16*(1), 32–39.

Son, K.-J., Son, H.-R., Park, B., Kim, H.-J., & Kim, C.-B. (2019). A community-based intervention for improving medication adherence for elderly patients with hypertension in Korea. *International Journal of Environmental Research and Public Health, 16*(5), 721. https://doi.org/10.3390/ijerph16050721

Spears, C. A., Abroms, L. C., Glass, C. R., Hedeker, D., Eriksen, M. P., . . . Wetter, D. W. (2019). Mindfulness-based smoking cessation enhanced with mobile technology (iQuit Mindfully): Pilot randomized controlled trial. *JMIR mHealth and uHealth, 7*(6), e13059.

For Further Reading

Bartlett, G., Dickinson, L. M., Meaney, C., Kwan, B., & Roper, R. (2015). Advanced methods for primary care research: The stepped wedge design. In *Advanced Methods for Primary Care Research*, Agency for Healthcare Research and Quality. Retrieved from https://pbrn.ahrq.gov/sites/default/files/docs/ Advanced Methods for PC Research Stepped Wedge Design 3-12-15 sxf.pdf

Brown, C. A., & Lilford, R. J. (2006). The stepped wedge trial design: A systematic review. *BMC Medical Research Methodology, 6*, 1–9. https://doi.org/10.1186/1471-2288 -6-54

Glasgow, R. E., Green, L. W., Klesges, L. M., Abrams, D. B., Fisher, E. B., Goldstein, M. G., . . . & Tracy Orleans, C. (2006). External validity: We need to do more. *Annals of Behavioral Medicine, 31*(2), 105–108.

Green, L. W., & Glasgow, R. E. (2006). Evaluating the relevance, generalization, and applicability of research: Issues in external validation and translation methodology. *Evaluation & the Health Professions, 29*(1), 126–153.

Hemming, K., Haines, T. P., Chilton, P. J., Girling, A. J., & Lilford, R. J. (2015, February 6). The stepped wedge cluster randomised trial: Rationale, design, analysis, and reporting. *BMJ* (Online), *350*, 1–7. https://doi.org/10.1136/bmj.h391

Shadish, W. R., Cook, T. D., & Campbell, D. T. (2002). *Experimental and quasi-experimental designs for generalized causal inference.* Boston, MA: Houghton-Mifflin.

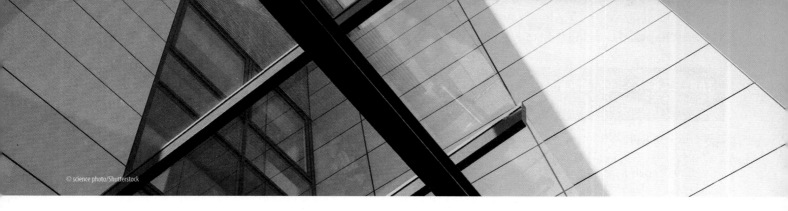

CHAPTER 9

Defining the Study Population

with Anne Marie Schipani-McLaughlin

LEARNING OBJECTIVES

1. Understand the meaning of population-specific research.
2. Interpret epidemiological studies that identify health disparities.
3. Define priority populations based on odds ratios.
4. Describe multiple methods of defining populations.
5. Understand intersectionality and its implications.
6. Recognize the value of studies conducted with populations of women and children.

▶ Overview

To begin this chapter, we first ask you to reflect on the nature of public health practice and how it differs from that of medicine and healthcare. In our experience as professors in the classroom, we have seen that students in public health programs often conflate public health with healthcare. This is a mistake of great magnitude. In fact, public health and healthcare are nearly at opposite ends of a spectrum. Healthcare is designed to be applied "one person at a time" and is typically applied once a disease process has begun. Conversely, public health is designed for application to *entire populations* and is focused on the prevention of disease rather than its treatment. The key word here is **population**. Because public health targets entire populations, it holds tremendous advantage over healthcare: It is much broader and thus highly efficient. Now that you understand the concept of **population health**, the next step is to become aware that vast disparities in health exist between and within populations.

An initial point to consider is that in the United States, health disparities "shape" the public health research agenda. To give you a quick example, we have taken a sample of research articles addressing diabetes control that were published in the *American Journal of Public Health* (**TABLE 9.1**). As you look through the article titles in this table, you will see that this journal (the flagship journal for public health) has published numerous studies focused on minority and underserved populations. It is these populations that warrant more intense study, which will ultimately foster improved prevention efforts. For any given disease (in this case, diabetes), public health priorities are given to those populations that are most at risk.

Ultimately, public health practice and the research informing that practice is one method of rectifying **health disparities**. Healthy People 2020 defines health disparity as

> a particular type of health difference that is closely linked with social, economic, [or] environmental disadvantage. Health disparities

TABLE 9.1 A Sample of Journal Articles Showing the Diversity of Populations Studied Relative to the Control of the U.S. Diabetes Epidemic

Priority Populations Relative to Diabetes

Cho, P., Geiss, L. S., Burrows, N. R., Roberts, D. L., Bullock, A. K., Toedt, M. E. (2014, June). Diabetes-related mortality among American Indians and Alaska natives, 1990–2009. *American Journal of Public Health, 104*(S3), S496–S503.

Ockene, I. S., Tellez, T. L., Rosal, M. C., Reed, G. W., Mordes, J., Merriam, P. A., . . . & Ma, Y. (2012, February). Outcomes of a Latino community-based intervention for the prevention of diabetes: The Lawrence Latino Diabetes Prevention Project. *American Journal of Public Health, 102*(2), 336–342.

Wilson, C., Gilliland, S., Cullen, T., Moore, K., Roubideaux, Y., Valdez. L., . . . & Acton, K. (2005, September). Diabetes outcomes in the Indian health system during the era of the special diabetes program for Indians and the government performance and results act. *American Journal of Public Health, 95*(9), 1518–1522.

Shea, S., Kothari, D., Teresi, J. A., Kong, J., Eimicke, J. P., Lantigua, R. A., . . . & Weinstock, R. S. (2013, October). Social impact analysis of the effects of a telemedicine intervention to improve diabetes outcomes in an ethnically diverse, medically underserved population: findings from the IDEATel study. *American Journal of Public Health, 103*(10), 1888–1894.

Robbins, J. M, & Webb, D. A. (2006, July). Hospital admission rates for a racially diverse low-income cohort of patients with diabetes: The Urban Diabetes Study. *American Journal of Public Health, 96*(7), 1260–1264.

Baptiste-Roberts, K., Gary, T. L., Beckles, G. L., Gregg, E. W., Owens, M., Porterfield, D., Engelgau, M. M. (2007, May). Family history of diabetes, awareness of risk factors, and health behaviors among African Americans. *American Journal of Public Health, 97*(5), 907–912.

Rothschild, S. K., Martin, M. A., Swider, S. M., Tumialán Lynas, C. M., Janssen, I., Avery, E. F., Powell, L. H. (2014, August). Mexican American trial of community health workers: a randomized controlled trial of a community health worker intervention for Mexican Americans with type 2 diabetes mellitus. *American Journal of Public Health, 104*(8), 1540–1548.

Melnik, T. A., Hosler, A. S., Sekhobo, J. P., Duffy, T. P., Tierney, E. F., Engelgau, M. M., Geiss, L. S. (2004, March). Diabetes prevalence among Puerto Rican adults in New York City, NY, 2000. *American Journal of Public Health, 94*(3), 434–437.

adversely affect groups of people who have systematically experienced greater obstacles to health based on their racial or ethnic group; religion; socioeconomic status; gender; age; mental health; cognitive, sensory, or physical disability; sexual orientation or gender identity; geographic location; or other characteristics historically linked to discrimination or exclusion. (U.S. Department of Health and Human Services, 2008)

Health disparities are prevalent throughout the world, including the United States (National Center for Health Statistics, 2019.

Much of public health research is devoted to identifying the most extreme health disparities and disseminating this information widely to inform and improve public health practice. For example, as shown in FIGURE 9.1, African Americans have the highest incidence of hypertension across all racial and ethnic groups in the United States (Centers for Disease Control and Prevention, 2015), and hypertension is but one of many health disparities experienced by racial and ethnic minorities. This ongoing effort to identify and prioritize demographically defined populations experiencing one or more forms of a health disparity is the catalyst for intervention development and

resource allocation; however, this effort must focus not only on *who* is affected but also on *why* and *how*. Also, great attention must be given to intergroup and intragroup differences, specific social positions, and the wider social processes and macrolevel factors that shape health (Hankivsky, 2012; Kapilashrami & Hankivsky, 2018). The who, why, and how approach is promising in bettering our understanding of the complex nature of health inequities, especially among the most vulnerable populations.

This chapter accentuates the point that population-specific research is paramount to public health practice. It also emphasizes the importance of moving beyond examining individual factors only such as biology, socioeconomic status, sex, gender, and race, which are important, to encompass a focus on the relationships and interactions between such factors and across multiple levels of society. By doing so, we can determine how health is shaped across population groups and geographical contexts. This expanded and more complex approach is referred to as *intersectionality* and will be covered in more detail. This chapter will also provide examples that illustrate the past use of studies that identified priority populations for the receipt of public health prevention programs.

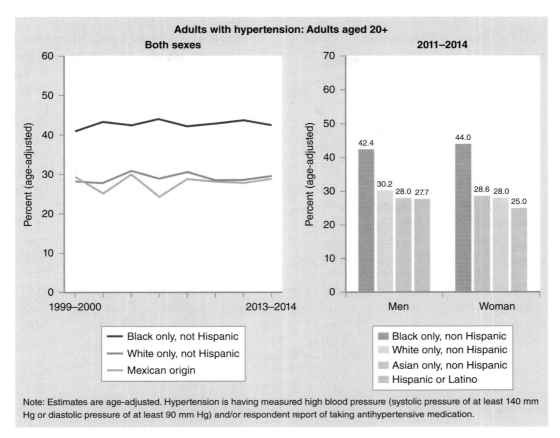

FIGURE 9.1 Hypertension Health Disparities in the United States.

CDC/NCHS, Health, United States, 2015, Figure 23. Data from the National Health and Nutrition Examination Survey (NHANES).

▶ What Is Population-Specific Research?

The complexity of public health is that "one size fits all" when it comes to public health programs is a rarely applicable description of how we can serve and protect the public. Although a one-size-fits-all approach is appropriate in many instances and can be extremely effective in reducing many public health issues when the approach involves a new policy—for example, seatbelt laws, adding iodine to table salt to avert goiter (an enlarged thyroid gland), tobacco policies prohibiting smoking, fortifying white bread with vitamins, and fluoridating water supplies to prevent tooth decay. Not all public health disparities, however, can be resolved with this approach. For many other issues that stem from risky health behaviors such as poor diet, lack of exercise, condomless sex, and so on, implementing a change in policy is not necessarily feasible. By definition, health disparities affect different segments of the population, so public health approaches to address them would only be effective by targeting individual behaviors plus the underlying social determinants (racism,

homophobia, poverty, etc.) that play a role. To more effectively do this, we first need to know who is most affected. It has become a common practice in public health research to use **demographic indicators** as the way to identify those populations and subpopulations most at risk and who experience disparities.

Accordingly, almost any action in public health that encompasses components related to minority status, income, and geographic location must be applied based on what is known to be the "best practices" for a demographically specified population. For example, using just three health behaviors—eating a diet high in fiber (e.g., vegetables and whole grains), using reliable methods of contraception, and engaging in daily exercise that benefits the cardiovascular system—along with five demographic indicators related to risk (race or ethnicity, gender, sexual orientation, geographic location, and socioeconomic status), one can readily imagine the complexity of developing effective programs to address two or more subpopulations. A "best practices" prevention program for any of these three health outcomes would involve having multiple versions to accommodate combinations of these five demographic indicators. For example, a public health program to address obesity by targeting exercise for African American women living in urban areas of Mississippi would most likely not be effective for White Appalachian women living in low-income areas of Kentucky. Thus, a population-specific approach that understands the unique needs and determinants underlying each subpopulation is needed to develop more effective programs.

How Do Public Health Studies Identify Health Disparities?

As a case study, consider an investigation conducted in Baltimore, Maryland, by O'Campo and colleagues (1997). Their objective was to identify whether individual-level factors interacted with macrolevel factors (factors in the social environment) such as *neighborhood of residence* relative to incidence cases of low birth weight babies. They found that prenatal care

interacted with *neighborhood of residence* such that women living in "risky neighborhoods" benefited less from prenatal care than those residing in less risk-prone environments. This serves as only one example of a health disparity, and it is one defined by the neighborhood. Risky neighborhoods were defined as having high levels of unemployment and low median income. In the event that you have an interest in preventing the occurrence of low birth weight, it may be practical to first do a records review tracking recent rates of low birth weight as a function of zip codes or census tracks. Indeed, as public health practice continues to advance as a discipline, the concept of disparity identification via zip codes has become increasingly popular.

FIGURE 9.2 provides a visual image of how zip code areas may serve as a proxy of risk (with life expectancy being the indicator in this example). As you can see, the mapping conveys a tremendous level of variation

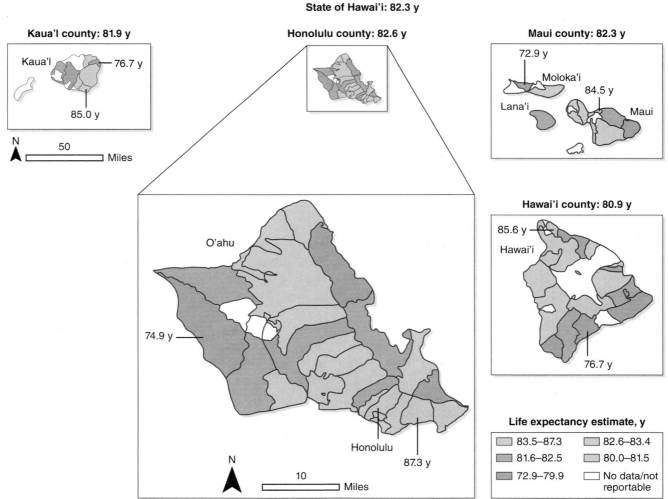

FIGURE 9.2 Life Expectancy Disparities in Hawaii.

2010 US Census, Office of Health Status Monitoring. Hawaii State Department of Health, 2008–2012.

between zip code areas in the state of Hawaii. Thus, if you were making resource allocation decisions for Hawaii now, using zip codes would prove a valuable method of selecting prioritized populations.

Although the use of **geographically defined populations** is increasingly common and valuable in selecting priority populations, this strategy implies that the ensuing intervention studies (designed to rectify the disparities) will occur on a community-wide basis. This assumption may not always apply. For instance, consider a possible gender-based violence risk-reduction program intended for young urban females. Imagine that the program could be designed for delivery entirely online, thus creating the possibility of intervention for any young woman with Internet access. In this case, you need to decide which sub-population of young women in the United States may benefit most from the program—that is, what are the demographic indicators of high risk for being a victim of gender-based violence? Consequently, you begin a literature review and soon learn that Black females 16 to 22 years of age and living in urban impoverished areas have a greater risk of experiencing this form of violence than any other subpopulation of young women. Now three indicators define your population, as shown in **FIGURE 9.3**. The section of this figure where the three circles overlap represents your new study population. Pragmatically, this sets up what is known as the **study-inclusion criteria**. Inclusion criteria operationally define who is eligible for study participation. At this juncture, a caveat is warranted. When creating interventions, it is important to develop programs for relatively defined and homogenous (similar) people. In this example, the violence-prevention needs of Black or African American women 16–22 years of age residing in an urban poverty area may be quite different from those of White women living in suburban environments. Thus, having multiple inclusion criteria sharpens what will eventually become an intervention program for the at-risk population.

What Is Intersectionality and Why Is It Important?

As a person dedicated to improving the health of the public, your primary goal should always be to serve those who can benefit the most. Once again, this is why carefully selecting the study population is so vital. The selection process, of course, is a function of the disease or health condition of interest. Preventing depression, for example, would entail a distinctly different high-risk population compared with preventing death from gun violence. Although White, middle-class suburbanites (for example) do have their share of health-related challenges and issues such as depression and obesity, you will find that the majority of threats to public health are primarily experienced by people who belong to multiple minority subpopulations as previously defined.

When a minority member (be it by race or ethnicity, sexual orientation, gender, gender expression, or living below the federal poverty level) is substantially more likely than his or her nonminority counterparts to experience a risk environment for any given disease or condition, this is a form of **oppression**. Furthermore, the concept of **intersectionality** refers to co-occurring oppressions and focuses attention on important differences within these population groups that are often portrayed as relatively homogenous such as women, men, sexual minorities, or racial or ethnic minorities. For example, intersectionality gives rise to a more nuanced understanding that a Black man from a lower socioeconomic group might be penalized for his race and class when accessing health and social care but has the relative advantage of gender over a Black woman. As the number of co-occurring oppressions increases, so does the risk of developing diseases or conditions that limit human potential and threaten well-being and overall quality of life. Thus, we cannot overemphasize the importance of examining heath disparities through an intersectional lens (see **FIGURE 9.4**).

BOX 9.1 provides a vignette to better convey the concept of intersectionality. In this example, you will read about two forms of co-occurring oppressions: (1) being foreign born and residing in the United States and (2) being a member of a racial or ethnic minority.

Although you may be tempted to equate the concept of multiple co-occurring oppressions with minority race and ethnicity, please bear in mind that public health priorities are vastly complex relative to how intersectionality applies to each one. Being a Latina, for example, neither equates with added risk for HIV infection (Centers for Disease Control and Prevention, 2016) nor equates with added risk for lung cancer or

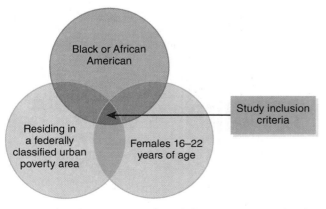

FIGURE 9.3 Inclusion Criteria for a Violence-Prevention Study.

AT A CROSSROAD OF OPPRESSIONS?

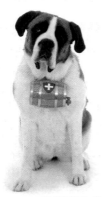 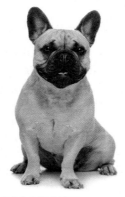

INTERSECT YOU MUST

FIGURE 9.4 Public Health Mascots Snow and Hamilton Advocate for Intersectionality.

© Eric Isselee/Shutterstock; © Svetography/Shutterstock

BOX 9.1 Uptake of HPV Vaccination Is a Function of the Intersection Between Race or Ethnicity and Being Born in the United States

A national, population-based study of U.S. women provided a succinct example of two co-occurring oppressions: being a member of a racial or ethnic minority and being born outside of the United States (i.e., foreign-born). Among foreign-born women living in the United States, Asian women were 57% less likely to be vaccinated than foreign-born White women. Similarly, foreign-born Latinas were 54% less likely to be vaccinated than foreign-born White women. All foreign-born women were significantly less likely than U.S.-born White women to be vaccinated, with Asian women and Latinas (72 and 71% less likely, respectively) being especially disadvantaged in this aspect of health protection. Foreign-born Black women (56% less likely) and foreign-born White women (36% less likely) were also disadvantaged in this regard, compared with U.S.-born White women (Agenor, Abboud, Delgadillo, et al. 2018).

---

lung cancer death (Miller et al., 2018)—in fact, for both HIV and lung cancer, Latinas have comparably low incidence rates compared with most other populations. Indeed, in many cases, a public health priority may be one that corresponds with disparities experienced by White populations. For instance, death rates from opioid overdose in the United States are highest among non-Hispanic Whites (19.4 per 100,000), followed by a much lower rate of 12.9 per 100,000 for non-Hispanic Blacks, and a substantially lower rate for Hispanics (6.8 per 100,000) (Han, Tuazon, Kunins, Mantha, & Paone, 2019; Kaiser Family Foundation, 2019).

Other examples include suicide and heart disease. Furthermore, note that being White and poor plays out much differently than being White and *not* poor. For example, returning to diabetes, consider the abstract we have featured in **BOX 9.2**. Regardless, the take-home message regarding intersectionality is that the goal of an intersectionality-informed approach is to map health disparities with more precision and then chart more effective directions in program development and policy.

BOX 9.2 An Example of a Disease Priority That Also Has a Disproportionate Impact on White Populations

The idea that race and ethnicity is always the mainstay of health disparities should be tempered by the idea that income levels may also be strong indicators of disparities in health as race and ethnicity. Consider, for example, the following abstract from a study published in the *American Journal of Public Health*. As you read this abstract, notice that "Black race" is a clear factor regarding this disparity; yet the role of poverty and living in high-poverty neighborhoods is also a vital factor—and one that implicates added risk for populations of White race.

Disparities in Diabetes: The Nexus of Race, Poverty, and Place

Objectives. We sought to determine the role of neighborhood poverty and racial composition on race disparities in diabetes prevalence.

Methods. We used data from the 1999–2004 National Health and Nutrition Examination Survey and 2000 U.S. Census to estimate the impact of individual race and poverty and neighborhood racial composition and poverty concentration on the odds of having diabetes.

Results. We found a race–poverty–place gradient for diabetes prevalence for Blacks and poor Whites. The odds of having diabetes were higher for Blacks than for Whites. Individual poverty increased the odds of having diabetes for both Whites and Blacks. Living in a poor neighborhood increased the odds of having diabetes for Blacks and poor Whites.

Conclusions. To address race disparities in diabetes, policy makers should address problems created by concentrated poverty—for example, lack of access to reasonably priced fruits and vegetables, recreational facilities, and healthcare services; high crime rates; and greater exposures to environmental toxins. Housing and development policies in urban areas should avoid creating high-poverty neighborhoods.

Darrell J. Gaskin et al. Disparities in Diabetes: The Nexus of Race, Poverty, and Place. *American Journal of Public Health* 104, no. 11 (November 1, 2014): pp. 2147–2155.

▶ Is There an Objective Measure of High Risk?

A standard statistical tool used in public health is known as the **odds ratio**. Briefly, this is nothing more than the added risk of a given outcome for people who have the risk factor compared with those without the risk factor (see Chapter 14 for more on odds ratios). In terms of selecting a priority population, the concept of risk can be operationalized as any given demographic factor. The most common demographic risk factors tend to be female biological sex, minority race and ethnicity, low income, and being a member of a sexual or gender minority group (SGM). Using just these risk factors, we have constructed **TABLE 9.2**, which provides examples from recent studies of the added risk experienced by people within these four populations.

▶ What Methods Are Used to Define Populations?

A study by Krieger and colleagues (2002) used a host of methods that can be applied to defining and classifying populations based on risk. In this study, the authors used all of the following indicators:

- Block census
- Zip code area
- Occupational class
- Unemployment
- Household income
- Income inequality
- Education level
- Crowded households in census tracts
- Gender
- Age
- Race and ethnicity

TABLE 9.2 Examples of Health Disparities Research Studies

Study	Disease or Event	Risk Group	Comparison Group	Odds Ratio
Unintentional cocaine overdoses in residents of New York (individuals aged 45–84) (Han, Tuazon, Kunins, Mantha, & Paone, 2019)	Cocaine overdoses	Residents aged 45–84	Residents aged 45–84	1.34
		Males	Females	1.3
		Bronx-specific residents	Other New York districts	1.29
		Non-Latino Black residents	Other races	2.37
Rural versus urban college-aged Kentucky students risk of developing high blood pressure (Abshire, Graves, & Dawson, 2019)	High blood pressure	Rural college students	Urban college students	0.32
Workplace clan culture and workplace health climate association with employee smoking rates (Kava et al., 2019)	Smoking rates	Improved workplace health climates	Unimproved workplace health climates	0.08
Infant hearing loss in Durham County, NC, both suburbs and rural communities (Lantos et al., 2018)	Hearing loss	Minority race	Majority races	2.45
Data from National Longitudinal Survey of Youth 1997 (Manlove, Steward-Streng, Peterson, Scott, & Wildsmith, 2013)	Teen pregnancy	American women	Caucasian women	2.1
		Foreign-born Hispanic women	Caucasian women	3.5
		Native-born Hispanic women	Caucasian women	1.9

Although we recognize that the bulleted list of options may feel like too much information, this menu of options may be valuable as you consider a somewhat different perspective when selecting a research population. Previously in this chapter, we provided information on selecting a priority population, with the assumption that you would subsequently seek out a method to locate and enroll the members of that population into a study. But what if you already have access to a geographically defined population and it is practical to conduct the study within that area? Indeed, the very nature of much public health research begins with a geographically defined population rather than a demographically defined population. This is especially the case for community-based participatory research—discussed in Chapter 4 and an emerging approach to public health practice (Wallerstein & Duran, 2003). This is true because once a researcher is embedded in a community, that "belongingness" becomes an asset for future research. So, the question now becomes, Within my given geographic community, how do I select a population that can benefit the most from my study? This question can be answered by conducting a **formal needs assessment** or **informal needs assessment**. The formal needs assessment typically involves conducting survey research used to gauge potential disparities in risk within a population. The survey can be constructed using the indicators shown in the preceding bulleted list. **BOX 9.3** presents an example of a formal needs assessment.

Alternatively, existing information (the informal needs assessment) may be all you need to identify the most salient disparities. For example, a study of pediatric asthma hospitalization rates in

Baltimore, Maryland, identified two primary factors—zip code area and household income—in the bulleted list as primary methods of predicting elevated asthma hospitalization rates (Environmental Integrity Project, 2017). Regardless of whether you use a formal or informal approach (or a combination of the two) to determine the needs of the community, the results will guide your development of the study-inclusion criteria and thus define the study population.

▶ Why Are Studies of Women and Children Vital to Public Health?

So far, this chapter has had a decidedly domestic (U.S.) focus. If, however, you are a student with an interest in practicing health promotion in developing nations, you should understand that women and girls experience the vast majority of health inequities in most parts of the world. Globally, these inequities range from social conditions (e.g., unequal pay, lack of the same education opportunities given to males, lack of legal protections given to males, laws prohibiting home ownership) to highly specific health-related forms of discrimination (e.g., lack of equal access to available food, healthcare, and vaccinations). We urge you to learn more by reading *Half the Sky: Turning Oppression into Opportunity for Women Worldwide*, a national best-selling book by Nicholas Kristof and Sheryl WuDunn.

Although not at all comparable to the social and health inequities faced by women in the developing

---

BOX 9.3 Example of a Needs Assessment That Identified Subpopulations at Heightened Risk for Diabetic Peripheral Neuropathy

This study investigated the prevalence of diabetic peripheral neuropathy (DPN) and identified populations at risk in medically underserved rural communities. A survey was administered among $N = 816$ type II diabetic patients located in five rural Arkansas counties who attended a diabetes education program from 2005 to 2009. The data were collected through a survey questionnaire and from medical records. Of the 816 patients studied, 9.6% had a DPN diagnosis, and 43% reported peripheral neuropathy symptoms (PNS). Among the patients with PNS, 79% had not been diagnosed with DPN. Multivariate analyses found that *being female, being White, having less than a college education;* having a longer duration of diabetes; having a history of smoking; having a professional foot examination; and performing self-examinations of feet were associated with a higher risk for having DPN or PNS. The study found that the prevalence of patients with PNS was high and that DPN was alarmingly underdiagnosed in these underserved rural communities. The high prevalence of PNS and underdiagnosis of DPN could influence the development of severe foot complications such as diabetic foot ulcers and even possibly increase the risk of lower-extremity amputation in these underserved communities. The at-risk population identified by this study would be a resource to help diabetes educators develop targeted education and intervention programs in underserved rural communities (Balamurugan, Biddle, & Rollins, 2011).

world, the oppression of women unfortunately continues in the United States. Inequalities experienced by U.S. women take the form of disadvantages inherent in the employment of women in high-income jobs, lack of adequate insurance coverage for reproductive health, and lack of adequately enforced protections against gender-based violence. To at least ensure minimal disparities in the selection of research populations, the National Institutes of Health (NIH) provides a requirement to all applicants of research funding awards to include women in all research studies. Grant proposals that do not include women in the study population must contain a thorough justification as to why women are not being included.

Just as women are so often treated inequitably regarding the social determinants of health, so too are children. NIH defines **children** as persons younger than 18 years of age. As noted in Chapter 3, this population is frequently neglected in research because of the added measures that must be taken to obtain and maintain institutional review board (IRB) approval. Yet, children so often bear an undue proportion of the nation's disease burden. A common example is sexually transmitted disease (STD), with one of every four teens acquiring an STD each year. Gun violence is also a common example; children ages five to 14 in the United States are 14 times more likely to be killed by gunshot than children of the same age in other developed nations (Grinshteyn & Hemenway, 2016). Based on these disparities and a multitude of others, NIH requires all applicants of research funding awards to include children. As is the case with women, proposals that do not include children in the study population must contain a thorough justification as to why not.

Think About It!

In the United States, one often-neglected population that experiences multiple health disparities is defined best by the term **rurality**. Although numerous definitions of what constitutes a rural area exist, a commonly accepted definition is a county with a population of fewer than 50,000 people outside the boundaries of a metropolitan area. Rural areas are often lacking in healthcare (i.e., they are often classified as medically underserved) and are highly likely to be economically poor and inhabited by a people of a high average age than nearby metropolitan counties or areas. Appalachia is one such partially isolated and economically depressed part of rural America (see **FIGURE 9.5**).

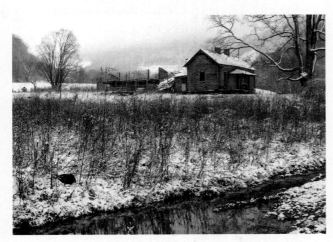

FIGURE 9.5 Abandoned Homestead in Appalachia.
© Joel Carillet/E+/Getty Images

Extending from Pennsylvania to the Mississippi Delta, the Appalachian region of the United States has experienced varying degrees of poverty and corresponding levels of being medically underserved since the 1960s. Since that time, many areas of Appalachia have experienced economic growth, with exceptions being largely found in southeastern Kentucky. A common barrier to healthcare in southeastern Kentucky is best characterized as *mountain culture*. This is a culture of tightly knit families and communities that have survived economic hardships for generations. A strong kinship exists within extremely large, extended families (greater than 100 people) and within geographically isolated communities (these are isolated by steep mountain terrain that is unsuitable for building roads or homes). This kinship defines a culture that is distrustful of persons not connected to recognized families or who are not long-standing members of a community. This distrust extends to many healthcare providers. A history of economic hardships in rural Appalachia further exacerbates barriers to healthcare through a common acceptance of undue morbidity and early morality. This type of fatalism has been documented in published studies coming from southeastern Kentucky (Mark, Crosby, & Vanderpool, 2018; Vanderpool, Dressler, Stradtman, &. Crosby, 2015).

Although overcoming a legacy of fatalism and medical mistrust in places like Appalachia is a formidable public health challenge, a more reasonable goal is to conduct research designed to better understand the fatalism and the medical mistrust. In turn, this improved understanding may inform structural changes to the current approaches promoting the use of the healthcare system and changes to the system

itself as a method of making healthcare more compatible with community values. Ultimately, the point to consider is that effective public health research is population specific.

Take Home Points

- Selecting a research population is an opportunity to contribute to larger efforts designed to rectify health disparities.
- The vast majority of public health practice depends on public health research conducted on a population-specific basis.
- Research to reduce health disparities requires an understanding of the intersection of multiple oppressions experienced by minority populations.
- Research populations can be demographically defined or geographically defined, with the latter being an approach that is consistent with

research conducted as part of a community-based effort.
- Odds ratios are an objective marker of inflated risk within defined populations.
- Disparities in social and health-related conditions are increasingly being identified through the use of census data and zip code areas.
- Women and children experience disparities throughout the world, including the United States. In the United States, federal policies help ensure the inclusion of women and children in health research.

Key Terms

Children
Demographic indicators
Formal needs assessment
Geographically defined
   populations

Health disparities
Informal needs assessment
Intersectionality
Odds ratio
Oppression

Population
Population health
Rurality
Study-inclusion criteria

For Practice and Discussion

1. How does the field of public health differ from the healthcare field? Explain the key differences between the two fields.
   a. Using the health problem of diabetes, explain how public health professionals would examine this problem compared with healthcare professionals.
2. Find a journal article that examines health disparities related to diabetes in the United States. Read the article and answer the following questions:
   a. What is the purpose of the study?
   b. How does this study address health disparities?
   c. What are the inclusion criteria for this study?

3. A public health professor wants to conduct a study to understand health disparities related to diabetes in metro Atlanta, Georgia. However, she wants to narrow her population to a specific geographic area within Atlanta that is experiencing disproportionate diabetes rates compared with others in the area. What method would you recommend she use to define her population and why?
4. Provide an example of an intersectional public health problem and explain why it would be considered intersectional based on the definition of intersectionality provided in this chapter.

References

Agénor, M., Abboud, S., Delgadillo, J. G., Pérez, A. E., Peitzmeier, S. M., & Borrero, S. (2018). Intersectional nativity and foreign born racial/ethnic disparities in human Papillomavirus vaccination initiation among United States women: A national

population-based study. *Cancer Causes and Control, 29*(10), 927–936.

Centers for Disease Control and Prevention (CDC). (2015). *Health, United States, 2015*, Figure 23. Data from the National Health and Nutrition Examination Survey (NHANES). Washington, DC: CDC. Retrieved from https://www.cdc.gov/nchs/hus/contents2015.htm#fig23

Centers for Disease Control and Prevention. (2016). *HIV and Hispanics/Latinos.* Washington, DC: CDC. Retrieved from https://www.cdc.gov/hiv/group/racialethnic/hispaniclatinos/index.html

Environmental Integrity Project. (2017, December 18). *Report documents impact of air pollution on asthma in Baltimore.* Retrieved from https://www.environmentalintegrity.org/news/baltimore-asthma/

Gaskin, D. J., Thorpe, R. J. Jr., McGinty, E. E., LaVeist, T. A., Bower, K., Rohde, C., . . . , & Dubay, L. (2014, November 1). Disparities in diabetes: The nexus of race, poverty, and place. *American Journal of Public Health*, 104(11), 2147–2155.

Grinshteyn, E., & Hemenway, D. (2016). Violent death rates: The U.S. compared with other high income OECD countries, 2010. *American Journal of Medicine*, 129(3), 266–273.

Han, B., Tuazon, E., Kunins, H., Mantha, S., & Paone, D. (2019). Unintentional drug overdose deaths involving cocaine among middle-aged and older adults in New York City. *Drug and Alcohol Dependence*, 198, 121–125.

Hankivsky, O. (2012). Women's health, men's health, and gender and health: Implications of intersectionality. *Social Science & Medicine*, 74(11), 1712–1720.

Kaiser Family Foundation. (2019). State Health Facts. Opioid overdose death rates by race/ethnicity. https://www.kff.org/other/state-indicator/opioid-overdose-deaths-by-raceethnicity/?currentTimeframe=0&sortModel=%7B%22colId%22:%22Location%22,%22sort%22:%22asc%22%7D

Kapilashrami, A., & Hankivsky, O. (2018). Intersectionality and why it matters to global health. *The Lancet*, 391(10140), 2589–2591.

Krieger, N., Chen, J. T., Waterman, P. D., Soobader, M.-J., Subramanian, S. V., & Carson, R. (2002). Geocoding and monitoring of U.S. socioeconomic inequities in mortality and cancer incidence: Does the choice of area-based measures and geographic level matter? *American Journal of Epidemiology*, 2002(156), 471–482.

Mark, K. P., Crosby, R. A., & Vanderpool, R. C. (2018). Psychosocial correlates of ever having a pap test and abnormal pap results in a sample of rural Appalachian women. *Journal of Rural Health*, 34(2), 148–154.

Miller, K. D., Goding Sauer, A., Ortiz, A. P., Fedewa, S. A., Pinheiro, P. S., Tortolero-Luna, G., . . . , Siegel, R. L. (2018). Cancer statistics for Hispanics/Latinos, 2018. *Cancer Journal for Clinicians*, 68, 425–445.

National Center for Health Statistics. (2019). NCHS data on racial and ethnic disparities. Hyattsville, MD: Author.

O'Campo, P., Xue, X., Wang, M. C., & Cauphy, M. (1997). Neighborhood risk factors for low birth weight in Baltimore: A multilevel analysis. *American Journal of Public Health*, 87, 1113–1118.

U.S. Department of Health and Human Services. (2008, October 28). The Secretary's Advisory Committee on National Health Promotion and Disease Prevention Objectives for 2020. Phase I report: Recommendations for the framework and format of Healthy People 2020 [Internet]. Section IV: Advisory Committee findings and recommendations. Retrieved from http://www.healthypeople.gov/sites/default/files/PhaseI_0.pdf

Vanderpool, R. C., Dressler, E. V. M., Stradtman, L. R., &. Crosby, R. A. (2015). Fatalistic beliefs and completion of the HPV vaccination series among a sample of young Appalachian Kentucky women. *Journal of Rural Health*, 31(2), 199–205.

Wallerstein, N., & Duran, B. (2003). The conceptual, historical, and practice roots of community based participatory research and related participatory traditions. Pp. 27–52 in M. Minkler & N. Wallerstein (Eds.), *Community-based participatory research for health.* San Francisco, CA: Jossey-Bass.

Wang, W., Balamurugan, A., Biddle, J., & Rollins, K. M. (2011). Diabetic neuropathy status and the concerns in underserved rural communities: Challenges and opportunities for diabetes educators. *The Diabetes Educator*, 37(4), 536–548.

For Further Reading

Gordis, L. (2013). *Epidemiology* (5th ed.). Philadelphia, PA: W. B. Saunders.

Kristof, N. D, & WuDunn, S. (2009). *Half the sky: Turning oppression into opportunity for women worldwide.* New York, NY: Vintage Books.

Marmot, M. (2015). *The health gap: The challenge of an unequal world.* New York, NY: Bloomsbury.

Treadwell, H. M., Xanthos, C., & Holden, K. B. (2013). *Social determinants of health among African-American men.* San Francisco, CA: Jossey-Bass.

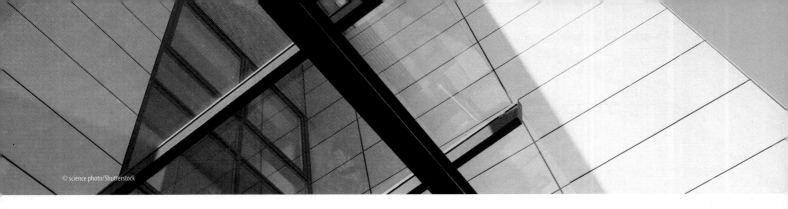
© science photo/Shutterstock

CHAPTER 10

Sampling Techniques

with Anne Marie Schipani-McLaughlin

LEARNING OBJECTIVES

1. Distinguish between probability and nonprobability sampling.
2. Understand generalizability of research findings and the effects of sampling techniques.
3. Describe the different probability-sampling techniques.
4. Describe the different nonprobability-sampling techniques.
5. Understand the lack of association between representativeness and sample size.
6. Understand how a sample can limit a study.

▶ Overview

A main goal of science is to generate usable knowledge that can be applied to the understanding and solving of various human problems and conditions. To use the knowledge that is generated, the research must be conducted in a way that will allow the results to be confidently applied to the population under study. Thus, one of the most important decisions to be made when conducting any kind of public health research involves determining the method to be used that will maximize the sample's representation of the **population** being studied. In this context, *population* refers to the defined segment of people your research targets. This major decision refers to choosing the most appropriate **sampling technique**. Stated simply, sampling describes the process of selecting a representative portion of the population. An analogy may be useful. Every 4 years in the United States, a presidential election draws people to their televisions on the first Tuesday evening in November. The news

shows typically predict which candidate will win each state well before most of the votes have been counted. How is this possible? The answer is complicated, but some predictions involve polling voters and the use of sampling techniques that theoretically allow accurate predictions based on a percentage of the actual votes. These predictions, of course, have been known to be wrong. Thus, sampling as a method of truly understanding the population has a degree of chance—meaning there is always some chance that the sample, which was surveyed, did not truly represent the population.

As is the case with most things, planning is key to successful sampling in a research study. Planning how your research participants will be selected starts with formulating an operationally defined goal using three vital questions that will drive this chapter:

1. What is the sampling element?
2. Is a sampling frame accessible?
3. What type of sampling technique should be employed?

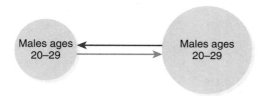

FIGURE 10.1 Does the Sample Represent the Population?

The usefulness of a research study depends on its **generalizability** to the target population. Simultaneously, the generalizability of a research study depends on how well the study sample represents the population. Generalizability refers to the sameness between a sample and the population from which the sample was drawn. This chapter provides you with fundamental concepts of research sampling as well as various sampling techniques that public health researchers use to overcome challenges that inhibit generalizability. In public health research, sampling methods can be divided into two categories: (1) **probability sampling**, which yields high generalizability; and (2) **nonprobability sampling**, which is weak in terms of generalizability.

FIGURE 10.1 visually shows what must occur for a sample to be generalizable to a population. If we were conducting a study among young adult males ages 20 to 29, age and gender are two important variables in the study. We would, therefore, want our sample to reflect the larger population. In this regard, the sample (smaller circle) has the same composition as the population (larger circle), although generalizability is not based solely on age and gender. The top arrow indicates that the sample was selected from the population. The bottom arrow indicates that, on assessing age and gender in the sample, the values did indeed match the known values of the population. Of course, this is something of an oversimplification because the example assumes a match (that is, generalizability) based only on two variables.

What Is the Difference Between Probability and Nonprobability Sampling?

First, understand that a high degree of generalizability of a sample can only be achieved by using probability-sampling techniques. Although there are various probability sampling techniques, at the most basic level, probability sampling involves selecting the sample with some degree of randomness or chance. Thus, opportunity for being selected is mostly fixed

and known, and all individuals from the targeted population get an equal opportunity to be selected. Nonprobability sampling contrasts sharply with probability sampling in that the former does not involve being randomly selected but is instead arbitrarily selected. With nonprobability sampling, there is no specific probability of an individual to be a part of the sample, thus there is bias in the resulting sample. For these reasons, you should always look for a possible **sampling frame** that will allow for probability sampling. This section of the chapter will slowly build to the point of defining the term *sampling frame*.

As you begin to think about a research question you have formulated, you will be able to discern many clues regarding sampling. For example, is the research question focused on testing a program? Is it focused instead on understanding a given health behavior? Is it the case that your research question involves prevalence rates of diseases among hidden populations to calculate trends? Further, as you consider the population you selected, you will have other clues, such as whether (1) the population can be easily accessed, (2) a list might exist that contains names of all people in this population, and (3) people in the population may be easily accessed in a given location. All of these clues help you to begin solving the puzzle, starting with selecting a technique. As with many puzzles, your first step is to narrow the options by making one basic decision. That decision comes down to your answer to this question: Is it possible to obtain an exhaustive list that includes all the elements in this population?

What Is the Sampling Element?

To answer this question, you must first understand what is meant by an **element**. An element is the basic unit that defines the study population. In this regard, the population refers to all the possible elements of a defined group. The elements used in different research studies vary based on the study's purpose. An element can be people, which is usually the case, such as children, adults, students, teachers, or employees, to name a few. Elements can also be well-defined units (or clusters). Some units that are important in public health are health departments, nongovernmental organizations, schools, hospitals, and health clinics.

Essentially, elements make up members of a target population. If people are the sampling element, the research question is focused on the person. An example of this would be, do women with a family history of breast cancer receive annual mammograms? However, when the sampling element is well-defined units, the research question is focused on the actions of the entire unit. For example, do hospitals provide breast cancer screening routinely for women over 40? One of the first steps is to determine whether the research question involves inquiry into the behavior of individuals or an entire system. Then it is up to the researcher to determine whether it is possible to access the sampling frame.

▶ Is a Sampling Frame Accessible?

Once you identify the type of sampling element in your study, the next step is to determine whether a *sampling frame* exists or can be created. A sampling frame is a formal, often exhaustive, list of the elements or units that make up the target population. *Exhaustive* is the key word here because the list must represent every possible element in the population. In turn, all elements of the target population make up the sampling frame for that study. The reality of research, though, is that few sampling frames are truly exhaustive. For example, let's say you are conducting a research study on alcohol use and mental health outcomes among college freshmen at a public university, and you plan to recruit participants by obtaining a sample from the registrar's office. However, some college students opt out of being in the registrar's system, so this list would not be exhaustive. Therefore, the question—Is this sampling frame exhaustive of the population?—can be answered by the degree to which it is exhaustive. Otherwise, the answer to this question would be simply "Yes" or "No."

Sampling frames also vary by the extent to which they represent the population or by whether they have *high generalizability* or *low generalizability*. Sampling frames with high generalizability are more representative of the population. Generally, sampling frames in which the sampling element constitutes units (e.g., churches, schools, health departments) rather than people are typically more exhaustive and therefore have higher generalizability. It is more difficult to achieve high generalizability with studies in which people are the sampling element because social structures and laws often protect individual identities unlike units, which are made public intentionally. Just think about nonprofit organizations, schools, colleges, churches, and places of work: You can easily look these up through a quick Google search. But you cannot simply look up the list of college students

enrolled at your school on the Internet; your school is required to protect students' information, and researchers must go through a process to have their research study approved by the institutional review board to obtain a sampling frame from this population. This goes hand in hand with an essential question: Can the sampling frame be accessed? As you can probably imagine, access to your population of interest is critical to a successful research study. Although it may be possible to obtain a list of college students from the registrar's office, in public health, we work with various populations from which it would not be possible to obtain a sampling frame. For instance, if we wanted to conduct a research study on injection drug users in Atlanta, Georgia, who are living with HIV or AIDS, it would not be possible to obtain a sampling frame of this target population. Because of this, the researcher needs to take two competing conditions into consideration: (1) the need for the sample to be generalizable to the target population and (2) the practical reality of obtaining a sampling frame. This compromise is often inevitable in research and shapes the research question because there is no research study without a sample.

▶ What Are the Common Techniques for Probability Sampling?

If your research question dictates that the sample is highly representative of the population, you must select a probability sampling versus nonprobability technique. The most common and user-friendly method of selecting a probability sample is known as **simple random sampling**. This technique is depicted in **FIGURE 10.2** and relies on the principle of *randomness eliminating selection bias*. A truly random-selection process gives every unit an equal and nonzero chance of being selected.

The most widely used strategy to achieve this randomness is the use of a software program (e.g., Excel) or the Internet to first create a computer-generated, sequenced listing of numbers that correspond to the numbered elements of your sampling frame and then selecting elements from the numbered list that correspond to those numbers. For example, if your sampling frame has 10,000 elements and your targeted sample size is 700, you could use a software program to generate a random sequence of 700 values between 1 and 10,000. So, the first number in the computer-generated sequence becomes your first

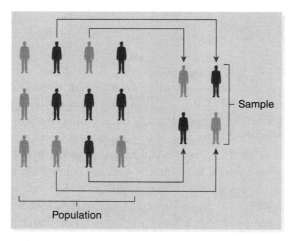

FIGURE 10.2 Simple Random Sampling.

TABLE 10.1 Steps to Generating a Systematic Random Sample
1. Determine your targeted sample size: (e.g., $N = 90$)
2. Determine the sampling interval (nth) by dividing the population size by the sample size: (e.g., 900/90 = 10th)
3. Choose a starting point or seed element at random and that falls below the interval (e.g., 1–9).
4. Recruit every nth element from the list into study.

selection of who you will recruit. The second number in the sequence becomes the second element selected, and the process repeats until you reach 700. See FIGURE 10.3 for an example of this. Of course, whether your element is people or units or entities, you still have to recruit the element once selected.

Another probability-sampling method is known as **systematic random sampling**. Systematic random sampling is similar to simple random sampling but does not ensure that each element has an equal chance of being selected, and selecting elements always begins with a **seed**. Here, the term *seed* refers to a randomly selected starting point in the sampling frame. It works by first determining the targeted sample size. Imagine that your planned sample size is 90 people and your sampling frame or population contains 900 people. Because you loved math in high school, you quickly divide 900 by 90 to obtain the quotient of 10, your sampling interval. You then select a number at random (i.e., the seed) that falls

below your interval and then this number becomes your first person to recruit. After choosing your initial seed as the starting point, you then select the 10th person from that point on from the list, and you keep going until you are back at your starting point and have selected 90 elements to be in the study. To simplify this process, we provide these steps in TABLE 10.1.

At this point, a logical question becomes, why would I use systematic random sampling rather than simple random sampling? The answer lies in the possibility that your sampling frame may be sequenced in a way or there is a pattern to the list that may bias your selected sample and ultimately your study results. For example, perhaps your sampling frame is ordered by age or some other characteristic. A practical application may be helpful. For example, a sampling frame of women receiving abnormal test results from mammograms may be organized by date of their tests—that is, women with abnormal results in 2017 might be

---

1 Set of 700 Unique **Numbers**

Range: From 1 to 10,000

Set #1

4702, 8692, 3998, 4681, 9187, 5756, 7849, 8285, 3401, 3953, 274, 5088, 3092, 1021, 9043, 8798, 4644, 3909, 9591, 1, 7396, 6641, 9682, 2988, 6046, 4539, 858, 6660, 7842, 6197, 6925, 1211, 962, 2454, 3322, 2544, 3793, 9653, 5281, 7646, 8124, 5645, 4459, 2710, 1564, 5190, 8282, 7880, 5686, 5761, 6407, 1287, 9914, 4786, 9841, 5173, 2678, 4823, 8670, 8027, 1140, 6731, 9543, 7016, 38, 5122, 4715, 637, 316, 937, 6492, 3836, 3534, 9697, 9292, 1256, 5983, 5426, 7405, 4514, 6987, 4332, 742, 7334, 3325, 6619, 5428, 7093, 2409, 8482, 1442, 6623, 3774, 6945, 5730, 3907, 2724, 7554, 9430, 1988, 7708, 3084, 6851, 8013, 6290, 8894, 5453, 1106, 997, 5337, 1810, 6426, 3464, 5739, 5460, 2127, 2983, 4964, 647, 1455, 3598, 3021, 2579, 7822, 1427, 7259, 4120, 1152,

FIGURE 10.3 Computer-Generated Random Numbers.

listed first, followed by those having abnormal results in 2018, and so on. If your research question was about whether advances in mammography technology made the test progressively more sensitive from 2017 through 2020, you would want proportional representation from all 4 years to minimize the chances of overselecting participants from 1 year. Accordingly, this inherent ordering of the elements by year has been referred to as **periodicity** and has the potential to greatly detract from the representativeness of the sample if simple random sampling were to be used. Systematic sampling from this sampling frame of abnormal mammography results would ensure that each year of diagnosis is proportionately represented in the selected sample and would enhance the generalizability. This technique is depicted in **FIGURE 10.4**.

The next technique is a **stratified simple random sample**. The word *stratified* implies that you have a good reason to again override randomness. A common example involves the predictor variable, racial or ethnic identity, used to assess disparities in health. Let's say your research study aims to compare reasons why people over age 50 do not have colonoscopies to detect early signs of cancer, and you suspect that race and ethnicity is a factor. The geographic area for the research shows that the population comprises three racial and ethnic groups: White non-Hispanic, Black or African American, and Asian. Left to chance (via simple random selection), one group may have vastly greater representation than the others in your final sample. Overriding chance would thus be a viable solution. So, to ensure your sample has equal representation across the three groups, you would

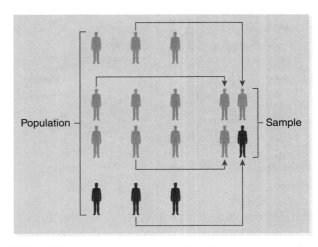

FIGURE 10.5 Stratified Simple Random Sampling.

start by separating your sampling frame into three lists. **FIGURE 10.5** depicts this sampling technique.

As shown in Figure 10.5, the three subframes made by stratifying the original frame based on racial or ethnic identity become the basis for three random-selection procedures. Random selection can also occur proportionately if necessary, thereby preserving the original ratio of the sampling frame. As you can see, this procedure relies on simple random sampling but begins with a division of the sampling frame, one that you create.

The final probability technique is called the **multistage cluster sampling**. To begin, recall earlier in this chapter that sampling elements may be people or units or entities. It is these units or entities that we now refer to as *clusters*. An easy example is a national survey, one that gives people in all 50 states an equal chance of being selected. In this example, your targeted sample size will consist of 1000 people. To recruit 1000 people, you will need to go through three steps:

Stage 1: Each state becomes a cluster, and you randomly select 10 of these.
Stage 2: Within each state, the zip code areas become clusters, and you randomly select 10 of these. This gives you 10 zip code areas in each of 10 states, so you now have 100 clusters.
Stage 3: In each cluster, you randomly select 10 people. This means you have a final sample of 1000 people.

Notice that the word *multistage* in this example refers to the use of random sampling to select clusters of states (stage 1) and zip code areas within states (stage 2). Notice also that the final stage 3 switched from selecting clusters to selecting people. With this example in mind, there are various combinations of clusters that could be sampled before reaching the

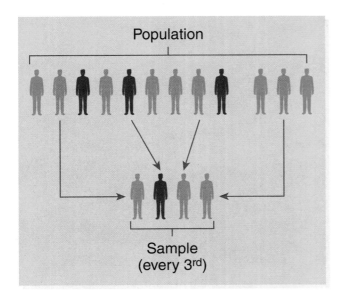

FIGURE 10.4 Systematic Random Sampling.

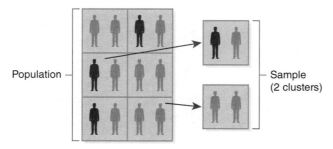

FIGURE 10.6 Multistage Cluster Sampling.

final stage of selecting people. However, the terminal point in a multistage cluster sample may consist of a smaller cluster. **FIGURE 10.6** illustrates this sampling procedure.

For another example, suppose you plan to recruit a nationally representative sample of nonprofit food banks located in urban areas. Your targeted sample size of these elements is 70, and your stages may look like this:

- Begin by randomly selecting seven states
- Within each state, randomly select 10 counties that are classified as urban for a total of 70 clusters
- Randomly select one nonprofit food bank from within each cluster

▶ What Are the Common Techniques Used for Nonprobability Sampling?

Ironically, the most common nonprobability technique is the one that offers the least generalizability. Instead, this first technique is used for the convenience of the researcher, so it is called **convenience sampling**. Stated succinctly, a convenience sample is a preexisting group of people who represent the pool of recruitment opportunities for the sample. Common convenience samples are college students taking psychology classes, people attending medical clinics, people in prison, high school students, and residents of in-house drug rehabilitation programs. Needless to say, a convenience sample at best may be a fair representation of the immediate population from which it was drawn. For instance, college students taking psychology classes may fairly reflect the entire population of psychology majors in that same college or university, but not other majors from that college or another college or university. Similarly, people attending medical clinics in one geographic area may be a

fair reflection of that population, but this would not extend to people attending medical clinics in other geographic areas.

Given the aforementioned limits of convenience sampling, the question arises, Why would this be used by anyone? For several reasons, convenience sampling is warranted. This technique is easy in that people are readily available to approach and recruit. It is also not expensive to implement as you neither have to obtain a sampling frame nor have to adhere to a strict random number sequence. Moreover, a sampling frame may not be available for the population. Finally, if the goal of the study is to test a public health intervention for efficacy, generalizability is not as important as internal validity. Thus, convenience sampling is justifiable when studies are meant to evaluate public health interventions, are exploratory in nature (meaning they are only testing basic ideas or are being used to generate testable research hypotheses for future more generalizable research studies), or sampling frames are not available.

A second option for a nonprobability sample is a derivative of convenience sampling. Known as **purposive sampling**, this option begins with preexisting groups, but it then specifies exactly who can be in the sample. For instance, people in the waiting area of a hospital emergency room are a type of preexisting group (see **FIGURE 10.7**). Imagine that you, however, are conducting a study of women ages 18 to 44. Your recruitment is on a prespecified basis—age (hence the term *purposive*)—and thus departs from the whole group concept of convenience sampling. To implement this technique, you would have to approach women only, excluding men and children, and screen the women for age to see if they are in the targeted age range.

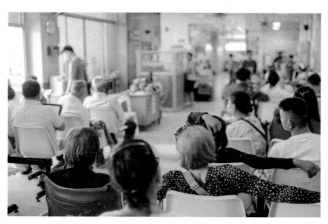

FIGURE 10.7 Hospital Waiting Room to Be Used for Convenience Sampling.

© Medicine-R/Shutterstock

A third option is known as **quota sampling**. Quota sampling mimics the properties of probability sampling by selecting the sample according to important but known demographic characteristics of the population. Quota sampling results in a highly tailored sample that is in proportion to some characteristic or trait of the population. Three steps are necessary: (1) determine the demographic characteristics for the matching process, (2) identify the distribution of these characteristics in the population (this sets the quotas), and (3) select the sample based on those characteristics and their proportion in the population.

Quota sampling can be useful if the researcher determines that demographic factors such as age, gender, and race or ethnicity are critical components of representativeness. Characterizing the population and matching the sample to these characteristics reduces the odds of sample bias. Studies of college students are a good example of an opportunity to apply this technique. Suppose the research question is to identify predictors of opioid use among undergraduates. Beginning with records from the registrar's office, you could identify the distribution of key demographic factors among the undergraduate population. Using these proportions, you would next develop a matrix containing cells that represent the intersections between two or more demographic characteristics. One cell in the matrix is needed for each possible combination. For example, "Hispanic females" would be one cell. The quota of undergraduates, then, who are female and Hispanic would be set, so the task becomes one of recruiting the corresponding number of female and Hispanic undergraduates that equates with their proportion. This process would then continue until all possible cells in the matrix have been filled, meaning that the sample size in each cell matches the set numbers. An example of a possible matrix is presented in **TABLE 10.2**.

A final option you may want to consider is known as **snowball sampling**. Snowball sampling involves obtaining referrals from participants. The name stems

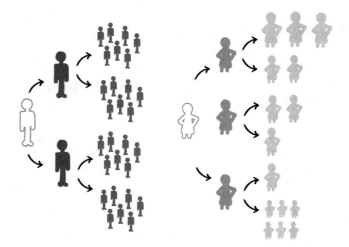

FIGURE 10.8 Snowball Sampling.
© Iamnee/Shutterstock

from the experience that children have if they grew up in places with snowfalls heavy enough to make snowmen. A small handful of snow is packed tightly and placed on the ground and then slowly rolled in the snow to gradually become larger and larger. The concept of starting small and becoming large quickly is very much the case when the people you enroll into a study help you to find others who also qualify. This concept is shown in **FIGURE 10.8**.

This technique is actually one that is commonly used for hard-to-reach and hidden populations for whom there is no sampling frame. People who inject drugs, for example, are not easy to identify. They may be of any race and ethnicity and be low income, middle income, or even high income in terms of social class and residence. So, how would you recruit a sample of 100 injection drug users? The answer begins with a seed. In this context, a seed is the primary data source, a person who is somehow found, screened for study eligibility, and enrolled to start the snowball chain. Finding just a few seeds may prove quite challenging; yet it may also prove to be enough to get you to 100. This is possible because you will ask each seed to assist you in

TABLE 10.2 Sample Matrix Constructed for Quota Sampling		
	Male (*N* = 7439)	**Female (*N* = 10,415)**
White	24% of enrolled students	32% of enrolled students
African American or Black	10% of enrolled students	14% of enrolled students
Asian	3% of enrolled students	8% of enrolled students
Hispanic	8% of enrolled students	5% of enrolled students

locating others who also inject drugs. This assistance may take on many forms such as a physical introduction, an e-introduction, or perhaps arranging a meeting place and time. Then, for each person you meet as a result of seed number 1, you repeat the process of asking for assistance in meeting others who may qualify for the study. So, if you begin with two seeds and each leads you to three other people, and each of those lead you to eight other people, you would already have 48 people! Thus, you can imagine how quickly you might make the goal of 100 by simply continuing this process.

Another form of nonprobability sampling that adds an element of randomness is known as **venue–day–time (VDT) sampling**. Randomness comes into play with a concept known as *time–space sampling*, which begins by counting three things: (1) the number of places (called *venues*) where recruitment might reasonably occur, (2) the days each week when those venues are available for use as a recruitment site, and (3) the times (assessed in blocks of 4 hours) within those days during which recruitment may occur. For example, let's say you wanted to recruit people who inject opioids for a cross-sectional study occurring in a large urban area. You have hired a staff of six former users (i.e., they had injected opioids), and these people know where all the drug spots are within a 2-mile radius, which you have determined should be the focal point of your sampling efforts. After some street surveillance work, staff members

inform you that the radius contains 13 currently active spots. They also make a list of which days these 13 spots are places of active sales. As it turns out, five spots are active 7 days each week, and the remaining eight are only active 4 days each week. After a great deal of street surveillance, your staff also identifies the corresponding time blocks for each day during which the spots are active. **TABLE 10.3** displays the final matrix showing the time blocks, within days, by venue. As you examine the 4-hour blocks available in 1 week for these five locations, you will see somewhat of a pattern that corresponds with weekdays, weekends, and nightfall. For instance, it may be that People's Park is a place where homeless people sleep and a norm exists relative to when drug sales occur so as not to cause issues at night. You will also see that two locations are simply not used on Sundays and that the matrix has a total of 67 4-hour time blocks. It is these 67 units that can therefore be subject to random selection. Thus, rather than assign research staff to all 67 units in this time–space sampling method, you might randomly select—for the first week of the study—12 units. For the second week of the study, you would then randomly select another 12 units using **replacement**, which simply means that units from week 1 are put back into the realm of all 67 possibilities. This approach would continue until your desired recruitment goals are met.

TABLE 10.3 Example of a Matrix for Venue–Day–Time Sampling

Venue Location or Name	Days When the Venue Is Accessible						
	M	**T**	**W**	**Th**	**F**	**S**	**S**
Corner of 3rd and Dunn	a, d	a, d	a, d	a, d	a, d, e	a, d, e	a, d, e
Lucky's hot dog stand	d, e	d, e	d, e	d, e	d, e	d, e	—
East 7th St. Subway entrance	c–f	c–f	c–f	c–f	c–f	c–f	—
People's Park	b, c	b, c	b, c	b, c	b–d	b–d	b–d
Alley behind 2nd St. gas station	f	f	f	f	a, f	a, f	f

a. Hours: midnight to 4 AM
b. Hours: 4 to 8 AM
c. Hours: 8 AM to noon
d. Hours: noon to 4 PM
e. Hours: 4 PM to 8 PM
f. Hours: 8 PM to midnight

As you can imagine, VDT sampling has several pros and cons. A key advantage is that it brings random selection into the technique that would otherwise be a simple purposive sample of injection drug users. A second advantage is that it provides an equal and nonzero chance that time of day and day of the week will be represented, thus potentially averting any selection bias based on time. A primary drawback is that research staff must be able and willing to work erratic shifts defined by 4-hour time blocks. A second drawback involves the shifting nature of the venues, days, and times when (in this case) drug sales occur and injection drug users can thus be recruited. Clearly, the type of matrix shown in Table 10.3 has a "limited shelf life" and must, therefore, be updated on a regular basis. On the balance, however, VDT sampling may have more pros than cons, especially for hard-to-reach populations.

As an example of the utility of VDT sampling, we provide the following paragraph from a grant proposal relative to the opioid epidemic.

> Data will be gathered from persons who inject drugs (PWID) using a venue-day-time (VDT) sampling method, as designed with input from the CDC for the National HIV/AIDS Behavioral Surveillance . . . system (McKellar et al., 2007). Clusters will be defined by a [two]-mile radius of drug copping areas. VDT has been used in several community level studies and offers a rigorous way of reaching more of the target population given likely round-the-clock space access. VDT involves randomly selecting and visiting venues on specific days and systematically intercepting and collecting information from consenting members of the target population. This allows researchers to construct a sample with known properties and make inferences to the larger populations. Venues are defined as public, semiprivate or private locations where PWID may be present. Examples include parks, public bathrooms, bridge underpasses, open fields, alleys, "trap" houses (where injection drug use is known to occur).

As you read the preceding paragraph, were you convinced this sampling procedure is worth funding? We hope your answer is "Yes," and we suggest that this nonprobability technique is a strong alternative to approaches that do not incorporate an element of random selection.

▶ What Is the Difference Between Representativeness and Sample Size?

All too often, people—including social and behavioral scientists—make the unfounded assumption that size matters when it comes to sampling and having a study with a large number of people is more valid than one with only a small number (see **FIGURE 10.9**). This thinking is unfounded because it is entirely possible to have a huge sample that is *not* representative of the population. The idea that small but highly representative samples are ideal for making generalizations is not new. In fact, this idea of smaller can be better predominates business and advertising practices in the United States.

Consider, for example, television ratings. These ratings are vital to advertisers as they inform the placement and cost of their ads based on a projected number of viewers for any given program. The Nielsen ratings are perhaps the most commonly known method used for this purpose. For 2017–2018, the Nielsen Corporation estimated that 120 million households had people who viewed television. Think of the 120 million as the population. So, how large do you suppose the Nielsen sample was for that year?

- ▪ Choice A = 12,000,000 households (i.e., 10%)
- ▪ Choice B = 6,000,000 households (i.e., 5%)
- ▪ Choice C = 1,200,000 households (i.e., 1%)
- ▪ Choice D = 600,000 households (i.e., .5%)
- ▪ Choice E = <60,000 (i.e., less than .05%)

The answer is 41,000, so if you were drawn to choice E, give yourself a pat on the back. The point here is

SIZE DOES *NOT* MATTER

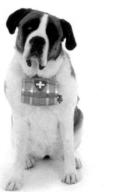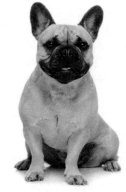

WHEN IT COMES TO SAMPLING

FIGURE 10.9 Public Health Mascots Snow and Hamilton Set the Record Straight on Sample Size.

that billions of dollars in advertising are allocated based on a sample size of less than one half of 1%. Given the success of advertising, this allegory provides a simple lesson for public health: Smaller can be better if the sampling technique minimizes bias.

Now that you are in the mood to answer multiple-choice questions, consider one more. Which sampling technique has the least chance of yielding a representative sample?

- Choice A = simple random sampling
- Choice B = multistage cluster sampling
- Choice C = quota sampling
- Choice D = systematic random sampling

As you look at the four options, we hope you will choose the one technique that does not belong in the list of probability techniques. That technique is quota sampling, so option C is the correct answer here. Please remember that representativeness can only be achieved with the use of a probability-sampling technique.

Finally, we ask you to consider one last but critical distinction between representativeness and sample size: **participation rate**. The rate is calculated by using the number of people who enrolled in a study as the numerator and the number asked to join the study as the denominator. As a wise consumer of public health research literature for studies involving people, you should always look to the reported participation rate. The lower the participation rate, the more likely the sample is biased and will have low generalizability. Of course, the opposite is true: The higher the rate, the less bias and the better generalizability. Thus, the size of the sample is not as important. But how do you know for sure what is considered a good or bad response rate? A useful heuristic to help you remember how to gauge a study's response rates in terms of the generalizability of results is an actual gauge. As shown in **FIGURE 10.10**, we categorized response rates into three classifications: high (green), medium (beige), and low (red) that align with accepted guidelines so you can know and understand how to interpret the results.

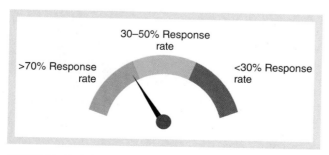

FIGURE 10.10 A Response-Rate Gauge for Judging the Generalizability of Research.

How Does the Sample Limit a Study?

Ultimately, your choice of a sampling method is potentially a make-or-break decision point regarding the generalizability of your study. As a rule, probability samples have high degrees of generalizability depending on response rate, whereas nonprobability samples yield far lower degrees of generalizability. This is not to say that studies based on nonprobability samples are of less value. Indeed, these studies may be far more important in public health. Consider, for instance, all of the hidden populations that are prioritized for public health interventions:

- Those who inject drugs
- Battered women living in shelters
- People living in food deserts
- Women engaged in sex work
- Men who have sex with men
- Cancer patients and survivors
- Socially marginalized people experiencing chronic daily stress
- People living with diabetes
- Children at risk of family violence
- Obese people attempting to lose weight
- People experiencing chronic depression

For each of these populations, having rigorous studies investigate the behavioral, social, and policy antecedents at play is clearly valuable as are more advanced studies that test possible structural-level and behavioral-intervention strategies. However, despite their importance to public health practice, none of these potential studies can realistically take advantage of the rigor added by a probability-sampling technique. The question then becomes, What does this mean in terms of public health research? The answer involves understanding the point that rigor has many components, with generalizability being only one. So, it is vital to develop your nonprobability study with as much rigor as possible and then be realistic about its generalizability once it is complete. This implies that your study conclusions should always be tempered by the limitations imposed by the sampling technique. A well-written conclusion should let the reader decide how much stock to put in the findings relative to their generalizability. Conversely, poorly written conclusions ignore the accompanying limitations and thus have a tendency to lead readers into a false belief about generalizability. **TABLE 10.4** provides examples of both well-written (i.e., fair) and poorly written (i.e., potentially misleading) conclusions.

TABLE 10.4 Examples of "Fair" and Potentially Misleading Conclusions from Studies Based on Nonprobability-Sampling Techniques

---

Fair Conclusions

Although limited by the use of a convenience sample, the findings from this longitudinal study suggest the possibility that people eat progressively more fresh produce as their level of income increases.

Based on a purposive sample of policy makers in Washington, D.C., this nonprobability sample of 53 people yielded findings that suggest climate change is the most common concern in the formulation of new policy related to the environment and to the economy as a whole.

Postprogram interviews with 199 people enrolled in weight-loss counseling programs found that the majority (79%) found the program to be "extremely helpful" in losing at least 10% of their body weight. This finding is limited by the use of a convenience sample of postprogram participants, so generalizability to all program participants is not ensured.

Snowball sampling was used to interview 33 women and 27 men diagnosed with opioid use disorder (OUD) and of reproductive age. Findings from these 60 people indicate that OUD was not a factor in their family-planning decisions. Given the limitations of a self-selected sample, it is possible that a disconnect may exist between OUD and contraceptive use among people of reproductive age.

Potentially Misleading

A telephone-based study of 212 congressional representatives found that those living in states nearest either coast were significantly more concerned about climate change compared with those living in noncoastal states. Noncoastal congressional representative may require added education and motivation before passing climate change legislation.

Based on quota sampling, we found that college students who are part of the Greek system are more likely to maintain a GPA above 3.0. Accordingly, the study findings support the ongoing existence and recognition of sororities and fraternities in the United States.

Our sample of homeless women yielded data showing that those living within 5 miles of a nonsecular shelter had significantly greater levels of optimism and hope for their future compared to those not living within five miles of a nonsecular shelter. Foundations, communities, and governmental agencies should allocate funds to create a greater geographic density of shelters for homeless women.

Think About It!

BOX 10.1 summarizes two studies that we quickly selected by looking only at one recent issue of the *American Journal of Public Health*. Read each study carefully and then consider the following questions.

- Is the sampling technique for study 1 adequate given the purpose of the study?
- Is either study relegated to only the individual level (meaning that the intervention is focused on changing knowledge, attitudes, beliefs, and behaviors)?
- Are the findings for study 1 compelling enough to place healthy food options in other tribally located stores in other states?
- Are the findings for study 2 compelling enough to engage in similar cleanup practices in other neighborhoods in both nearby and faraway neighborhoods (perhaps in other states)?

We suggest that the answers to the four questions just posed are, respectively, yes, no, yes, and yes. The larger point here is that public health is progressively becoming more centered on interventions that occur in an ecological framework—meaning that environments (including social, legal, and policy environments) are the focal point of change. As this shift away from centering efforts on individuals continues, it is likely that the universe of possible sampling techniques will shift in a corresponding manner. It may be, for instance, that probability methods become a staple for the selection of places rather than people and that nonprobability methods are expanded to encompass new techniques of sampling people within structures (meaning, for example, customers of grocery stores who provide healthy foods at a low cost).

BOX 10.1   Two Studies That Target Higher Levels in the Socioecological Model: Implications for Sampling

Study One: The Tribal Health and Resilience in Vulnerable Environments Study
Abstract

Objectives. To assess a healthy retail intervention in Tribal convenience stores in Oklahoma.

Methods. We adapted healthy retail strategies to the context of [eight] Tribally owned stores. We assessed individual- and store-level outcomes in a cluster-controlled intervention trial (April 2016–June 2017). We measured fruit and vegetable intake, store environment perceptions, and purchases before and after the intervention among a cohort of 1637 Native American shoppers. We used mixed-effects linear regression to estimate pre- to postintervention changes in and between groups.

Results. We followed 74 percent of participants ($n = 1204$) nine to 12 months. Intervention and control participants perceived healthier stores after intervention. Higher shopping frequency was related to purchases of fruits, vegetables, and healthy items.

Conclusions. Intervention exposure was associated with healthy purchasing but not fruit and vegetable intake. Research is needed to further assess impacts of environmental interventions on intake.

Public health implications. As the first healthy retail intervention in Tribally owned stores, our results contribute evidence for environmental and policy interventions to address obesity in Tribal Nations. Multicomponent interventions, led by Tribal leaders from diverse sectors, are needed to create healthy environments and sustainable improvements in Native American health.

Valarie Blue Bird Jernigan et al. "A Healthy Retail Intervention in Native American Convenience Stores: The THRIVE Community-Based Participatory Research Study", *American Journal of Public Health, 109*, no. 1 (January 1, 2019): pp. 132–139.

Study Two: Remediating Blighted Vacant Land
Abstract

Objectives. To determine if remediating blighted vacant urban land reduced firearm shooting incidents resulting in injury or death.

Methods. We conducted a cluster randomized controlled trial in which we assigned 541 randomly selected vacant lots in Philadelphia, Pennsylvania, to 110 geographically contiguous clusters; these clusters were randomly assigned to a greening intervention, a less-intensive mowing and trash-cleanup intervention, or a no-intervention control condition. The random assignment to the trial occurred in April and June 2013 and lasted until March 2015. In a difference-in-differences analysis, we assessed whether the two treatment conditions relative to the control condition reduced firearm shootings around vacant lots.

Results. During the trial, both the greening intervention, −6.8 percent (95-percent confidence interval [CI] = −10.6 percent, −2.7 percent), and the mowing and trash-cleanup intervention, −9.2 percent (95 percent CI = −13.2 percent, −4.8 percent), significantly reduced shootings. There was no evidence that the interventions displaced shootings into adjacent areas.

Conclusions. Remediating vacant land with inexpensive, scalable methods, including greening or minimal mowing and trash cleanup, significantly reduced shootings that result in serious injury or death.

Public Health Implications. Cities should experiment with place-based interventions to develop effective firearm violence–reduction strategies.

Ruth Moyer, John M. MacDonald, Greg Ridgeway, Charles C.Branas, "Effect of Remediating Blighted Vacant Land on Shootings: A Citywide Cluster Randomized Trial", *American Journal of Public Health, 109*, no. 1 (January 1, 2019): pp. 140–144.

Take Home Points

- Sampling can make or break the generalizability of a research study.
- The goal of sampling is perfect representativeness.
- Probability-sampling techniques provide the highest level of generalizability.
- Nonprobability-sampling techniques are warranted when there is no sampling frame or for studies that are not concerned with generalizability such as experiments that are evaluating public health interventions.
- Sampling selects elements, which can be people or organized units or entities (clusters). The selection of people versus clusters is dictated by the nature of the research question.
- The size of the sample does not equate with representativeness.
- Generalization is enhanced when study participation rates exceed 70%.

Key Terms

Convenience sampling
Element
Generalizability
Multistage cluster sampling
Nonprobability sampling
Participation rate
Periodicity

Population
Probability sampling
Purposive sampling
Quota sampling
Replacement
Sampling frame
Sampling technique

Seed
Simple random sampling
Snowball sampling
Stratified simple random sample
Systematic random sampling
Venue–day–time (VDT) sampling

For Practice and Discussion

1. Why is sampling so critical to the generalizability of a study? Explain the difference between probability and nonprobability sampling and provide an example of a situation when it would be appropriate to use each.

2. A public heath professor is planning a research study to examine the effects of an antibullying intervention on students' mental health and academic performance that is being implemented in middle schools in a New York school district.
   a. Explain what sampling elements the researcher would need to consider when planning the sampling for this study.
   b. Based on the study purpose, what would be the most appropriate sampling unit to use as the basis for the study sample?
   c. Would it be possible to obtain an exhaustive sampling frame for this sampling unit? Explain why or why not.

3. For each of the following sampling methods, explain whether it is a type of probability or nonprobability sampling and provide an example of a situation in which it would be appropriate to use this sampling method.
   a. Simple random sampling
   b. Multistage cluster sampling
   c. Convenience sampling
   d. Snowball sampling

4. What is a participation rate, and how does it relate to the representativeness and sample size of a population? Why is a participation rate important to the generalizability of a study?

References

Jernigan, V. B. B., Salvatore, A. L., Williams, M., Wetherill, M., Taniguchi, T., Jacob, T., . . . Noonan, C. (2019, January 1). A healthy retail intervention in Native American convenience stores: The THRIVE Community-Based Participatory Research Study. *American Journal of Public Health, 109*(1), 132–139.

McKellar, D. A., Gallagher, K. M., Finlayson, T., Sanchez, T., Lansky, A., & Sullivan, P. S. (2007). Surveillance of HIV and prevention behaviors of men who have sex with men: A national application of venue-based, time-space sampling. *Public Health Reports, 122*(Suppl. 1), 39–47.

Moyer, R., MacDonald, J. M.,. Ridgeway, G., & Branas, C. C. (2019, January 1). Effect of remediating blighted vacant land on shootings: A citywide cluster randomized trial. *American Journal of Public Health, 109*(1), 140–144.

For Further Reading

Crosby, R. A., Salazar, L. F., Holtgrave, D. R., & Head, S. (2007). Homelessness and HIV-associated risk behavior among African American men who inject drugs and reside in the urban south of the United States. *AIDS and Behavior, 11*, 70–75.

Shirani-Mehr, H., Rothschild, D., Goel, S. & Gelman, A. (2018) Disentangling bias and variance in election polls, *Journal of the American Statistical Association*, 113:522, 607–614.

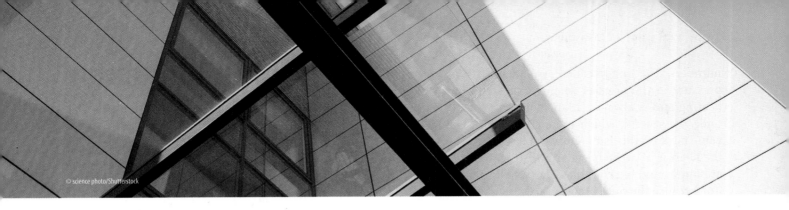
© science photo/Shutterstock

CHAPTER 11

Measurement

▶ Overview

Think about a typical day in your life. Chances are that your phone served as a way to sound an alarm designed to wake you this morning. Any hot foods or liquids you consumed throughout the day were most likely heated or cooled to the ideal temperature. If you drove or rode in a car or bus to work or school, the speed of that vehicle was constantly measured with a speedometer. As the day went on, you encountered countless other forms of measurement that you may not have given any thought to (e.g., how much data you have used on your cell phone plan, your Internet connection speed, or the size of the T-shirt you purchased). Just as measurement surrounds us in our daily lives, it is also ubiquitous in all public health research.

One common characteristic of public health research is its reliance on **triangulation** of measurement. As the term implies, triangulation of measurement facilitates validation of data through cross verification *from more than two sources*. The reason for triangulation involves understanding a basic premise of primary prevention, which is to focus public health interventions to improve quality of life, overall health, and wellness to avert disease and associated conditions. This ostensibly simple premise translates into a need for measurements across three levels. For example:

1. Self-reported measures of knowledge, attitudes, beliefs, and practices
2. Measures from clinical records of biological and physiological functions
3. Measures specific to the research study that are assessed based on specimen collection and analysis

Consider, for example, the common public health problem of hypertension (high blood pressure). To begin, you should know how this is defined. As you may or may not know, a blood-pressure reading (a type of measurement) involves two readings or numbers. The first is called *systolic* and refers to the pressure in the arteries when the heart pumps or is beating and is always a higher number than the second. The second, which is called *diastolic*, is a lesser value because this is the pressure in the arteries when the heart is between beats or is resting. Both numbers are important, but diastolic is especially vital to monitor because the only time the arteries have to recover is between heartbeats. The previous definition of what constituted high blood pressure used to be 140/90, however, this number has been changed to 130/80 as public health practice evolved. The leading causes of hypertension are sodium consumption, tobacco use, alcohol use, fatty plaques in the arteries that narrow the passageway, and chronic daily stress. Thus, numerous behaviors offer prevention opportunities for this condition. The behaviors, however, are linked to the causes, and the causes are linked to the actual outcome of blood pressure. **FIGURE 11.1** illustrates this chain of causation.

Looking carefully and thoughtfully at Figure 11.1, you can quickly see where the three levels of measurement previously noted come into play. To accentuate this, **TABLE 11.1** provides an example of the cause-and-effect model integrated into the three levels of measurement. As shown in the table, *behaviors* and *physical changes* are what public health researchers would want to measure to better understand the risk factors for hypertension and to evaluate interventions designed to reduce or prevent it. The measures are the different types of measurements we would use. Clinical records and tests from specimens are relatively straightforward and easy to understand.

TABLE 11.1 An Integration of Causal Chains and Levels of Measurement

Measures	Behaviors	Physical Changes
Self-report	Daily sodium intake	Enlarged ventricle
Clinical records	Frequency of tobacco use	Arterial edema
Tests from specimens	Frequency of aerobic exercise	Catecholamines
	Consumption of foods causing plaques	Lipid profiles
	Treatment for hypertension	Blood CO levels
	Use of cholesterol-lowering drugs	

This leaves the **self-reported measures**. Self-reported measures are survey items that ask people to report their behavior, but it also includes knowledge, intentions, attitudes, perceptions, beliefs, and so on, all forerunners to behavior change. In this context, self-report of health behaviors shown in the table is the most immediate indicator we can use to determine whether public health intervention efforts to

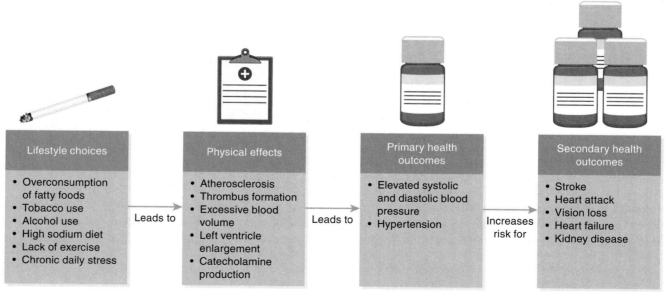

FIGURE 11.1 Chain of Causation Relative to Hypertension.

leverage behavior change actually worked. So, as you can imagine, at this stage, the entire research process becomes reliant on your ability to accurately assess behavior change via self-report. Because of the wide range of possibilities within measurement in the field of public health, the learning objectives for this chapter are broad.

▶ What Is a Construct?

Do you believe in things you cannot see? Your first answer might be a hesitant "No," but what about something such as self-confidence? When applied to changing health behaviors, the concept of self-confidence is often reconceptualized as a task-specific perception known as **self-efficacy**. Indeed, self-efficacy is a widely applied theoretical **construct**. A construct is an indicator variable that represents a hidden characteristic or a trait. In the example of hypertension, one important belief that may be measured by self-report is "self-efficacy to consume a low-sodium diet." This is, of course, "something you cannot see"—it is, instead, a term used by psychologists, sociologists, and others to represent this hidden trait. The term *self-efficacy* is important given that a first logical step in the primary prevention of hypertension would be to help people gain sufficient confidence in their ability to switch to a low-sodium diet. Without this confidence (operationalized now as "self-efficacy to consume a low-sodium diet"), it is unlikely that people will even attempt to make this all-so-important dietary change.

The reason why constructs are vital to understand and thus measure is that these are the stepping-stones to leveraging behavior change. Numerous examples exist in this regard, as shown in **FIGURE 11.2**. To summarize so far, a construct represents something that is not otherwise tangible, and it serves as an intermediate step between an intervention program and actual behavior change.

▶ How Do I Measure Constructs?

Because constructs are not directly observable, their accurate definition and measurement is an important aspect of valid and rigorous research. As an example, consider the construct of perceived risk for alcoholism. Let's say that you have operationalized this construct as: "beliefs about whether current drinking patterns will lead to problem drinking within the next 12 months." Notice also that a time frame is attached

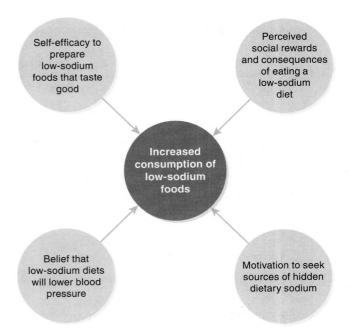

FIGURE 11.2 Common Constructs of Health Behavior Change.

to this definition (e.g., "within the next 12 months"). The most important word to notice, however, is *beliefs*. The plural use of this word implies that the measure will have to include multiple questions using a prescribed response format (this provides uniformity). The most common response formats are set up as five-point **Likert scales** like those shown in **FIGURE 11.3**, although some measures have seven-point or nine-point scale response options. A Likert scale is a type of rating scale used to measure constructs such as attitudes, beliefs, and perceptions. With this scale, respondents are asked to rate items on a level of agreement. For example:

Strongly Agree   Agree   Neutral
Disagree   Strongly Disagree

The scale doesn't always have to state "agree" or "disagree"; dozens of variations are possible on themes like agreement, frequency, quality, and importance. For example:

Agreement: Strongly Agree to Strongly Disagree

Frequency: Often to Never

Quality: Very Good to Very Bad

Likelihood: Definitely to Never

Importance: Very Important to Very Unimportant

These responses are called *Likert scale response anchors*. Once respondents have answered, numbers are assigned to the responses and then the

On a scale from 1 to 5, please indicate how much you agree or disagree with the statement shown below.

	Strongly disagree	Somewhat disagree	Neither agree nor disagree	Somewhat agree	Strongly agree
I drink heavily when I am depressed.	○	○	○	○	○

On a scale from 1 to 5, please indicate the extent to which you find the following statement easy or difficult.

	Very easy	Somewhat easy	Neither easy nor difficult	Somewhat difficult	Very difficult
Please indicate how easy or difficult it would be for you to not drink alcohol for 30 days in a row.	○	○	○	○	○

FIGURE 11.3 Examples of Scale Items and Corresponding Response Options.

responses are summed across all items to provide an overall score. This enables you to assign meaning to the responses and perform statistical analyses. For example,

Strongly Agree = 5   Agree = 4   Neutral = 3
Disagree = 2   Strongly Disagree = 1

As you can see in Figure 11.3, two different response anchors are used (i.e., "Strongly Agree" and "Very Difficult"), thus allowing you to tailor the anchor to the question asked. The one inflexible requirement is that you can only use one response anchor for the measurement of one construct. If, for instance, you are measuring the perceived risk of becoming a problem drinker in the next 12 months using seven items or statements, each item must have the same response anchor.

Now that you understand the basics, your next task is to understand what is meant by the type of measure known as a **scale**. In the parlance of measurement, a scale is a selected set of correlated questionnaire items created to assess a specific construct that has been operationally defined. Returning to the example, your seven questionnaire items that assess the "problem drinker" construct might be:

1. I rely on alcohol to provide psychological comfort.
2. I rely on alcohol for daily happiness.
3. Alcohol is embedded into my social life.
4. Alcohol is a part of my romantic or sexual relationships.
5. Alcohol leads me into decisions I later regret.
6. Alcohol use causes me to regret drinking.
7. Alcohol makes me feel more attractive.

Thinking back to Figure 11.3, you would use a response anchor for this set of seven questions that ranged from 5 ("Strongly Agree") to 1 ("Strongly Disagree"). At this point, you have a scale that is ready to be tested for what is known as **reliability**. If that scale passes the reliability test, you would feel confident it would perform consistently for the same sample, but you would still need to subject it to a test of **validity**. Reliability refers to the *consistency* of the scale. A good analogy here is an old-fashioned bathroom scale. A bathroom scale is considered reliable if it consistently tells you what your weight is. So, given that you have not gained or lost any weight, the scale should tell you the same weight every time you step on it. With a scale measure of a construct, the scale should also provide the same or a similar score for a person on multiple assessments given no change in the construct being measured. For example, if you fill out a survey that measures your self-efficacy to exercise, given no intervention or no changes, you should have the same score more or less for each time you fill out the survey. Another issue related to reliability is that scale measures are also expected to consist of correlated questionnaire items, meaning your response on one item should correlate highly with your response on other items. Now let's turn our attention to an **index** and how this differs from a scale.

Unlike a scale, an index is typically *not* a set of correlated questionnaire items. Instead, an index is a set of questionnaire items that independently add to the measure of something that may, in fact, be tangible. Please notice two points from this last sentence: (1) *independently add* and (2) *something that may, in fact, be tangible*. To the first point, index items are not expected to be correlated with one another. Instead, each item in an index provides its own unique contribution to explaining the construct at hand. This means that how someone responds to one item ("most of the time") does not necessarily correlate with responses on the other items. To the second point, an index may be assessing something that is a composite of observable quantities. To better explain both the first and second points, consider the Life Events Checklist (LEC). The LEC assesses people's exposure to certain events that are considered stressful such as experiencing a natural disaster, a life-threatening illness or injury, a divorce, a sexual assault or any other type of assault, exposure to a toxic substance, and so on. As you can imagine from thinking about this example of an index, it is more objective than a scale because it involves measurement of more tangible factors: life events. Also, because these items are not necessarily related to each other, they are more heterogeneous, meaning they are not necessarily correlated. For example, experiencing a natural disaster is not necessarily related to experiencing a divorce. Reliability is infrequently assessed for an index. On the other hand, because the items on a scale measure should be correlated, reliability needs to be assessed to determine whether the items consistently provide the same results when assessing the target construct.

▶ How Can Scale Reliability and Validity Be Assessed?

One critical note before we describe the different methods of assessing reliability and validity for scale measures is that reliability and validity for a scale or index (or both) is *sample dependent*. This means that the reliability and validity for a scale or index or both are not intrinsic characteristics of the scale or index, but instead are a function of the sample with which these statistics were assessed. Thus, for one sample drawn, the scale or index might be reliable and valid; however, for a sample drawn from a different population, the same may not be true. Thus, if you use an existing measure that has established reliability and validity for a particular population, you will need to reassess both with your sample because they may differ, especially if your sample represents a different population.

There are three basic methods to assess the reliability of a scale measure. Each involves administering the scale and collecting a data set of responses with those responses being represented typically as numbers ranging from 1 to 5. With data from at least 30 people, a software program can then calculate the internal consistency of the items, which evaluates the degree to which different test items probing the same construct produce similar results. Internal consistency involves assessing the interitem correlations among all items in the scale and then taking the average. The ideal range of **average interitem correlation** is 0.15 to 0.50; less than this means the items are not well correlated and are not measuring the same construct or idea well (if at all). More than 0.50, and the items are so close as to be almost repetitive. Another reliability method is calculating a statistic called **Cronbach's alpha**, which takes into its formula the number of items in the scale, the average covariance between item pairs, and the average variance. Because Cronbach's alpha is sensitive to the number of items in the scale, its value will be much larger for scales that consist of a large number of items. A computer-generated value (ranging from 0 to 1.0) for Cronbach's alpha provides an indication of reliability. As a general rule, a Cronbach's alpha coefficient greater than 0.70 supports the reliability of the measure.

A third method of testing scale reliability is called **test–retest** and involves administering the scale measure on two occasions separated by a time span of days or weeks. As an example, you might have 40 people complete the seven-item problem-drinking scale and then invite each one to complete this same set of questions again in 30 days. Your data set would then double in size, but this allows you to apply a computer test that correlates the score from each person at time 1 to his or her score 30 days later. Again, if this correlation were greater than 0.70, you would have support for reliability of the scale.

Once reliability is established, your next step is to assess the measure for validity to determine whether it is measuring what it is supposed to measure. Going back to the bathroom scale analogy, even if your scale is reliable—meaning it says you weigh the same amount day after day given no real change in your weight—it still should be valid. Unfortunately, when you go to the doctor for an annual physical, the scale at the doctor's office says you weigh 10 pounds more. A sad *tale of two scales* indeed (see **FIGURE 11.4**). Thus, your bathroom scale has been consistent but not valid. With measuring intangible constructs, your scale must be not only reliable but also valid. A general rule is that you can have a scale that is reliable but not valid (like the bathroom scale), but you *cannot* have a scale that is valid but not reliable.

BOX 11.1 provides you with further practice in this regard by summarizing a study that tested the reliability and the validity of a scale measure. Please notice in this example that the scale being tested did indeed achieve reliability but not validity. Thus, we included

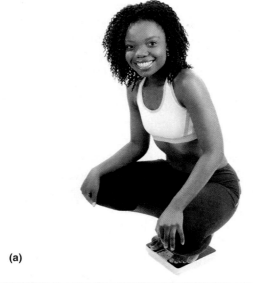

(a)

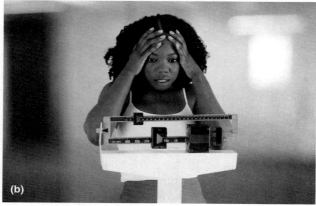

(b)

FIGURE 11.4 A Tale of Two Scales: **(a)** A Reliable But Not Valid Scale Measure of Weight; **(b)** A Valid Scale Measure of Weight.

(a) © Norman Pogson/Shutterstock; (b) © Rocketclips, Inc./Shutterstock

this example to accentuate the point that, despite being reliable, validity may or may not be established. Clearly, as you read about this study featured in Box 11.1, you will see that the research team devoted ample time, attention, and resources to this psychometric study—yet the resulting measure is simply not valid.

We describe two forms of validity, although there are many more. The first type is known as **construct validity**. Construct validity means that your measure indeed measures what it is supposed to based on the theory behind it and evidenced by its correlation with another existing scale measure of the same construct. Consider, for example, that you locate another scale that consists of 44 items measuring problem drinking. The measure is described in a peer-reviewed journal article, and evidence of its reliability and validity are presented. The issue for you, however, is that 44 items is long and would overwhelm your study sample, so you would rather use your newly developed seven-item short measure. To reconcile this issue, the solution lies in trusty data collection. You would administer both the 44-item version and the seven-item version of the scales to a small study sample of 30 or more people. The resulting data set would then give you the ability to obtain a correlation coefficient indicating the ability of the seven-item scale to represent the 44-item measure fairly. If favorable (0.70 or more), you would be the proud developer of a brief measure that reliably and accurately (i.e., valid) measures problem drinking.

The second type of validity is known as **criterion validity**. Criterion validity is how well your scale measure predicts an outcome that it should be associated with. Once again, this method involves a correlation coefficient. As the word *criterion* implies, the method relies on a different but objective measure to validate your scale measure (remember, a scale measure assesses a construct, something that is not tangible). Returning to our problem-drinking example, consider for a moment the possible objective behaviors that could be used to test our seven-item measure for criterion validity. These might include:

- Number of drunk-driving arrests
- Low grade-point average

BOX 11.1 Summary of a Psychometric Study of the Treatment Expectations in Chronic Pain Scale

In a 2019 journal article, Page and colleagues described the development of the Treatment Expectations in Chronic Pain (TEC) scale. The need for this measure pertained to noncancer patients who were considering treatment for long-term chronic pain. The research team carefully developed scale items and used a panel of clinicians and patients to help with item wording. The final scale comprised nine items. This scale was then tested for interitem reliability using Cronbach's alpha, with the obtained coefficient being 0.87. Given this established reliability, the scale was then tested for construct validity. This test took the form of assessing the correlation between the TEC scores (based on a sample of 522 patients experiencing chronic pain) and a measure of optimism, with the expectation of a significant and positive correlation between the two constructs. Unfortunately, the obtained correlation coefficient was low ($r = 0.24$), so the article could not conclude that the scale was valid (Page, Ziemianski, Martel, & Shir, 2019).

BOX 11.2 Summary of Study Establishing the Reliability and Validity of Scale

Given the urgency of the HIV epidemic among young Black men who have sex with men (YBMSM) in the United States, it is imperative to apply the full strength and weight of behavioral science to the prevention of this epidemic. The ultimate goal of applying behavioral science principles to this challenge is to promote an ethic of consistent and correct condom use among YBMSM at risk of HIV acquisition or transmission. A preliminary step to this goal is to measure the barriers to condom use as experienced by this population. A recent study described the test of the Condom Barriers Scale (CBS) for an extremely high-risk population of YBMSM residing in the southern United States; the scale had not been previously assessed for reliability or validity with any population of men having sex with men.

The CBS is a 26-item scale measure that was developed for heterosexuals. In previous studies of heterosexuals, it obtained strong evidence of reliability and validity. In the study summarized here, however, the researchers tested a much shorter version of the CBS, one comprising only 14 items. Each item was scored on a five-point Likert scale ranging from 1 (strongly disagree) to 5 (strongly agree). Because each question was worded as a barrier to condom use, lower scores suggest fewer barriers, and higher scores suggest a greater number of barriers.

The 14-item CBS was first adapted with changes in wording for the population of YBMSM. As is true for its 26-item counterpart, the 14-item version contained three subscales: partner-related barriers, sensation-related barriers, and motivation-related barriers. Each subscale was first tested for reliability using Cronbach's alpha and then tested for criterion validity. The tests for criterion validity comprised measures of association between each subscale and several different measures of condom use.

First, the researchers reported that all three subscales were reliable: (1) The partner-related barriers subscale had a Cronbach's alpha of 0.73, (2) the sensation-related barriers subscale had an alpha of 0.70, and (3) the motivation-related barriers subscale had an alpha of 0.81. Second, subscales were each significantly (all = $P < 0.001$) associated with reporting *any* condomless sex (a set of dichotomous variables assessed using several different measures). Further, the subscales were each significantly (all = $P < 0.001$) associated with a set of measures of condomless sex preserved at a continuous level. Moreover, the subscales were each significantly associated with reporting any condom use problems (all = $P < 0.001$) and a measure of condomless oral sex (all = $P < 0.001$, except for partner-related barriers = 0.31). Finally, the sensation-related barriers subscale was significantly associated with testing positive for chlamydia or gonorrhea ($P = 0.049$). Thus, the shortened version and its subscales demonstrated acceptable reliability and validity with the targeted population of YBMSM.

Modified from Crosby, R. A., Sanders, S. A., Graham, C. A., Milhausen, R., Yarber, W. L., & Mena, L. (2017). Evaluation of the Condom Barriers Scale for young black MSM: Reliability and validity of three sub-scales. *Sexually Transmitted Disease, 44*, 91–95.

- Binge drinking
- Absences from class or work

Let's say that you select the first option in this bulleted list. Your task would then be to ascertain the number of arrests that involved an alcohol-related behavior among study volunteers who also complete the seven-item measure of problem drinking. With these data, you could then ask your computer to faithfully calculate a correlation coefficient between the sum of the seven-item scale measure and number of arrests. As you may have guessed, a value of 0.70 or greater means you are good to go.

BOX 11.2 provides an example of a psychometric study that used multiple outcome measures to establish the criterion validity of a scale measure (please note that the study began by establishing reliability because that is the obligatory first step in achieving validity). Please also notice as you read Box 11.2, that criterion validity was established through the use of multiple tests of association with the expected behavioral outcomes, with all except one of these tests being significant. Even more important, one of the subscales

was also significantly associated with an expected biological outcome.

How Can I Optimize the Precision of Self-Reported Data?

So far in this chapter we have focused on *what* to measure rather than *how* to measure. The *how* is now our focus. Although paper-and-pencil assessment methods are still in use for taking tests and filling out surveys, this method is fraught with issues. These include literacy issues, survey burden, not following skip patterns, and being afraid that answers will be linked with your name. The first three of these possibilities are, fortunately, ameliorated by the use of a **computer-assisted self-interview (CASI)**. CASI is a technique for survey data collection in which the respondent uses a computer to complete the survey questionnaire without an interviewer administering it to the respondent. This assumes the respondent can read well enough to complete the questions. In the event that literacy may be an issue with your population, optional audio is available in which the audio is played for the respondent one question at a time (i.e., audio computer-assisted self-interviewing—A-CASI). Both CASI and A-CASI can be programmed to automatically navigate skip patterns, thereby ensuring 100% compliance with rules and simultaneous reduction of the survey burden, meaning the survey takes less time for participants to read (or to listen) and complete. With carefully designed messages, it is also possible to assure study participants that their responses are linked to their names only through a study ID code (a code known only to you as the investigator). A great advantage of A-CASI is that it can be administered online, thereby negating a need for study participants to meet with you in person, as is the case with paper-and-pencil methods.

Yet another method of increasing the precision in self-reported measure involves *when* the measures are taken. Known as **ecological momentary assessment (EMA)**, this method relies on various forms of technology to take measures on a frequent basis (anyone who has used a wrist device to measure the number of miles they move, walk, or run per day is already familiar with this method). An EMA can take on many forms. One popular form involves texting survey questions. This method sends a select few questions to study participants on a planned basis (see **FIGURE 11.5**). By sending the same set of questions on a repeated basis—once per week for example—the data for any given measure accumulate over time. Let's begin with the simple example of marijuana use. Rather than ask a question such as, "In the past 60 days, how many times have you used

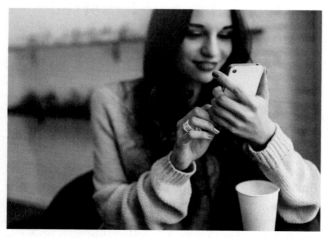

FIGURE 11.5 Young College Student Completing Texting Survey.

© Svitlana Sokolova/Shutterstock

marijuana to get high?" either by paper-and-pencil survey or by CASI, you could text the question, "Did you use marijuana to get high today?" every day over 60 days. By adding the response values for each text message, you would know exactly how many times they used marijuana and would have a 60-day total. This total would ideally be a more valid indicator of the number of times marijuana was used because forgetting and guessing would be minimized in contrast to having people recall how often they used marijuana over an entire 60-day period. Note, however, that this facilitation of accuracy and recall applies to people who use marijuana frequently rather than those who may get high just once every month or every few months.

One key consideration in using an EMA-type of approach to assessment involves the question of how often to send the survey items containing the set of repeated questions. The planned sequence could be, for example, once each week for 2 months, with the "once" being a day of the week agreed on by the researcher and the study participant. Alternatively, the planned sequence may not be linear in time: It may be random. The use of a random pattern is best suited to capturing complex and unpredictable outcomes such as experiencing anger, depression, or binge eating. In addition, innovative studies involving assessment of substance use or tobacco, use EMA to assess exposure to advertising, for example, and then subsequent behaviors and risk perceptions to document associations in real time (e.g., Hébert et al., 2017; Setodji, Martino, Scharf, & Shadel, 2014).

A final how-to strategy we would suggest you learn to employ is known as the **timeline follow-back method**. This method facilitates recall in studies that may not have the advantage of using a form of EMA. This method involves a face-to-face interview and it can be used (and most often is used) at study enrollment. It is best suited for measures that are difficult for most people to remember with accuracy. For instance, imagine you were conducting a study of medication adherence for people with high blood pressure. Your task at study enrollment is to accurately assess how often people have missed days of medication in the past calendar month. You would begin the assessment with an actual calendar in front of both of you. You would then begin the interview by asking, "Can you remember which days on the calendar may have been days when you completely forgot to take your blood pressure medication?" The person may need time to reflect and prompting on your part to encourage a response. For example, you could ask, "What about a day during a weekend when you were not at home?" As the person begins to identify 1 or 2 days of missed medication you would look for patterns. For example, are the days the person missed his or her medication on the same day of the week? Was it the case that the 2 days the person missed medication, for example, were a consecutive Saturday and Sunday? Once you develop a working theory as to why people may miss days, you can then ask follow-up questions. Let's say, for instance, that the person selects two Sundays on the calendar as days he or she definitely forgot to take meds. You might then ask, "Is there something about Sundays that makes you forget to take medication?" The point here is less about being right in your hunches and more about encouraging the person to think about and talk openly about what may trigger his or her lack of adherence to medication. This may prompt the person to think of other days of the month they forgot to take their medication; together, you would mark these days as missed on the calendar in front of you both.

▶ What Are the Two Main Types of Measurement Error?

Ultimately, all measures have some degree of error. As this degree of error increases, our confidence in the validity of the measure decreases. Measurement error can stem from numerous sources and can be classified as either **random** or **systematic**. As its name implies, random error is caused by any factor that randomly affects the measurement of the variable. For example, the way a person *feels* (e.g., mood, energy level, attention level) on a certain day may influence how he or she answers a particular question on a survey and could conceivably affect his or her score upward or downward. The good thing about random error is that it does not have consistent effects across the entire sample because its effects are likely to be evenly distributed around the mean score for any given questionnaire item. Essentially, this form of error pushes observed scores up or down randomly. If we plotted the random errors in a distribution, they should sum to zero because there would be as many negative errors as positive ones. Unfortunately, random error cannot be controlled, and it reduces the reliability of the measurement resulting in a loss of statistical power; however, it does not affect the average for the group. Random error is sometimes referred to as **noise**.

Another form of measurement error is **systematic error**. Systematic error is any kind of measurement error that leads to systematic (that is, nonrandom) differences between the observed measurement and

its true value, and it will influence the true mean (in either direction). Unlike random error, the effect of systematic error is not reduced when observations are averaged. Systematic errors are introduced by an inaccuracy involving either the observation or the measurement *process*, factors that will affect the entire sample. Unlike random error, systematic errors:

- Tend to be consistently either positive or negative
- May be predictable and, therefore, attenuated or eliminated
- Result in bias in the measurement of the variable
- Reduce the accuracy of measurements, or
- Yield potentially erroneous conclusions

When the data have been collected and it is time for analysis, it is important to know that systematic error can act to either attenuate (decrease) or inflate measures of association (e.g., correlation coefficients, odds ratios) between two variables or an exposure and a disease, depending on your research question. Thus, systematic error is a serious issue (see FIGURE 11.6) that necessitates creating procedures for addressing it. Although there are multiple forms of systematic error, one specific and problematic type that affects public health research is **recall bias**, which occurs when participants are asked about events, behaviors, and so on that have occurred in the past. Differences in the accuracy or completeness of the recollections retrieved ("recalled") by study participants regarding events or experiences from the past introduce bias or error into the measurement of the variable. Recall bias is a serious concern especially in case-control studies or retrospective cohort studies (Coughlin, 1990).

To accelerate your learning of random versus systematic error, consider two different studies of the

DON'T GET CAUGHT WITH

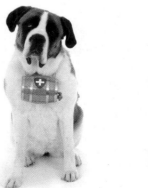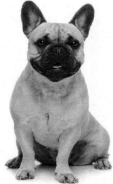

SYSTEMATIC ERROR—CONTROL IT!

FIGURE 11.6 Public Health Mascots Snow's and Hamilton's Words of Wisdom on Measurement Error.

© Eric Isselee/Shutterstock; © Svetography/Shutterstock

same population of people and of the same health behavior. The population is people 30 to 44 years of age (defined as young adults), and the health behavior is the consumption of refined sugars. The measurement aspects of these two studies are described in **BOX 11.3**.

Given the phenomenon of **social desirability bias** (a form of systematic error that occurs when people want to avoid embarrassment and project a favorable image to others and want to appear better than they really are), as you look at the wording of the items and the two modes of administration, you can imagine that the scores would most likely be lower for people in Study 2 compared with people in Study 1. This does not mean that the two questions are *perfectly* reliable—indeed, random error could affect each study. Given the mode of administration, however, it is likely (highly likely) that systematic error was operating in Study 2. To illustrate this point, we have fabricated possible answers for 12 people in Study 1 and 12 more in Study 2. **BOX 11.4** displays theses values, using two columns for each study (one is the "true" score and the other is the actual score).

As you inspect Box 11.4, please look carefully at the means. You will see that the 12 people enrolled in Study 2 underreported their sugar consumption by around three servings on average. In contrast, the true mean and the obtained mean in Study 1 are off by only one serving. Once again, this is because random error occurred in Study 1; however, it is apparent that Study 2 was most likely a victim of systematic error from social desirability bias.

▶ How Does It All "Fit Together"?

We fully recognize that what you have been learning in this chapter is far from easy. In many ways, learning about the principles regarding measurement in public health is a bit of a piecemeal exercise. To help you gain some practice in moving from a basic understanding of the principles to a sense of how to blend these into a coherent set of actions, we have created the following vignette. In what follows, we have left key notes for you.

The vignette begins with you being an evaluation researcher in a state department of public health.

BOX 11.3 Two Modes of Survey Administration: SAQ Versus IAQ

Study One

This study used a self-administered questionnaire (SAQ) to assess the average weekly consumption of refined sugars. Because it was given online, study volunteers completed the SAQ at a time and location of their choosing. Three questions were asked.

In the past 7 days, about how many servings have you consumed of:

1. Foods classified as desserts (puddings, pies, cakes, chocolates, cookies, or ice cream).
   Write in the number of servings: _____
2. Foods classified as condiments or sauces such as ketchup, barbeque sauce, sweetened salad dressings, meat glazes, or whipped toppings.
   Write in the number of servings: _____

Study Two

This study used an interviewer-administered questionnaire (IAQ) to assess the average weekly consumption of refined sugars. The same two questions were asked in a private, face-to-face setting. Because the study is principally about the emerging problem of adult-onset diabetes, the interviews were conducted in clinical settings.

Interviewer: Begin by asking the following question and then prompt people to provide an answer in the form of a number.

"In the past 7 days, about how many servings have you consumed of foods classified as desserts—such as puddings, pies, cakes, chocolates, cookies, or ice cream?"

Interviewer: Continue by asking the following question and then prompting people to provide an answer in the form of a number.

"In the past seven days, about how many servings have you consumed of foods classified as condiments or sauces—such as ketchup, barbeque sauce, sweetened salad dressings, meat glazes, or whipped toppings?"

BOX 11.4   Hypothetical Data for Two Studies Varying Mode of Survey Administration: Study 1 (Self-Administered) Versus Study 2 (Interviewer Administered)

Please note that in Study 1, different days (Sunday versus Wednesday) and times (6 PM versus 2 AM) in which people completed their survey resulted in answers that were either slightly over- or underreported. By contrast, in Study 2, social desirability bias led people to always underreport their response to the nearest value of 5. Hypothetically, the two study populations should be approximately the same in their food habits (i.e., their "true" scores). However, given these two forms of error (one random and one systematic), their scores are quite different ($M = 11.66$ versus $M = 8.75$) and would suggest different conclusions.

"True" Scores	Study One Scores	"True" Scores	Study Two Scores
14	12	14	08
12	14	12	07
19	17	19	13
11	13	11	08
07	06	07	03
13	14	13	09
14	12	14	11
13	16	13	09
04	02	04	01
12	14	12	10
06	05	06	04
14	15	14	10
10.58	11.66	10.58	7.75

You have been asked to evaluate a statewide program designed to promote responsible drinking. You begin by developing an instrument that will assess current practices of people in your state before the program begins. You have unlimited funds for this, so your options are open in terms of how you administer this instrument.

> *Note*: So far, you have the word *instrument* (this is a collection of the items constituting your assessment) and the word *administer* (this is the method for collecting the data).

Your intuition tells you to collect quantitative data that represents frequency of behaviors and would range from zero onward, thus avoiding the use of Likert scales or categories. So you begin to develop items that will measure how often people engage in behaviors such as binge drinking, daily drinking, driving while drunk, and so on.

> *Note*: These items are all assessing behaviors; they are not getting at intangible things (i.e., constructs). Things may get a bit more complicated as you keep working on the instrument.

Next, you want your instrument to measure (1) attitudes toward binge drinking, (2) beliefs about alcoholism, and (3) beliefs about drinking alone as a sign of alcoholism. You realize that each of these three variables is considered a construct; therefore, you know that each one can only be measured by a scale instrument. You look for reliable and valid scale measures; fortunately for you, you find an existing measure for each.

Note: Although the previous research with the scale measures shows that the Cronbach's alpha was 0.70 or greater, indicating scale reliability, and there was support for the validity of the scale, you understand that for your study, you must reassess both with your sample because reliability and validity of scales vary from one population to another.

Next, you decide you want to measure *neighborhood cohesion* as a variable for your evaluation. You create a five-item index that you also include in the instrument. With that, you decide the instrument is ready. Then you debate whether this will be self-administered or interviewer administered. You ultimately realize that recall bias may be an issue that introduces measurement error, so you go with the interview-administered option. You train a team of interviewers in a technique known as *cognitive interviewing*, a method used to facilitate recall. You justify the added expense of this training as a way to enhance validity. You also decide to enhance validity by declaring that interviews can only be done in the setting of a private phone call because interviewing people in groups, in places that lack privacy, or in places that may skew the responses (such as a bar or place of worship) will introduce bias.

Note: You have now made major decisions about the method. Your choice was a good one, but it does not entirely eliminate measurement error. You were wise to take precautions against both a respondent factor (i.e., recall bias) and a setting factor (i.e., privacy and physical places that may introduce systematic error. Think about this: Interviews in bars might inflate answers regarding drinking behaviors, and interviews in places of worship might consistently underestimate true drinking behaviors.)

After a pilot test of your instrument and your method, you suspect that recall bias may still be an issue even with the trained interviewers. To help resolve this, you change the items assessing drinking behavior so they use a 7-day recall period rather than 30 days (as you had initially written). You wisely also build in a timeline follow-back method into the interview. Before you finally launch the massive statewide survey, you make one last big decision. You decide you want to take a subsample of the respondents (at random) and ask them to carry and use a self-test for blood alcohol level, on a daily basis for 7 days. This is thus a second method, and now you have a strategy.

Note: Please notice three key terms in this vignette—(1) Items are the questions used to measure something, (2) a method is the way you administer a given set of items, and (3) a strategy is used when you need more than one method to complete the assessments. Remember that the strategy is the collection of methods. The biological measure in this vignette adds validity to your evaluation.

Think About It!

As you learned in this chapter, ecological momentary assessments are often used to help reduce measurement error. One important side note to an EMA is that this approach is somewhat of a constant reminder to people that they are enrolled in a study. This point raises the question of whether simply being enrolled in a study and completing repeated assessments may actually be a type of intervention because it alters behavior. For example, have you ever been asked to keep a food consumption diary for a week or more? If so, did the mere act of recording on paper whatever you ate or drank affect your dietary habits? We bet your answer is "Yes," and the reason we are making this bet has to do with a phenomenon known as the *Hawthorne effect*.

So, now you are asking yourself, What is the Hawthorne effect? Simply stated, the Hawthorne effect is a type of reactivity in which people who are aware they are being observed modify some aspect of their behavior. The effect is named after a somewhat famous study occurring in the 1940s that sought to determine whether improved lighting conditions in a factory setting would increase worker productivity. The irony of the study was that workers in the experimental group (building with increased lighting) and the control group (building *without* increased lighting) both demonstrated greater productivity. Thus, behavior was altered regardless of lighting, leading researchers to conclude that simply being observed led to behavior change. Although we are not suggesting this scenario would equate with changes to health behavior practices as a function of being studied (because the Hawthorne study occurred in a place of employment), it is typically accepted that the perception of being observed or measured has the potential to alter health behavior, albeit temporarily.

Given the Hawthorne effect, a few logical questions become of direct relevance to public health promotion efforts: "Would an ongoing EMA be an effective method to change health behaviors?" "Can we make use of the real-time assessments to provide real-time tailored feedback for intervention purposes"? Indeed, a systematic review by Heron and Smyth (2010) examined studies that implemented *ecological momentary interventions* (EMIs) and documented the efficacy of these EMIs in various fields such as weight control, anxiety regulation, and diabetes management. Furthermore, a recent meta-analysis by Wang and Miller (2019) documented moderate to large effect sizes for what are called *just-in-time, adaptive interventions* (JITAIs). JITAIs are similar to EMIs and are an emerging type of intervention that provides *tailored support at the exact time of need*. JITAIs do so by using new technologies (e.g., mobile phones, sensors) that capture the changing states of individuals. Thus, from a practice perspective (as opposed to a measurement method), using EMIs or JITAIs to provide real-time tailored feedback as an effective behavior-change strategy holds great potential and should be further investigated for possible applications in future public health programs. We strongly encourage you to think about it.

Take Home Points

- Reliable and valid measures are the basis of any rigorous research study.
- Reliability and validity are sample dependent and need to be reassessed for each new population studied.
- Measures should ideally be triangulated, meaning that you should use a combination of biological measures, measures from clinical records, and self-reported measures.
- Self-reported measures are especially susceptible to both random error and systematic error.

- In the social and behavioral sciences, an important type of self-reported measure is one that assesses something that is intangible; this is a construct.
- Constructs are assessed by scales that need to be tested for reliability (i.e., consistency) and validity (i.e., accuracy) with each new population.
- There are multiple options available for designing studies that collect self-reported data: Choosing the appropriate method for the research study is an obligation of the researcher.

Key Terms

Average interitem correlation
Computer-assisted self interview (CASI)
Construct
Construct validity
Criterion validity
Cronbach's alpha
Ecological momentary assessment (EMA)

Index
Likert scales
Noise
Random
Recall bias
Reliability
Scale
Self-efficacy
Self-reported measures

Social desirability bias
Systematic
Systematic error
Test–retest
Timeline follow-back method
Triangulation
Validity

For Discussion and Practice

1. Consider the public health problem of HIV prevention and the measurement concept of triangulation. What three sources of measurement could be used to assess HIV prevention, according to the three types described in this chapter? Be specific about what each type of measurement will assess and how it will be assessed.

2. What is the difference between validity and reliability, and why are both important in the measurement of constructs? Explain how scale reliability and validity can be established. Explain what is meant by "reliability and validity are sample dependent."

3. The scale that you developed has a Cronbach's alpha of 0.61. Does this sufficiently support the reliability of your scale? Explain why or why not. What are other ways you can assess the reliability of your scale?

4. You develop a scale to assess self-efficacy for condom use and find that it is highly correlated with condom use attitudes. Identify which type of validity applies to this situation and explain why.

5. You are conducting a new research study that will assess illicit behaviors among a sample of college students. Students will be recruited online and will be asked to answer questions about their tobacco use, opioid use, alcohol use, and cannabis or marijuana use. What time-referent period should you use to assess these behaviors? What are the different sources of random and systematic errors? What are the ways in which you can potentially control for the systematic errors?

References

Coughlin, S. S. (1990). Recall bias in epidemiologic studies. *Journal of Clinical Epidemiology, 43*(1), 87–91.

Crosby, R. A., Sanders, S. A., Graham, C. A., Milhausen, R., Yarber, W. L., & Mena, L. (2017). Evaluation of the Condom Barriers Scale for young black MSM: Reliability and validity of three sub-scales. *Sexually Transmitted Disease, 44,* 91–95.

Hébert, E. T., Vandewater, E. A., Businelle, M. S., Harrell, M. B., Kelder, S. H., & Perry, C. L. (2017). Feasibility and reliability of a mobile tool to evaluate exposure to tobacco product marketing and messages using ecological momentary assessment. *Addictive Behaviors, 73,* 105–110.

Heron, K. E., & Smyth, J. M. (2010). Ecological momentary interventions: Incorporating mobile technology into psychosocial and health behaviour treatments. *British Journal of Health Psychology, 15*(1), 1–39.

Page, M. G., Ziemianski, D., Martel, M. O., & Shir, Y. (2019). Development and validation of the Treatment Expectations in Chronic Pain scale. *British Journal of Health Psychology, 24,* 610–628.

Setodji, C. M., Martino, S. C., Scharf, D. M., & Shadel, W. G. (2014). Quantifying the persistence of pro-smoking media effects on college students' smoking risk. *Journal of Adolescent Health, 54*(4), 474–480.

Wang, L., & Miller, L. C. (2019, September 5). Just-in-the-Moment Adaptive Interventions (JITAI): A meta-analytical review. *Health Communication,* 1–14.

For Further Reading

Heale, R., & Twycross, A. (2015). Validity and reliability in quantitative studies. *Evidence Based Nursing, 18*(3), 66–67.

Jones, A., Remmerswaal, D., Verveer, I., Robinson, E., Franken, I. H. A., . . . , & Field, M. (2019). Compliance with ecological momentary assessment protocols in substance users: A meta-analysis, *Addiction, 114,* 609–619.

Rowe, C., Hern, J., DeMartini, A., Jennings, D., Sommers, M., . . . , & Santos, G.M. (2016). Concordance of text message ecological momentary assessment and retrospective survey data among substance-using men who have sex with men: A secondary analysis of a randomized controlled trial. *JMIR Mhealth Uhealth, 4*(2), e44.

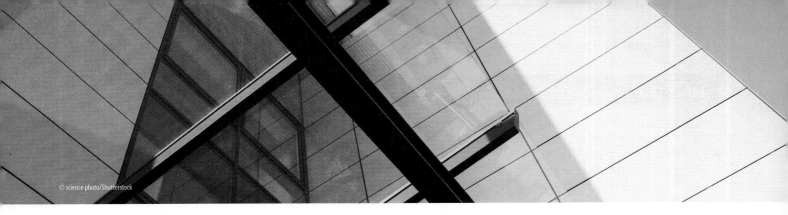

CHAPTER 12

Data Management and Cleaning

LEARNING OBJECTIVES

1. Understand the three basic tasks of data management.
2. Understand the concept of central tendency and associated attributes such as the mean, median, and mode.
3. Describe the concept of variability, specifically variance, and standard deviation, and explain their overall importance to statistical analysis.
4. Explain why proportionally smaller standard deviations are preferred to those that are proportionally large.
5. Learn the basic properties of a normal curve.
6. Understand the basics of graphing data.

▶ Overview

If you have conducted your study—meaning you identified the gaps, developed the research question, chose your study design, selected your sampling strategy, recruited your sample, collected the data, and organized it into a data set (phew!)—you are ready for data analysis. The data set is the product of all this arduous work; as such, it deserves a great deal of time and attention, which comes in the form of data management. A key aspect of the data-management process involves what is known as data *cleaning*, a term used to denote multiple tasks designed to ensure validity of your data. Once your data have been cleaned, the next steps involve running basic statistical procedures related to ensuring the data are cleaned and to answering your research questions. This chapter will teach you basics of data management

and cleaning skills. Although these tasks are not glamorous compared with the excitement and discovery of data analysis, they are nonetheless vital, essential, and absolutely indispensable for all subsequent discoveries produced by the study.

▶ Why Is Data Management So Critical?

A critical step in data management is ensuring that your data are protected during the entire data-collection period. You must have a process in place that adheres to standard guidelines for data-collection storage, sharing, and use. **TABLE 12.1** provides 10 guiding principles to help with this process for securing your data, keeping your data confidential, and guarding against loss or accidental destruction

TABLE 12.1 Ten Guiding Principles for Data Collection, Storage, and Use to Ensure Data Security and Confidentiality

1. Public health data should be acquired, used, disclosed, and stored for legitimate public health purposes.
2. Programs should collect the minimum amount of personally identifiable information necessary to conduct public health activities.
3. Programs should have strong policies to protect the privacy and security of personally identifiable data.
4. Data-collection and use policies should reflect respect for the rights of individuals and community groups and minimize undue burden.
5. Programs should have policies and procedures to ensure the quality of any data they collect or use.
6. Programs have the obligation to use and disseminate summary data to relevant stakeholders in a timely manner.
7. Programs should share data for legitimate public health purposes and may establish data-use agreements to facilitate sharing data in a timely manner.
8. Public health data should be maintained in a secure environment and transmitted through secure methods.
9. Minimize the number of persons and entities granted access to identifiable data.
10. Program officials should be active and responsible stewards of public health data.

of your data. Following these guidelines will protect not only the human subjects who contributed the data, which is first and foremost, but also your data file so that your study's aims are fulfilled.

Also critical is the extensive documentation of all these procedures, including data management. Especially important in this regard is the task of creating a codebook that contains all of the items, scales, and associated labels that were used to measure the different variables in your study. In addition, your codebook should also document the response options for each questionnaire item and assigned numerical values. For instance, response options to any five-point scale measures used should be consistently coded as 1 = Strongly disagree through 5 = Strongly agree. This information is necessary in creating the scale scores that will be used when analyzing these data. It is also important to include in your codebook documentation of any scale items that need to be reverse coded before creating a scale. For example, two of the eight items measuring self-efficacy are worded such that a "Strongly agree" response corresponds to low self-efficacy, whereas for the other six items, "Strongly agree" corresponds to high self-efficacy. Thus, two items need to be recorded so that "Strongly agree" now equals 1 versus its original value of 5. These processes will ensure consistency. All these types of information are essential to include in a codebook to ensure future data analyses are valid. An appendix to this chapter provides an example of a codebook. This is designed with three columns of information to streamline the data analysts' (and data managers') tasks. The first column is simply the variable name. The second is a special column, unique to this data set, that provides variable names for a subset of the 106 variables shown in the first column. The third and final column is the most important: This is where you, as the data manager or analyst, can

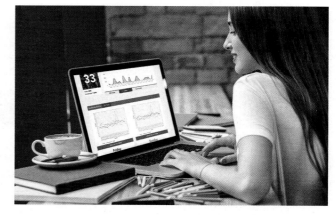

FIGURE 12.1 Data Manager for Research Study Performing Data-Monitoring Activities.
© RossHelen/Shutterstock

"translate" the answers provided in the data (which are in the forms of numbers) into meaning. Without this key column, you would not know what a 0 or 1 meant, for example.

As part of the routine process of data management, at least three steps related to data cleaning should be followed: (1) conduct checks for out-of-range values, (2) monitor missingness, and (3) monitor study identification numbers. This process does not have to be daunting (see **FIGURE 12.1**), but it does need careful attention to detail.

▶ Conducting Checks for Out-of-Range Values

One great advantage of collecting data using an electronic format is that it can be uploaded directly into a database. This prevents data-entry errors that are largely inevitable when data are transferred by hand from paper formats to a database. Regardless, out-of-range values may still be a problem with electronic data-collection systems simply because of errors made by study participants responding to questions. Although the vast majority of these errors can be averted through careful programming rules when designing electronic surveys, avoiding all errors is seldom possible. Thus, for each variable (in this context, variables equate with an item that was measured such as *age, race, and ethnicity*; *gender*; or *self-efficacy*), it is a wise practice to routinely do a simple frequency analysis to see the range of values for each variable. Numbers that are not possible represent out-of-range values. For instance, let's say a variable is based on the following question: "Generally, how often do you think about eating?" The response options are (1) never, (2) rarely, (3) sometimes, (4) often, and (5) very often. Given this range of possibilities, a number in your frequency distribution of zero or six, for example, would be an error. Correcting this error is not as easy as identifying its existence. Typically, data should never be altered, but exceptions to this dictum involve the creation of a set of "rules" that will be applied to the out-of-range values or for certain errors that need correction. These changes should be applied consistently and to all incoming data and made available to any users of the final database.

▶ Looking for Implausible Values

In our experience, a common issue in cleaning a data set involves the problem of having recorded values that simply are not possible. For instance, consider a set of questions such as the following (from a study of marijuana users).

1. In the past 60 days, how many times have you been high on marijuana?
   Write in number of times: _____
2. In the past 60 days, how many times have you been alone when you were high on marijuana?
   Write in number of times: _____

Now, what would you do in a case where the value provided to question 1 was 12, and the value provided to question 2 was 15? Clearly, of course, the answer to one of these is not correct, and even both may be incorrect. This is a situation that lacks a fair method of resolution, so the sad reality becomes that the data must be recoded as "missing." As you may not be aware, data are difficult and costly to collect. Consequently, losing data through this cleaning action is tragic. Given, however, that we (like you) are in public health, a prevention alternative here must be considered but at the programming stage rather than at the data-cleaning stage.

The prevention alternative here is to collect data with electronic survey software that includes programmed *logic checks*. When a logic check is violated (as in the two preceding questions), the software is triggered to force the respondent to provide an answer within a mathematically plausible range. Another programming fix would be to have the software automatically insert or "carry forward" the previous response to the first question into the second question, so that it reads like, "In the past 60 days, of the 15 times you reported that you got high on marijuana, how many of those times were you alone?" This use of programming is also valuable to prevent yet another form of implausible data stemming from *skip patterns*.

An example of a skip pattern follows, using the old-fashioned paper-and-pencil method.

1. In the past 30 days, have you injected opioids?
   _____ No (if no, skip to Q6)
   _____ Yes
2. How many times did you do this?
   Write in number of times: _____
3. How many times was a clean needle or syringe used?
   Write in number of times: _____
4. How many times did you inject alone?
   Write in number of times: _____
5. How many times did you inject with a needle or syringe used by somebody else?
   Write in number of times: _____
6. In the past 30 days, have you been arrested for drugs?
   _____ No (if no, skip to Q12)
   _____ Yes

Notice that questions 2 through 5 should be answered by people saying "Yes" to question 1 and should not be answered by people saying "No" to question 1. This seems simple enough, but without electronic (i.e., automatic) navigation, the data will be compromised. This could occur in two ways: (1) People who said "No" to question 1 might provide answers to questions 2–5, and (2) people who said "Yes" to question 1 might skip directly to question 6. Either way, this reliance on the study volunteers to accurately navigate their way through skip patterns may open the door to incorrect data. Again, technology comes to the rescue. With software-programming methods, anyone who responds "No" to question 1 is automatically skipped to question 6. Similarly, anyone who responds "Yes" to question1 is automatically taken to questions 2, 3, 4, and 5.

▶ Monitoring Missingness

Missing data can sometimes be the bane of existence for people who have a passion for data analysis. Depending on the type and degree of missing data, the results of your study could be greatly affected and you will be unable to see the bigger picture that your study was designed to provide (see **FIGURE 12.2**). **Statistical power** is but one issue that is affected by missing data. Being able to detect an effect if one exists is a function of sample size. When data are missing for some participants, these participants are typically excluded from data analysis, so each missing data point for any given variable is seen as a liability for maintaining statistical power.

In general, there are three types of missing data according to the mechanisms of missingness:

1. **Missing completely at random (MCAR)** is when the probability that the data are missing is not related to its value or to the value of other variables in the study. Missing values are randomly distributed across all observations. MCAR is an ideal but *unreasonable* assumption for many studies performed in the field of public health. However, if data are missing by design, because of equipment failure (e.g., responses to an online survey got dropped by the server), or were lost in transit (e.g., data were stored on a hard drive that crashed), such data are regarded as being MCAR. The advantage of MCAR is that data analysis remains unbiased, although power may be lost and no steps need to be taken.

2. **Missing at random (MAR)** is a more realistic assumption for studies conducted in public health. Data are regarded to be MAR when the probability that the responses are missing is unrelated to its value after controlling for other variables in the analysis. Under MAR, the data are not missing randomly across *all* observations but are missing randomly only within subsamples of data. For example, if high school income data are missing randomly across all schools in a district, those data will be considered MCAR. However, if data are randomly missing for students in specific schools of the district, the data are MAR.

3. **Missing not at random (MNAR)** is when the missing values *do* depend on unobserved values. If the characters of the data do not meet those of MCAR or MAR, they fall into the category of MNAR. When the missing data have a structure to them, we cannot treat them as missing at random. In the preceding example, if the data were missing for *all* students from specific schools, the data cannot be treated as MAR. The cases of MNAR data are problematic. The only way to obtain an unbiased estimate of the parameters in such a case is to model the missing data. The model may then be incorporated into a more complex one for estimating the missing values.

Several common techniques are used to address missing data. The first two techniques involve not using the missing data, but to different degrees and are **listwise deletion** and **pairwise deletion**. One caveat here is that these two techniques should be used only when data are deemed MCAR. Listwise deletion drops all cases from the analysis for which there is at least one value missing from one of the variables in the model. Pairwise deletion allows you to use more of your data and involves using cases that contain some missing data. The procedure cannot include a particular variable when it has a missing value, but it can still use the case when analyzing other variables with nonmissing values. For example, a case may contain three variables—VAR1, VAR2, and VAR3—and have a missing value for VAR1, but this does not prevent some statistical procedures from using the same case to analyze variables VAR2 and VAR3. Both techniques result in a loss of statistical power because cases for which data are missing are excluded from statistical analyses, so neither technique may be the most feasible option. Also, if the missing data are deemed MAR or MNAR, these forms of correction will result in bias in the sample.

If the frequency of missing data is great, or if missing data are MAR or MNAR, using **imputation**

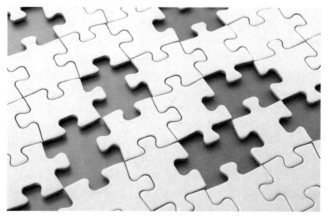

FIGURE 12.2 Missing Data Affect the Bigger Picture.
© tadamichi/Shutterstock

DO YOU HAVE MISSING DATA?

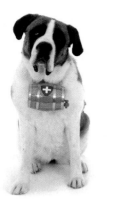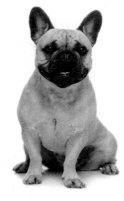

YOU MUST IMPUTE!

FIGURE 12.3 Public Health Mascots Snow's and Hamilton's Directive on Missing Data.

© Eric Isselee/Shutterstock; © Svetography/Shutterstock

is a better approach (see **FIGURE 12.3**). For example, depending on the amount of missing data, replacing the missing values with the mean or median of the nonmissing values is one type of imputation approach. However, the main weakness of this technique is the loss of variation in your data, so it may be better to use more sophisticated imputation methods.

The scope of this textbook does not allow us to describe all of them, but most involve estimating the missing values based on statistical modeling and more complex algorithms (Dong & Peng, 2013; Kang, 2013; Patrician, 2002). Diagnosing systematic missingness

early in the course of data collection allows the research team to make the corresponding corrections or alterations to the questionnaire or protocols needed to reduce this problem for future study participants. However, if NMAR occurs, there are several ways to address and increase the validity of your findings, depending on the type of data (see **FIGURE 12.4**).

▶ Monitoring Study Identification Numbers

Oddly, an often-challenging task in collecting data involves assignment and the recording of coded identification numbers designed to protect the confidentiality of study participants. The task itself is simple in principle: By assigning all participants code numbers, their names do not need to appear in the database (this is vital for multiple reasons relevant to the protection of human subjects). The problem is that assigning these numbers may be a process fallible to human error. This form of staff error is especially likely when more than one staff member is responsible for data collection. Because the coded identification number is a key variable for so many forms of analysis, its entry at the time of data collection should be made by the research assistant if data are collected in person. If data are self-collected via an online survey, you can program the software to generate the study ID. The procedure for assigning study IDs varies, but one way is to reserve banks of

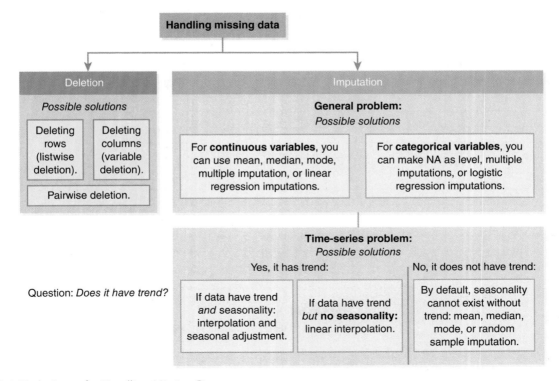

FIGURE 12.4 Techniques for Handling Missing Data.

ID numbers and thereby let the research assistant know exactly which numbers have and have not been used so far in the study. For computer-generated ID numbers, you can create a range of values for the number (e.g., 1000–5000) and then program the software to generate a random number for each participant that falls within the range. Yet it is common to have this process break down occasionally or to have the electronic data-collection software fail, which necessitates starting over and triggers an automatic assignment of a second code number to the same person. Clearly, finding and correcting duplicate code numbers is an important task, one that requires constant vigilance and perhaps some detective work on the part of the data manager.

▶ How Can Data Be Entered Most Efficiently?

Data entry is a rule-governed process that begins with some general principles:

- Name the variables using eight or fewer characters and develop a simple naming convention rather than trying to impress others (for instance, a variable capturing age can be called "Age").
- For each variable, you can also develop a label. Labels can be much longer and consist of entire phrases (for instance, "Age of Participants at Study Enrollment").
- Each variable also requires you to designate whether the metric of measurement is nominal, ordinal, interval, or ratio. This is vital because the statistical software programs typically recognize these designations and may disqualify certain variables from tests that are not consistent with the named metric.

Although many statistical software programs are user-friendly for data entry, one of the most popular programs is known as IBM's SPSS Statistics for Windows or Macintosh (IBM, Armonk, New York), and it works the same as most other statistical software programs relative to data entry. FIGURE 12.5 displays the basic SPSS data-entry screen. As you can see, the top of each column is marked *var*, which is a placeholder for what will become the actual variable

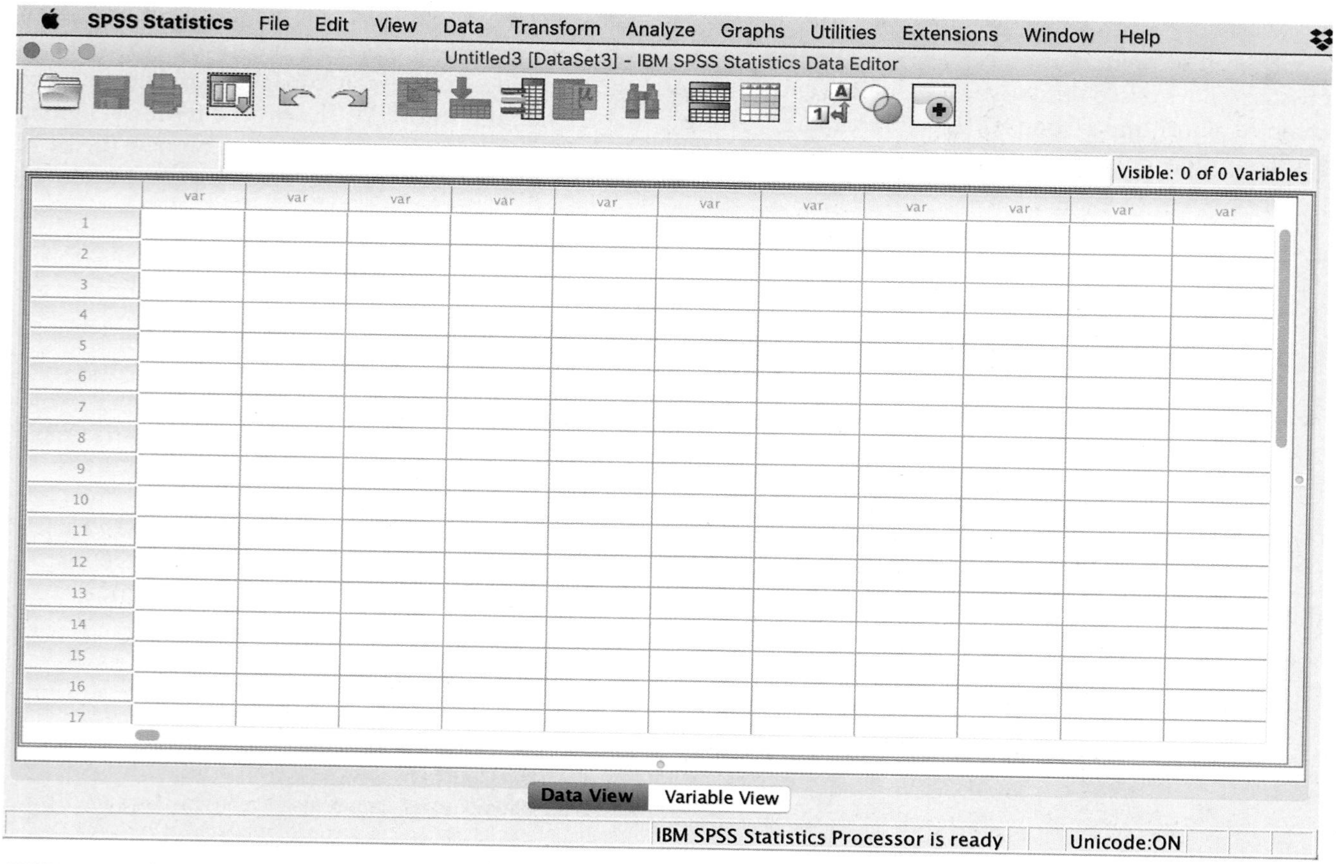

FIGURE 12.5 Blank Data File from SPSS Statistical Software Program.
Courtesy of IBM/SPSS.

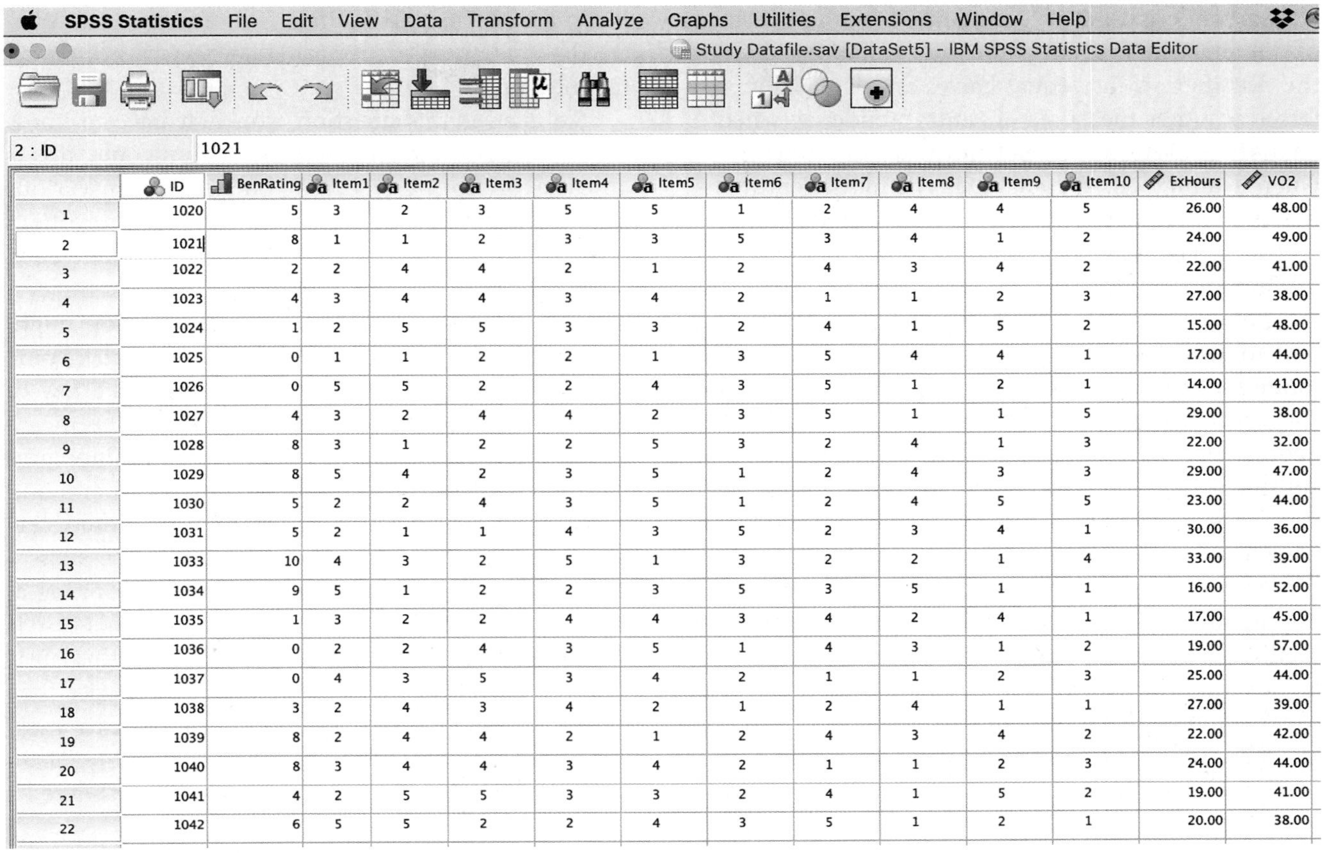

	ID	BenRating	Item1	Item2	Item3	Item4	Item5	Item6	Item7	Item8	Item9	Item10	ExHours	VO2
1	1020	5	3	2	3	5	5	1	2	4	4	5	26.00	48.00
2	1021	8	1	1	2	3	3	5	3	4	1	2	24.00	49.00
3	1022	2	2	4	4	2	1	2	4	3	4	2	22.00	41.00
4	1023	4	3	4	4	3	4	2	1	1	2	3	27.00	38.00
5	1024	1	2	5	5	3	3	2	4	1	5	2	15.00	48.00
6	1025	0	1	1	2	2	1	3	5	4	4	1	17.00	44.00
7	1026	0	5	5	2	2	4	3	5	1	2	1	14.00	41.00
8	1027	4	3	2	4	4	2	3	5	1	1	5	29.00	38.00
9	1028	8	3	1	2	2	5	3	2	4	1	3	22.00	32.00
10	1029	8	5	4	2	3	5	1	2	4	3	3	29.00	47.00
11	1030	5	2	2	4	3	5	1	2	4	5	5	23.00	44.00
12	1031	5	2	1	1	4	3	5	2	3	4	1	30.00	36.00
13	1033	10	4	3	2	5	1	3	2	2	1	4	33.00	39.00
14	1034	9	5	1	2	2	3	5	3	5	1	1	16.00	52.00
15	1035	1	3	2	2	4	4	3	4	2	4	1	17.00	45.00
16	1036	0	2	2	4	3	5	1	4	3	1	2	19.00	57.00
17	1037	0	4	3	5	3	4	2	1	1	2	3	25.00	44.00
18	1038	3	2	4	3	4	2	1	2	4	1	1	27.00	39.00
19	1039	8	2	4	4	2	1	2	4	3	4	2	22.00	42.00
20	1040	8	3	4	4	3	4	2	1	1	2	3	24.00	44.00
21	1041	4	2	5	5	3	3	2	4	1	5	2	19.00	41.00
22	1042	6	5	5	2	2	4	3	5	1	2	1	20.00	38.00

FIGURE 12.6 Data Screen Capture from SPSS Statistical Software.
Courtesy of IBM/SPSS.

names that you assign. Thus, variables are found in the columns. Looking now at the rows, each one is numbered, so only a single row will serve as the entire record for any one study participant.

Although data entry seems simple enough so far, it becomes a bit complex when entering data from a longitudinal study in which you have multiple assessment points for each person enrolled. An easy method is to add a letter or number to each variable name for data collected after the first time period, which many times is called *baseline*. For instance, at baseline, a measure of stable housing might be named *stabhou*, whereas at the first follow-up assessment you can create a new variable for the same measure and name it *stabhou2*. As you can readily see, this naming procedure tells the data analyst that stabhou2 is the second assessment point of the same baseline construct. Pay close attention to these types of naming conventions because these procedures are critical to good data management. **FIGURE 12.6** depicts a data-entry screen with an accumulation of data. Based on this data set, SPSS can be used to easily run simple descriptive statistics such as the mean, range, standard deviation, and variance.

▶ What Are Measures of Central Tendency and Variability?

Statisticians rarely agree on best practices or top priorities in data analysis, but the one point they all agree on is that the first step of most data analyses is to describe the data in terms of their central tendency and variability. Of course, this step applies only to continuous data. Continuous data describe the quantity measured and typically use a scale measurement; the metric is interval or ratio. This step would not apply to categorical data, which describe the quality of the data and are not from a normal distribution.

Measures of **central tendency** are some of the most basic and useful statistical functions, and they form the basis for most other statistical tests. Measures of central tendency summarize a sample or population by a single typical value. The two most commonly used measures of central tendency for numerical data are the **mean** and the **median**, although in some instances, the **mode** may be determined. The mean is simply the arithmetic average of all recorded scores or observations and is the mostly widely used measure of central tendency, but it is influenced by the presence of outliers. The median is the data value that divides the distribution into equal halves and is usually preferred to other measures of central tendency when a data set is skewed (i.e., not normally distributed) or when dealing with ordinal data. The mode represents the data value that is the most frequent in the data set and should be used when data are nominal or categorical in nature.

Before we proceed, it is well worth thinking about how to decide whether to select the mean, median, or mode for your measure of central tendency. First, we suggest that the mode is really never a measure that people select if they are engaged in research, so we can eliminate that from the lineup of possibilities. That leaves the median and the mean. The question you have to ask here has two parts: (1) Are the data continuous? (2) If so, are there outliers? If the answer to the first question is "No," you are obligated to use the median. However, if the answer to the first question is "Yes" and the answer to the second question is also "Yes," you may also want to use the median. As always, an example may be helpful. FIGURE 12.7 provides data from the U.S. Census Bureau regarding the median income of various U.S. cities. The question is, "Why are the median values reported here—why not report the means?"

To answer this question, you first have to know the meaning of the term *outlier*. With income, this is an easy concept. As you may be aware from various political campaigns, it is often said that more than 90% of the wealth in the United States is controlled by less than 3% of the population. In this example, it is this 3% who would be the outliers. As you might imagine, a 3% person could have an annual income of far greater than $1 million. It would take few of these extreme values to artificially inflate the mean. What would happen if, for instance, multimillionaires (and billionaires) suddenly moved out of Miami and began living in Portland, Oregon? This would certainly change the means and, therefore, necessitate a new graph as opposed to the one you are looking at now. Thus, the eloquence of the median in this case is that these extreme values do not influence this measure of central tendency. Similarly, a given city may have a preponderance of people with no or extremely low income, and these values would reduce the mean. Consequently, the mean has always been considered a

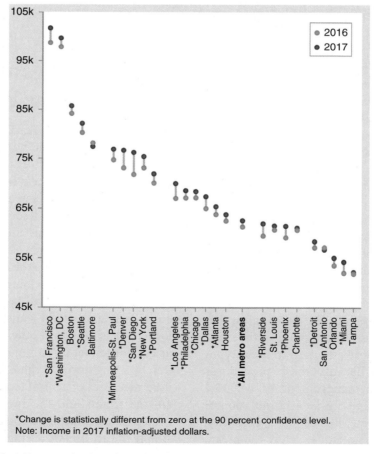

*Change is statistically different from zero at the 90 percent confidence level.
Note: Income in 2017 inflation-adjusted dollars.

FIGURE 12.7 Median Household Income by Populous Cities in the United States.

2016 and 2017 American Community Survey. www.census.gov/acs

poor measure of central tendency for income. Turning to public health measures, it is likely that outliers may also be a common problem relative to several measures (listed in the following), thus making the mean a less-than-perfect choice:

- The frequency of getting high among 12th graders
- The number of alcoholic beverages consumed in an average week among employees of a small factory
- The number of times in the past year people have been in a therapy session for mental health reasons
- The number of miles per week that people 60 years of age and older walk or run

After generating your measure of central tendency, we hope that your data are not skewed and that you are able to report the mean rather than the median or mode. The great advantage to using the mean lies at the heart of all statistics involving continuous data. It is only with continuous data that you would interact with the concept of **variance**, a term used to denote

the diversity or variability of scores for a given variable within the population of study. Before learning about this term from a statistical viewpoint, it is a bit easier to begin with a common example.

Consider that you have a chance to live in only one of two places, and your primary concern is having a temperate climate. You quickly learn that both options have the same mean yearly temperature of 72°F. The first city is in Southern California, and the second one is on the East Coast of the United States in an area prone to snow and ice during the winter months. So, are you to assume that the two climates are the same? The answer, of course, is no. Clearly, you need more information before you can make a decision. The information you need is simply the variance—meaning how much do the daily temperatures on average depart from 72 degrees? However, before we go further, it is important to know a related term called **dispersion**. Dispersion is the distance, in units of measure, that scores or observations (in this case, daily temperature readings) deviate from a midpoint. The defined midpoint used in nearly all statistical applications is the mean. **TABLE 12.2** displays

TABLE 12.2 Dispersion of Fahrenheit Temperatures Recorded at Noon on the First Day of Each Month for 1 Year in Two U.S. Locations

Date	Southern California	Distance from the Mean	East Coast	Distance from the Mean
January 1	66	−6	26	−46
February 1	64	−8	43	−29
March 1	69	−3	65	−7
April 1	71	−1	84	+12
May 1	71	−1	90	+18
June 1	73	+1	93	+21
July 1	84	+12	95	+23
August 1	81	+9	97	+25
September 1	79	+7	91	+19
October 1	72	0	73	+1
November 1	69	−3	55	−17
December 1	67	+5	47	−25
Mean	72.17		71.58	

the dispersion of temperatures recorded at the start of each month for a 1-year period.

As shown in Table 12.2, the temperatures recorded for the East Coast city span 71 degrees from 26°F to 97°F, whereas the temperatures for the Southern California city had a much narrower range of 20 degrees (from 64°F to 84°F). The range alone, however, does not provide a valuable sense of the dispersion because it is influenced by extreme scores. The solution to this is take a simple mathematical approach to measuring dispersion, which is done by subtracting the mean from each score. So, for example, subtracting the mean of 72 degrees from the January 1 temperature in Southern California of 66 gives a value of –6 (see Table 12.2). Similarly, subtracting the mean from the September 1 temperature of 79 degrees gives a value of +7. Note that once this process of subtracting the mean from each score is complete, the values obtained from summing these answers will always add up to zero (you can see for yourself by performing this math

in Table 12.2). This is because of the fact that the mean is indeed the true mathematical midpoint of the distribution of scores, so the distance from this midpoint has to be equal on both sides of the midpoint. So at this juncture, the logical question becomes, How is it possible to generate a measure of dispersion based on a value of zero? The answer to this question brings us back to the mathematical equation of *variance*. Variance uses squared values; it is, therefore, a transformed metric. By squaring the values obtained by subtracting the mean from the obtained scores, all values become positive (recall from your early training in math that squaring a negative value produces a positive value).

TABLE 12.3 provides a completed set of mathematical calculations relative to our example of the temperatures in the two cities. As you can see, the squared scores add up to a positive number, which is far greater for the East Coast city compared with the city in Southern California. The total of the squared values, however, cannot yet be compared with each

TABLE 12.3 Dispersion and Standard Deviations of Fahrenheit Temperatures Recorded at Noon on the First Day of Each Month for 1 Year in Two U.S. Locations

Date	Southern California	(Mean - Score)^2	East Coast	(Mean - Score)^2
January 1	66	36	26	2116
February 1	64	64	43	841
March 1	69	9	65	49
April 1	71	1	84	144
May 1	71	1	90	324
June 1	73	1	93	441
July 1	84	144	95	529
August 1	81	81	97	625
September 1	79	49	91	361
October 1	72	0	73	1
November 1	69	9	55	289
December 1	67	25	47	625
Totals	866	420	859	6345
Totals/12	Mean = 72.2	VAR = 35.0	Mean = 71.6	VAR = 528.75

other until we account for the natural occurrence of unequal numbers of scores or observations when comparing two or more groups. This is done simply by dividing the total of each distribution by the number of scores or observations in that distribution. In our example of temperatures, for both sets of temperatures, the number used is 12, representing the total number of months in the year. You can now see that the sum of the squared values divided by 12 for the East Coast city is astronomically higher (more than 15 times greater) than the corresponding total for the Southern California city. Hence, in addition to the old saying that it never rains in Southern California, it is obvious from this example that the temperatures never stray too far from that all-so-perfect 72 degrees. So, which city will you pick? Incidentally, what we have just compared—that is, the 528.75 versus the 35.0—is known as the *variance*. Variance is a measure of variability or spread that remains in the transformed metric of squares and tells us how far a set of numbers are spread out from the average value or the mean.

That last step (as you might imagine) is to return our obtained values back to their original metric. At this point, recall that we have been working with squared scores (i.e., they were transformed by squaring—this is the special definition of variance mentioned previously). To return to the original metric, the final move is to unsquare the values, a task easily done by taking the square root. So, in our example, we take the square root of the variance, which is known as the **standard deviation**. The standard deviation is widely used in public health research. In fact, it is obligatory to report the standard deviation whenever a mean is reported.

A simple and memorable way to learn about the standard deviation is to think about a guessing game that involves one person predicting the weight of a complete stranger, using only sight to make this guess. The rules of this game are a bit rigged, however, because they specify "plus or minus" 7 pounds. If you were to play this game as the person whose weight is the topic, you might think that it would be fairly difficult for the person to guess correctly. What you may not consider is that this person does not have to be correct at all—any answer within a range of 14 pounds would count as winning. Give this game a try sometime as the person making the guess; you will find that such a wide standard deviation makes this relatively easy when the guessing game involves people of low weight. So, why would this be the case? Let's say we have a 10-year old boy who is of average height and weight in appearance. His weight is 70 pounds. Thus, the standard deviation in this case (i.e., + or –7 lbs) represents around 10% of the actual weight, which we

can think of now as the mean. In this case, you have a 20% range where you will still be correct (i.e., 63 lbs to 77 lbs); this makes the game easy (especially now that you can quickly use Google to check on the average weight of a nonobese 10-year-old boy). Next, let's say you have to guess the weight of a 40-year old man who is noticeably obese for his height (weighing in at 210 pounds). Now your standard deviation is just barely above 3%, making your range of correct guesses only around 6%. The point here is that the width or narrowness of a standard deviation is defined by it proportional relationship to the mean. Proportionally wide standard deviations are of little predictive value. Conversely, proportionally narrow standard deviations are of great predictive value. The take-home point here is to look for—and put your trust in—studies that report proportionally narrow standard deviations.

A key utility of the standard deviation is its application to a **normal distribution** curve. By definition, graphed normal distributions are (1) symmetrical around the mean, meaning that the mean is at the middle and divides the area into halves where each half is a mirror image; (2) the mean, median, and mode are all equal; and (3) determined by their mean and standard deviation. In addition, as shown in **FIGURE 12.8**, a distribution that is normal will have properties such that all values that fall between one standard deviation above the mean and one standard deviation below the mean will constitute 68% of the total distribution. Further, and of great importance, 95% of all scores will fall between the points marked by two standard deviations below the mean through two standard deviations above the mean.

Diving deeper into the data from the two cities, **FIGURE 12.9** depicts a bar chart comparison between Southern California temperatures and East Coast temperatures each month. The data are also displayed as separate histograms showing the mean and standard deviations for each set of temperatures. Notice the difference in the normal distribution curve between the two data sets. The East Coast data set has a standard deviation of 24, whereas the Southern California set has a significantly smaller standard deviation of 6.1.

BOX 12.1 provides further examples of how vital the standard deviation is to understanding and judging the precision of point estimates made by mean values.

Now that you have a firm understanding of how the standard deviation is a useful measure of dispersion in a distribution, you are ready to apply this knowledge to data obtained from studies applied to public health. When you read (or write) peer-reviewed

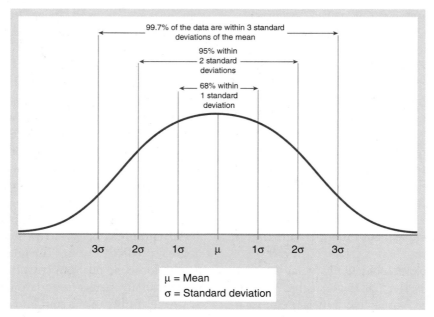

FIGURE 12.8 A Normal Distribution Curve.

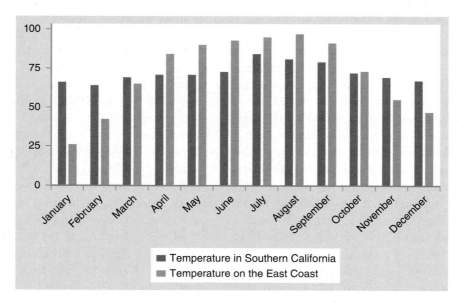

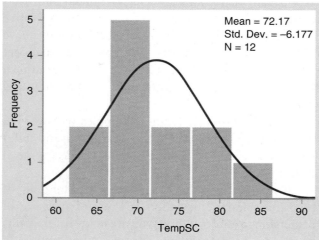

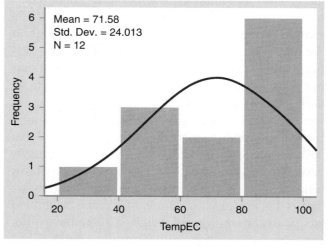

FIGURE 12.9 Deeper Dive into Temperature Data: Bar Chart and Histograms.

BOX 12.1 Can the Mean Be Trusted?

Academics are often fond of saying, "The mean only applies to the group as a whole." This saying has only a partial grain of truth, however. When the standard deviation is small (tight), the mean is highly applicable to all people in the population. Conversely, when the standard deviation is large (wide), the mean has little value for any one person. Thus, a mean only has meaning in the context of its respective standard deviation.

A study of positive sexual experiences while using condoms was conducted among young Black men by Crosby, Mena, and Smith (2018) and reported the following: "The baseline scale yielded a mean of 18.0 (sd = 5.1), and the same measure at the 12-month assessment yielded a mean of 18.5 (sd = 5.6). The mean of the difference score (12-month score minus baseline score) was 0.56 (sd = 6.4)." The measure referred to here yielded possible scores from 5 to 25. Armed with what you now know about the standard deviation, you can apply that knowledge to judge the precision of these means. With a range of 20, a standard deviation of 5.1, for example, represents a fair portion of the distribution. To represent ~34% of the scores, a single standard deviation will occupy 5.1 units in this 20-unit range. Thus, ~68% of the scores would be located between one standard deviation below the mean and one standard deviation above the mean, a distance of 10.2 units in this range of 20 units. So, the question becomes, "Is the mean a strong representation of this measure of positive sexual experience?" Had this ~68% interval been shorter—for instance, spanning only 3 units in this range of 20—we would have more confidence that the mean is truly capturing the measure. The quest then is to have narrow intervals relative to the number of units below and above the mean that capture most scores in the distribution. By tradition, it is ~95% of the scores that are desirable to define by relatively narrow intervals. This is known as the *95% confidence interval*.

---

journal articles, always ask, what are the basic descriptive characteristics of the sample? We ask that you look closely at these values when reading research with the following questions in mind:

- Which characteristic has the least dispersion?
- Which mean is the best estimate of the distribution?
- Which mean is the worst estimate of the distribution?
- Which standard deviation has the greatest potential for not being valid?

▶ How Can Descriptive Data Be Summarized?

Graphs are one of the most efficient methods of summarizing descriptive data. For instance, **histograms** are a traditional method of describing continuous data measured by an interval metric (data that represent numerical values of a construct where zero does not necessarily equate with an absolute absence of the construct) or a ratio metric (data that represent numerical values of a construct where zero equates with a complete absence of the construct), whereas **bar charts** are especially useful for categorical or nominal (data that are categorical in nature and represent a quality—e.g., sex or race and ethnicity) or ordinal data (data that are numerical and ordered, although distance between points may not be equal). **FIGURE 12.10** displays an example of a histogram. These

are interval data taken from a study that assessed body image among a sample of 162 women. Higher scores on this measure equated with a more favorable body image. The variable for body image was named *zbody*, and this is shown on the *x*-axis. The *y*-axis shows the frequency of women with the various scores shown along the *x*-axis. For instance, you can see that around 17 women had a score of 35 (highest score obtained for this sample of women). The key to understanding a histogram is knowing that it reports the approximate shape of a continuous distribution. In this case, the distribution as depicted is far from normal—in fact, it has what is called a **negative skew**, meaning that it has few scores on the left-hand side, with the preponderance of scores on the right-hand side. As you

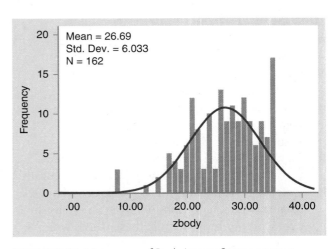

FIGURE 12.10 Histogram of Body Image Scores among Women.

imagine then, a **positive skew** is the term used when a distribution is not normal but has the preponderance of scores on the left-hand side and few scores on the right-hand side.

FIGURE 12.11 displays an example of a bar chart. Bar charts look similar to histograms, but the difference is that the categories are shown along the *x*-axis along with the percent or count of individuals falling into the categories along the *y*-axis, so this is *not a true distribution of scores* and the question of whether it is normal or skewed does not apply. For these types of data, you can readily see the value of graphing the data with a bar chart because it shows that people mostly selected either the third or fourth option.

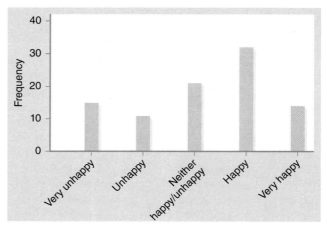

FIGURE 12.11 Bar Chart of "Happiness" Categories.

Think About It!

As noted in this chapter, data can be expensive to collect. It is, for example, not at all uncommon for studies funded by the National Institutes of Health (NIH) to cost the taxpayers several million dollars. When a study is completed, the only tangible product is the data set. Of course, that tangible product can be used to generate journal articles that may ultimately have a large impact on public health policy and practice, yet the true product remains as a data set stored in a computer. Recognizing this point, federally funded research projects are often awarded under a data-sharing agreement. This implies that another researcher (not the grant recipient) could ask for and receive the data. In fact, data sharing itself (without a specific plan submission) continues to be a requirement of all NIH-funded grants. This practice is extremely useful. For example, in an open access journal article, Adjemian, Volpe, and Adjemian (2015) reported findings from a large (and thus expensive) study regarding the relationship between diet and alcohol consumption with two health outcomes—diabetes and heart disease. The authors made the following declaration:

> Data Availability: Data were collected from the National Consumer Panel, a joint venture between IRI and Nielsen. Access to these data requires a negotiated contract, specifying use, and terms and conditions under which the sensitive data can be made public. This type of statement invites other researchers to take full advantage of this all-so-valuable data set. Indeed, the idea of analyzing data, under a shared data agreement, may be an option for you someday!

Take Home Points

- Safety, security, and confidentiality of your data should be a major priority, and rules and procedures should be developed and implemented to ensure this.
- Data management is fundamental to the research process. It involves ongoing attention and maintenance as data accumulate.
- Having clear and cohesive data-management procedures will assure that the data are accurate.
- Assessing the data for missing values and out-of-range values in addition to having an established protocol for how to handle these values will enhance the statistical power of your study.
- As part of the data-management process, it is important to assess your data for basic statistical properties such as central tendency (mean) and variability (variance and standard deviation).
- Proportionally narrow standard deviations provide optimal predictive ability.
- Generating graphs is a vital part of data analysis. Graphs will help depict the underlying frequencies of continuous variables, the normal distribution (or lack of normality) of the data, or the percentage of people classified into categories.
- Data management and its secondary obligation of descriptive data analysis lay the foundation for an extensive array of possible data-analytic strategies.

Key Terms

Bar chart
Central tendency
Dispersion
Histogram
Imputation
Listwise deletion
Mean

Median
Missing at random (MAR)
Missing completely at random
  (MCAR)
Missing not at random (MNAR)
Mode
Negative skew

Normal distribution
Pairwise deletion
Positive skew
Standard deviation
Statistical power
Variance

For Practice and Discussion

1. You are a project coordinator for a research study on mental health that just finished the data-collection phase, and you cannot wait to start analyzing the study data. Then you take a step back and remember to begin the data-management process. What does data management involve? Explain why data management is so critical to the research process.

2. You are currently going through the electronic data set of data collected from the mental health study referred to in question 1 and are preparing for data cleaning. Explain why each of the following three steps is valuable, and how you will adhere to each of these three steps as you go through these data:
   a. Conduct checks for out-of-range values
   b. Monitor missingness
   c. Monitor study identification numbers

3. Read a journal article on a quantitative study and look closely at the descriptive statistics, which include the measures of central tendency and variability. Answer the following questions about the sample:
   a. Which characteristic has the least dispersion?
   b. Which mean is the best estimate of the distribution?
   c. Which mean is the worst estimate of the distribution?
   d. Which standard deviation has the greatest potential for not being valid?

4. What is a normal distribution, and what does it represent? Explain how a normal distribution relates to the data for a study. How can a normal distribution of your data be summarized?

References

Adjemian, M. K., Volpe, R. J., & Adjemian, J. (2015). Relationships between diet, alcohol preference, and heart disease and type 2 diabetes among Americans. *PLoS ONE, 10*(5): e0124351. https://doi.org/10.1371/journal.pone.0124351

Crosby, R. A., Mena, L., & Smith, R. V. (2018). Promoting positive condom use experiences among young Black MSM: A randomized controlled trial of a brief, clinic-based intervention. *Health Education Research, 33*(3), 197–204.

Dong, Y., & Peng, C. Y. (2013, May 14). Principled missing data methods for researchers. *Springerplus, 2*(1), 222.

Kang, H. (2013). The prevention and handling of the missing data. *Korean Journal of Anesthesiology, 64*(5), 402–406.

Patrician, P. A. (2002). Multiple imputation for missing data. *Research in Nursing & Health, 25*(1), 76–84.

For Further Reading

Allison, P. D. (2000). Multiple imputation for missing data: A cautionary tale. *Sociological Methods & Research, 28*(3), 301–309.

Gerstman, B. B. (2014). *Basic biostatistics: Statistics for public health* (2nd ed.). Burlington, MA: Jones & Bartlett.

Osborne, J. W. (2013). *Best practices in data cleaning: A complete guide to everything you need to do before and after collecting your data.* Newbury Park, CA: Sage.

Sinharay, S., Stern, H. S., & Russell, D. (2001). The use of multiple imputation for the analysis of missing data. *Psychological Methods, 6*(4), 317.

APPENDIX

Codebook Sample

1.	Participant	Repeat FIT Study Data Master Copy	None
2.	Phone#		None
3.	Phone#2		None
4.	Comments		None
5.	DOB		None
6.	Gender	Gender	0 = Male 1 = Female
7.	Zip Code		None
8.	Distribution Date		None
9.	Distributed to		None
10.	Assigned to		None
11.	Reminder Call_2		None
12.	Reminder Call_2_Result		None
13.	Reminder Call_3		None
14.	Reminder Call_3_Result		None
15.	Date Mailed		None
16.	Kit Returned	Kit Returned	0 = No 1 = Yes
17.	Date of 1st Specimen		None
18.	Date of 2nd Specimen		None
19.	Process Date		None
20.	Result	FIT Results	0 = Negative 1 = Positive/reactive
21.	Delivery Status	Delivery Status	0 = No 1 = Yes 2 = Provider given results

22. Delivery Date		None
23. Accepted/Declined	Joined Study	0 = Declined 1 = Accepted 2 = Ineligible
24. Control/Intervention	Randomization	0 = Control 1 = Intervention
25. Navigation Status	Accepted Navigation	0 = No 1 = Yes
26. Colonoscopy	Colonoscopy Performed	0 = No 1 = Yes
27. Results	Colonoscopy Results	0 = Clean 1 = Polyps benign 2 = Precancerous 3 = Cancer 4 = Other diagnosis
28. V28		None
29. V29		None
30. V30		None
31. V31		None
32. V32		None
33. ID	Participant's ID	None
34. Age	Participant's Age	None
35. Sex	Participant's Gender	0 = Male 1 = Female
36. County	County Participant Resides In	0 = Knott 1 = Lee 2 = Leslie 3 = Letcher 4 = Perry 5 = Owsley 6 = Wolfe 7 = Breathitt
37. Zip	Participant's Zip Code	None
38. Race	Participant's Race	0 = White 1 = Black 2 = Asian 3 = Native American 4 = Other
39. Hispanic	Participant's Ethnicity: Hispanic	0 = Yes 1 = No

40. Marital Status	Participant's Marital Status	0 = Married 1 = Divorced 2 = Widowed 3 = Separated 4 = Member of an unmarried couple 5 = Single
41. Education	Participant's Education	0 = Never attended school or only kindergarten 1 = Grades 1 through 8 (elementary) 2 = Grades 9 through 11 (some high school) 3 = Grade 12 or GED (high school graduate) 4 = College, 1 year to 3 years (some college or technical school) 5 = College, 4 years or more (college graduate)
42. Employment	Participant's Employment Status	0 = Employed for wage 1 = Self-employed 2 = Out of work for more than 1 year 3 = Out of work for less than 1 year 4 = Homemaker 5 = Student 6 = Retired 7 = Unable to work
43. Household Income	Participant's Yearly Household Income	0 = Less than $10,000 1 = $10,000 to less than $15,000 2 = $15,000 to less than $20,000 3 = $20,000 to less than $25,000 4 = $25,000 to less than $35,000 5 = $35,000 to less than $50,000 6 = $50,000 to less than $75,000 7 = $75,000 or more
44. Healthcare Coverage	Participant's Healthcare Coverage	0 = Yes 1 = No
45. Type of Coverage	Participant's Type of Healthcare Coverage	0 = Self-purchased 1 = Provided by employer or spouse's employer 2 = Medicaid 3 = Medicare 4 = TRICARE 5 = VA 6 = Other
46. Healthcare Provider	Participant's Regular Healthcare Provider	0 = Yes 1 = No
47. Years of Care Received	Number of Years Participant Has Received Care from Healthcare Provider	0 = Less than 1 year 1 = 1 to 2 years 2 = 3 to 5 years 3 = More than 5 years
48. Number of Visits to Healthcare Provider	How Often Participant Visits Regular Healthcare Provider	0 = Monthly 1 = Quarterly (every 3 months) 2 = Semi-annually (every 6 months) 3 = Once per year 4 = Less than once per year

49.	Tobacco Use	Participant's Tobacco Use	0 = Every day 1 = Some days 2 = Not at all
50.	Type of Tobacco Product	Tobacco Products Participant Uses	0 = Cigarettes 1 = E-cigarettes 2 = Smokeless tobacco (chewing tobacco, snus, snuff) 3 = Other 4 = Not applicable
51.	Smoked 100 Cigarettes	Has Participant Smoked at Least 100 Cigarettes in His or Her Lifetime?	0 = Yes 1 = No
52.	Past Year Tried to Quit Smoking	Has Participant Tried to Quit Smoking?	0 = Yes 1 = No 2 = Never smoked regularly
53.	Time Since Last Cigarette	Duration Since Participant Last Smoked	0 = Within past month (less than 1 month ago) 1 = Within past 3 months (1 month but less than 3 months ago) 2 = Within past 6 months (3 months but less than 6 months ago) 3 = Within past year (6 months but less than 1 year ago) 4 = Within past 5 years (1 year but less than 5 years ago) 5 = Within past 10 years (5 years but less than 10 years ago) 6 = 10 years or more 7 = Never smoked regularly
54.	Daily Number of Drinks	Participant's Weekly Average Drink Intake	0 = 0 drink 1 = 1 drink 2 = 2 drinks 3 = 3 drinks 4 = 4 drinks 5 = 5 drinks 6 = 6 drinks 7 = 7 drinks
55.	Average Number of Drinks per Day	Participant's Daily Average Drink Intake	0 = Not applicable 1 = 1 2 = 2 3 = 3 4 = 4 5 = 5 6 = 6 7 = 7 8 = 8 9 = 9 10 = 10

56.	Number of Drinks by Gender	Participant's Drink Intake by Gender at One Sitting	0 = Not applicable 1 = 1 2 = 2 3 = 3 4 = 4 5 = 5 6 = 6 7 = 7 8 = 8 9 = 9 10 = 10
57.	Most Drinks on Occasion	Participant's Average Number of Drinks per Occasion	0 = Not applicable 1 = 1 2 = 2 3 = 3 4 = 4 5 = 5 6 = 6 7 = 7 8 = 8 9 = 9 10 = 10
58.	Low-Dose Aspirin Therapy	Is the Participant on a Low-Dose Aspirin Therapy?	0 = Yes 1 = No
59.	Body Type	Participant's Description of His or Her Body Type	0 = Underweight 1 = About right for my height 2 = Overweight 3 = Obese
60.	Weight	Participant's Weight (in pounds)	0 = No answer
61.	Height	Participant's Height (in feet and inches)	None
62.	Weekly Fruit Juice Intake	Participant's Weekly 100% Fruit Juice Intake	None
63.	Weekly Fruit Intake	Participant's Weekly Fruit Intake	None
64.	Weekly Dark Green Vegetable Intake	Participant's Weekly Dark Green Vegetable Intake	None
65.	Weekly Orange-Colored Vegetable Intake	Participant's Weekly Orange-Colored Vegetable Intake	None
66.	Weekly Other Vegetable Intake	Participant's Weekly Other Vegetable Intake	None
67.	Monthly Physical Activity	Does the Participant Engage in Physical Activity?	0 = Yes 1 = No
68.	Number of Times per Week Physical Activity	Participant's Monthly Physical Activity Engagement	None

69.	Duration of Physical Activity	Duration of Participant's Physical Activity (in minutes)	None
70.	Experience with Blood Stool Sample Test	Has Participant Used an At-Home Blood Stool Sample Kit?	0 = Yes 1 = No 2 = Don't know
71.	Duration Since Last Blood Stool Sample Test	Duration Since Participant's Last At-Home Blood Stool Sample Kit	0 = Within the past year (any time less than 12 months ago) 1 = Within the past 2 years (more than 1 year but less than 2 years ago) 2 = Within the past 3 years (more than 2 years but less than 3 years ago) 3 = Within the past 5 years (more than 3 years but less than 5 years ago) 4 = 5 or more years ago 5 = Not applicable
72.	Sigmoidoscopy or Colonoscopy Test	Has Participant Ever Received a Sigmoidoscopy or Colonoscopy?	0 = Yes 1 = No 2 = Don't know
73.	Most Recent Sigmoidoscopy or Colonoscopy	Participant's Most Recent Test Either a Sigmoidoscopy or a Colonoscopy?	0 = Sigmoidoscopy 1 = Colonoscopy 2 = Not applicable
74.	Duration Since Last Test	Duration Since Participant's Last Sigmoidoscopy or Colonoscopy	0 = Within the past year (any time less than 12 months ago) 1 = Within the past 2 years (more than 1 year but less than 2 years ago) 2 = Within the past 3 years (more than 2 years but less than 3 years ago) 3 = Within the past 5 years (more than 3 years but less than 5 years ago) 4 = Within the past 7 years (more than 5 years but less than 7 years ago) 5 = Within the past 10 years (more than 7 years but less than 10 years ago) 6 = More than 10 years ago 7 = Not applicable
75.	Family Diagnosed with Colorectal Cancer	Does Participant Have a Full Biological Family Member Who Has Ever Had Colorectal Cancer?	0 = Yes 1 = No 2 = I'm not sure what type of cancer my family member had
76.	Age Family Member Was Diagnosed	Age Family Member Was Diagnosed with Colorectal Cancer	None
77.	Believed Causes of Colorectal Cancer	Participant's Beliefs of Causes of Colorectal Cancer	0 = Eating lots of red or processed meats (sandwich meat, hotdogs, beef) 1 = Excessive alcohol consumption 2 = Lack of exercise 3 = Being overweight or obese 4 = Eating lots of bleached flour and processed sugar 5 = Not eating lots of fruits or vegetables

78.	Likelihood of Developing Colorectal Cancer	Participant's Belief of His or Her Likelihood of Developing Colorectal Cancer	0 = Strongly disagree 1 = Disagree 2 = Slightly disagree 3 = Slightly agree 4 = Agree 5 = Strongly agree	
79.	Worried About Colorectal Cancer	Is Participant Worried About Developing Colorectal Cancer?	0 = Strongly disagree 1 = Disagree 2 = Slightly disagree 3 = Slightly agree 4 = Agree 5 = Strongly agree	
80.	If It Was Meant to Be, Nothing to Do	Participant's Belief That There Is Nothing to Be Done If It Was Meant to Be to Develop Colorectal Cancer	0 = Strongly disagree 1 = Disagree 2 = Slightly disagree 3 = Slightly agree 4 = Agree 5 = Strongly agree	
81.	Nothing to Reduce Risk of Colorectal Cancer	Participant's Belief That Nothing Can Be Done to Reduce His or Her Risk of Developing Colorectal Cancer	0 = Strongly disagree 1 = Disagree 2 = Slightly disagree 3 = Slightly agree 4 = Agree 5 = Strongly agree	
82.	FIT Test Use	Was the FIT Test Easy to Use?	0 = Strongly disagree 1 = Disagree 2 = Slightly disagree 3 = Slightly agree 4 = Agree 5 = Strongly agree	
83.	Collection Process	Was the FIT Test Simple?	0 = Strongly disagree 1 = Disagree 2 = Slightly disagree 3 = Slightly agree 4 = Agree 5 = Strongly agree	
84.	Specimen Hesitation	Participant's Hesitation to Collect Specimen Sample	0 = Strongly disagree 1 = Disagree 2 = Slightly disagree 3 = Slightly agree 4 = Agree 5 = Strongly agree	
85.	FIT Test Diagnose Colorectal Cancer or Polyps	Participant's Belief That FIT Test Can Provide Colorectal Cancer or Polyp Outcome	0 = Strongly disagree 1 = Disagree 2 = Slightly disagree 3 = Slightly agree 4 = Agree 5 = Strongly agree	

86.	Positive FIT Result Healthcare Follow-up	If Participant Had a Positive Result on FIT Test, Likelihood He or She Would Follow up with Healthcare Provider	0 = Strongly disagree 1 = Disagree 2 = Slightly disagree 3 = Slightly agree 4 = Agree 5 = Strongly agree
87.	Duration Before First Specimen Collected	Number of Days Since Participant Collected First Specimen	None
88.	Best Thing About FIT Test	Best Thing About FIT Test?	0 = Simple; easy to use 1 = Clean collection process 2 = Convenient; didn't have to go to doctor's office 3 = Private; could use it at home 4 = To find out about my health status 5 = Painless; noninvasive test 6 = Other
89.	Worst Thing About FIT Test	Worst Thing About FIT Test?	0 = Nothing; I didn't have any problems with the test 1 = Collecting stool sample 2 = Finding the right time to do the test/ remembering to do it 3 = Wondering if I am doing the test correctly 4 = Worrying about test results 5 = Other
90.	Possibility of Completing FIT Once a Year	Likelihood of Participant Completing Fit Test Annually	0 = Yes 1 = No 2 = Not sure
91.	Variables More Likely to Complete FIT Annually	Variable That Would Make a Participant More Likely to Complete a FIT Test Annually	0 = If I could pick one up at my doctor's office 1 = If it was paid for by my insurance 2 = If a kit was mailed to me 3 = If I received a reminder by mail 4 = If I received a reminder via Facebook/Twitter 5 = If I received a reminder via phone call 6 = If I received a reminder via text message 7 = If someone I know also takes a FIT test once a year 8 = If a family member or friend also takes a FIT test every year 9 = If a family member or friend reminds me 10 = Other
92.	Likelihood of Recommending FIT	Participant's Likelihood of Recommending FIT	0 = Highly likely 1 = Likely 2 = Unsure 3 = Unlikely 4 = Very unlikely

93.	Reminder_1	Method of Contact	0 = In person 1 = Postcard 2 = Facebook 3 = Email 4 = Phone call 5 = Text message 6 = Timed out
94.	Reminder_2	Method of Contact	0 = In person 1 = Postcard 2 = Facebook 3 = Email 4 = Phone call 5 = Text message 6 = Timed out
95.	Reminder_3	Method of Contact	0 = In person 1 = Postcard 2 = Facebook 3 = Email 4 = Phone call 5 = Text message 6 = Timed out
96.	Reminder_4	Method of Contact	0 = In person 1 = Postcard 2 = Facebook 3 = Email 4 = Phone call 5 = Text message 6 = Timed out
97.	Reminder_5	Method of Contact	0 = In person 1 = Postcard 2 = Facebook 3 = Email 4 = Phone call 5 = Text message 6 = Timed out
98.	Reminder_6	Method of Contact	0 = In person 1 = Postcard 2 = Facebook 3 = Email 4 = Phone call 5 = Text message 6 = Timed out
99.	Reminder_7	Method of Contact	0 = In person 1 = Postcard 2 = Facebook 3 = Email 4 = Phone call 5 = Text message 6 = Timed out

100. Reminder_8	Method of Contact	0 = In person 1 = Postcard 2 = Facebook 3 = Email 4 = Phone call 5 = Text message 6 = Timed out
101. Reminder_9	Method of Contact	0 = In person 1 = Postcard 2 = Facebook 3 = Email 4 = Phone call 5 = Text message 6 = Timed out
102. Reminder_10	Method of Contact	0 = In person 1 = Postcard 2 = Facebook 3 = Email 4 = Phone call 5 = Text message 6 = Timed out
103. Reminder_11	Method of Contact	0 = In person 1 = Postcard 2 = Facebook 3 = Email 4 = Phone call 5 = Text message 6 = Timed out
104. Repeat_2	Participant Did 2nd FIT	0 = No 1 = Yes
105. Repeat_3	Participant Did 3rd FIT	0 = No 1 = Yes
106. Repeat_4	Participant Did 4th FIT	0 = No 1 = Yes

Codebook used for study titled, "Repeat Use of the Fecal Immunochemical Test Among Rural Appalachians" supported by Dr. Richard A. Crosby's Rural Cancer Prevention Center: Early Detection of Colorectal Cancer and Polyps (5U48DP005014) funded by the Centers for Disease Control and Prevention's, National Center for Chronic Disease Prevention and Health Promotion.

CHAPTER 13

Parametric Data Analysis

with Anne Marie Schipani-McLaughlin

LEARNING OBJECTIVES

1. Know the assumptions for using parametric tests.
2. Understand the principles of an independent groups *t*-test.
3. Distinguish between a Type I and Type II error.
4. Understand why variance is important in parametric statistics.
5. Understand the meaning of alpha for significance testing.
6. Learn the basis of correlation and understand its applications.
7. Apply the principles of correlation to linear regression.
8. Describe the concept and application of one-way analysis of variance.

▶ Overview

Even more vital than data management—and ultimately more enjoyable—is the process of data analysis. Data analysis can be conceptualized as a process of discovery; it is, therefore, exciting and fulfilling to determine study findings that will guide and shape public health practice. This chapter will teach you basic parametric data-analysis skills. The first thing to know is that statistical tests can be classified as either **parametric** or **nonparametric**. In the literal meaning of the terms, a parametric statistical test is one that makes assumptions about the parameters (i.e., defining properties) of the population distribution from which one's data are drawn, whereas a nonparametric test is one that makes no such assumptions. Parametric tests generally assume that the data follow a normal distribution; nonparametric tests do not make this assumption. In the last chapter, you learned how to assess central tendency and variability so that you can determine which type of statistical tests would be most appropriate. The math behind parametric tests involves variance, means, and standard deviations, all of which provide you with clues to the distribution of your data. Thus, using what you have already learned about these basic tools, you can now advance to the basic parametric analytic skills most frequently applied to public health. Throughout this chapter, we want you to be at ease with the math involved (we promise it will be simple), and we urge you to disregard any fears you may have about the word *statistics* (these fears, as you will see, are unfounded). We understand that fear of statistics is common among college students, but rest assured that statistics can be relatively easy and does not warrant excessive worry. Instead, you can worry about things that are worth worrying about such as choosing the right major

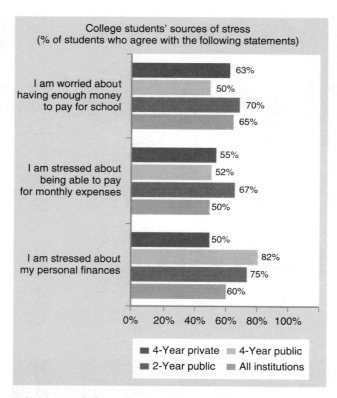

FIGURE 13.1 College Students' Financial Stress Results.

McDaniel, A., Montalto, C.P., Ashton, B., Duckett, K., Croft, A. (2014). National Student Financial Wellness Study. Ohio State University, Office of Student Life College of Education and Human Ecology.

and student debt. In fact, let's use stress over college finances (see **FIGURE 13.1**) as an example of how to determine whether to apply parametric or nonparametric statistics. In looking at the data in the figure, you would want to know whether you can calculate a mean and plot the data and compare it with a normal distribution or calculate standard deviations. Alas, we have fooled you because you cannot determine any of these things by examining the data in this

figure. The types of analyses that correspond with the data in the figure will be covered in Chapter 14. Alternatively, having data that are, in fact, amenable to parametric tests opens up a host of possible statistical procedures (whereas, nonparametric options are relatively limited). In basic terms, parametric tests assume the data follow a normal distribution, and the data are measured at the interval or ratio levels of measurement whereas nonparametric tests do not make these assumptions and are more appropriate for nominal or ordinal data. This chapter is devoted to helping you capitalize on the opportunity to use parametric tests to analyze data.

▶ What Does *Significance* Mean, and How Is It Determined?

To begin, we first want you to thoroughly understand what is meant when a person says (or writes) that "a significant relationship was found." To begin, please take a long and careful look at **FIGURE 13.2**.

The figure depicts two populations, from which we drew two samples and collected data on an outcome measure and were used to form two normal distribution curves. The first population (on the left) has a mean of 71. The second (on the right) has a mean of 86. In everyday life, we would certainly claim that "86 is greater than 71." But, in the language of science, words such as *greater* must only be used when they can be prefaced by the term *significantly*, thus the question posed by Figure 13.2 would read like this: "Is the mean of 86 significantly greater than the mean of 71?" This question can begin to be answered by thinking back to what you learned in Chapter 12 regarding the concept of a normal distribution. In a normal distribution,

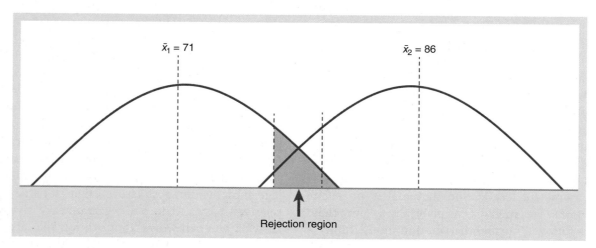

FIGURE 13.2 Comparison of Means of Two Samples' Distribution Curves.

the distance of almost two (1.96) standard deviations away from the mean on both sides encompasses 95% of the scores. Using the standard deviation, we can create a 95% confidence interval that will essentially tell us "with 95% confidence, the mean 'outcome' of the population is between these two values based on my sample data." The 95% confidence interval equates to the sample statistic (such as the mean) plus or minus 1.96 times the standard deviation. A general rule is that if the two confidence intervals do *not* overlap, the two means are significantly different. Unfortunately, the opposite is not always true (Schenker & Gentleman, 2001). In looking at overlapping confidence intervals, notice there is a caveat for when there may be a *slight* overlap, although we would like to conclude that there is *not* a significant difference, there could be a statistically significant difference between the means. For instance, let's say the 95% confidence interval around the mean of 71 is 61–81. Also, let's say the interval for the distribution with a mean of 86 has a 95% confidence interval of 76–96. In this example, the confidence intervals do overlap, suggesting that the two means do not differ significantly, but we cannot be 100% sure. Thus, although this information is useful, examining confidence intervals only when there is some overlap should not be considered a definitive test.

Nonetheless, armed with this information and looking at Figure 13.2, looking at their normal distribution curves is another method that can help you answer conceptually whether these two populations may be different (Snedecor & Cochran, 1989). Notice there is, indeed, some overlap between the two populations indicated by the overlapping areas of the distributions. In and of itself, that gives you information and suggests that the populations may not be different. However, another area of the figure shown is deemed the **critical region** or the **rejection region** and provides information to either reject or not reject the null hypothesis. The rejection region refers to the total area under the curve representing the level of **alpha**. The alpha level is the probability of rejecting the null hypothesis (e.g., "there are no differences," "$\mu_1 = \mu_2$," or "there is no effect of program X") when the null hypothesis is true. In essence, when performing significance tests, the alpha level represents the odds of making a wrong decision. Typically, the standard alpha level set by the investigator for each statistical test is 0.05. You want to minimize the chance of making a wrong decision; thus, given that the null hypothesis is true, the probability of obtaining the statistical result is less than 0.05. Deeming that there is an effect (rejecting the null) when in reality there isn't one is also known as a *false positive* or a **Type I error**. In fact, alpha level equates with the Type I error for a significance test. The inverse of this error would be to make a **Type II error**, which equates with a *false negative* because the null hypothesis is incorrectly accepted. **FIGURE 13.3** presents a matrix that may help you with these two types of errors.

	Null hypothesis true	Null hypothesis false
Reject	Type I error	Correct
Fail to reject	Correct	Type II error

FIGURE 13.3 Matrix of Hypothesis Testing Decisions and Outcomes.

Now that you understand hypothesis testing, refer back to Figure 13.2 in trying to judge whether these two means differ. To reject the null, we should see that there are scores from the distribution on the right that fall in the extreme left-side tail *and* that also overlap with the distribution on the left but exceed the rejection region. Although rejecting the null is "every researcher's hope" (because this is partly the philosophy of empirical research), we urge you to look closely at Figure 13.2. What do you see just to the left of the rejection region? You will notice that the extreme left-hand tail of the distribution on the right (the one with a mean of 86) actually crosses over the rejection region slightly and thus violates the idea that the two populations are significantly different. In this case, you cannot reject the null hypothesis. Although this exercise is helpful for you to understand significance testing for determining whether two means differ, there are better, more sophisticated ways of approaching significance testing other than generating and comparing distribution curves. We describe a fundamental statistical test called the **independent groups *t*-test** in the next section.

▶ What Is the Independent Groups *t*-Test and When Do You Use It?

Now that you have a basic understanding of the mean and standard deviation and a conceptual understanding of hypothesis testing, you are ready for the next step in data analysis. One of the most fundamental statistical tests is the independent groups *t*-test. The independent groups *t*-test is a parametric test that compares the means of two independent groups to determine whether there is statistical evidence that the associated population means are significantly different. The independent groups *t*-test is much more powerful and reliable than looking at the overlap of confidence intervals or of normal distribution curves. You would use this test if your data meet several assumptions such as the following:

- Dependent variable is continuous (i.e., interval or ratio level).
- Independent variable that is categorical (i.e., two or more groups).
- There is no relationship between the subjects in each sample. This means that:
    - Subjects in the first group cannot also be in the second group
    - No subject in either group can influence subjects in the other group
    - No group can influence the other group
- Normal distribution (approximately) of the dependent variable for each group.
- Homogeneity of variances (i.e., variances approximately equal across groups).

To begin our discussion, consider a fictional study of 900 adults newly diagnosed with type II diabetes. The mean age in which diabetes was diagnosed among this sample is 62.9 years (sd = 1.7). As you can judge from the relatively small standard deviation, this mean value is a good estimate of the age when type II diabetes may occur. However, an additional goal of this study was to identify the significant health behaviors that are related to this occurrence. In essence, you want to identify risk and protective behaviors based on an extensive set of survey questions that has been collected from the sample of study participants. You can do this by thinking of a risk or protective factor as a "yes versus no" variable. For example, does the person spend more than 3 hours each day in a sitting position? Does the person consume meat? Does the person exercise for

at least 5 hours each week? Is the person experiencing chronic daily stress? Is the person consuming a diet that includes sweetened beverages? Does the person have a family history of diabetes? Is the person's body mass index above the level classified as obesity? Each question lends itself to the forming of two groups (e.g., those classified as obese vs. those not classified as obese). For each **grouping variable**, your simple question then becomes, Do the two groups have a different mean age when type II diabetes was diagnosed? **TABLE 13.1** displays the means for each grouping variable.

Looking carefully at the means within each grouping variable, you will see that some comparisons barely depart from the overall mean age of 62.9 years. For example, the two grouping variables of sitting and consuming meat. If you look at the table, you can see that there is no **statistically significant** difference between the two groups for these two variables. This is because the *P*-value in the table is greater than the cutoff value of 0.05. (We will get to the other information in the table soon.) Thus, you can think about these two grouping variables as being "unable to split a mean apart." In other words, knowing whether people sit for more than 10 hours per day or eat red meat does not give us meaningful information about age of being diagnosed with type II diabetes. The goal in many studies is to find variables that clearly split the mean apart. Consider, for instance, the grouping variable of consuming sweetened beverages. For those who do not, the mean age of onset was quite late (71.3 years). Conversely, as you would then expect, for those who do consume sweetened beverages, the mean age was lower at 58.7 years. These two means are significantly different, so knowing about the behavior (sugar-sweetened beverage consumption) provides predictive ability regarding adult type II diabetes. Ignoring for a moment the *P*-values in the table that tell us it is significant, would you be sure that 71.3 and 58.7 are means that truly differ? You may recall from our previous example in which we wanted to determine the difference between two means, more information was needed to answer this question. It is not surprising that the answer comes back to the variance and a normal distribution. The independent groups *t*-test uses variance to compare the difference score between two groups and tells you how significant the differences are. The formula for the *t*-test is a ratio of (1) the difference between the two means to (2) the pooled variances and sample sizes of the two sample distributions. From this ratio, you can see that the resulting **test statistic** would increase as

TABLE 13.1 Independent Groups *t*-test Findings from a Fictional Study of Type II Diabetes				
Grouping Variable	**Mean Age of Onset**	**t-Value**	**df**	**P**
Does this person sit for more than 10 hours each day?				
Yes	61.7			
No	63.0	1.11	888	0.86
Does the person consume red meat?				
Yes	60.1			
No	62.5	0.97	891	0.77
Does the person exercise >5 hours each week?				
Yes	69.1			
No	60.0	2.44	896	0.001
Is the person experiencing chronic daily stress?				
Yes	60.5			
No	69.0	2.99	898	0.001
Does the person consume sweetened beverages?				
Yes	62.7			
No	74.0	3.42	889	<0.001
Is there a family history of diabetes?				
Yes	57.7			
No	66.1	1.99	878	0.04
Is the person considered obese?				
Yes	60.7			
No	66.9	2.12	880	0.02

the variance-adjusted difference between the means increases. A larger *t*-value equates with more confidence that the two means are indeed different from a smaller one. Once you have your *t*-statistic, using the **degrees of freedom** (i.e., *N1* + *N2* − *2*) for your analysis, you then compare your value with a distribution of *t*-values to determine whether it is significant. Generally, for studies with high degrees of freedom with alpha = 0.05 (two-tailed), a *t*-value of 1.96 or greater indicates that the mathematical difference in means was not likely the result of chance, leaving only a 5% likelihood of chance playing a role. Thus, for all the grouping variables in Table 13.1 with *P*-values of <0.05, you can reasonably say that these variables are statistically associated with but do not necessarily *cause* adult type II diabetes. One note related to this last statement is that although with a *t*-test you are determining whether group means differ from each other, if one of the variables has only two values (in this example, the grouping variable has two values, although the outcome variable age does not), the two variables can be deemed *to be associated*. Thus, it is appropriate to state that there is an association between the two variables. As you are most likely aware, another word for association is **correlation**, which we cover more in depth in this chapter.

Furthermore (although it requires other testing), you can judge the strength of any significant association by the magnitude of the *t*-value. For instance, the consumption of sugar-sweetened beverages has the greatest *t*-value in the table; thus, from a public health perspective, trying to reduce the amount of sugar-sweetened beverages people consume may be a primary leverage point for the prevention of adult type II diabetes. As previously indicated, the independent groups *t*-test is one of the most widely used parametric statistical tests because it provides so much important information that can be used to inform public health interventions. An example of a study is provided in **BOX 13.1**.

▶ Why Does Variance Matter?

To understand variance, you must first understand the concept of dispersion. Fortunately, you learned in Chapter 12 that dispersion is the distance, in units of measure, that scores or observations (in this case, daily temperature readings) deviate from a midpoint. You may also recall from Chapter 12 that squaring this distance gives us the metric known as *variance*. Variance is important because it relates to the ability of one variable to predict another variable. As an example, consider body mass index (BMI) and the amount of blood (expressed as a percentage) that is pumped in a single contraction of the heart and is known as the *ejection fraction*. For your study, you have collected data on BMI and the ejection fractions of 200 adults recruited from a workplace. The mean

BOX 13.1 Example of Study that Used Independent Groups *t*-Tests

Recently, it has become common for children to specialize in only one sport beginning at a young age. A Columbia University study was performed to determine both the motivations behind sports specialization and when athletes decide to specialize in one sport. A 50-question Likert-style survey was distributed among 303 collegiate athletes, 174 females and 129 males, from two National Collegiate Athletic Association Division I institutions. The collegiate athletes represented 19 different sports and collegiate athletes from both individual and team sports. The results showed 94.7% of specialized athletes played more than one sport before college, but only 45% of these athletes played multiple sports up to age 16. Roughly 17.4% of the participants reported specializing at age 12 or younger. The mean age for specialization among individual sport athletes was 14 years old, and the mean for an athlete within a team sport was 15.5 years old. A *t*-test was performed ($P = 0.008$). Overall, the mean age of specialization, including both individual and team sport athletes combined, was 14.9 years old. Further analysis determined male athletes in individual sports specialized earlier than did male athletes participating within team sports ($P \leq 0.001$). The motivation for sports specialization results indicated personal interest, skill level, time constraints, and potential scholarship opportunities were the top-ranked reasons a collegiate athlete decided to specialize in a single sport. Individual sport athletes reported wanting to compete at both collegiate and professional levels as significantly more influential factors ($P < 0.001$). The study provided insights into the age trend of early sports specialization and the differences between athletes within individual and team sports. In addition, the results indicated motives for specialization may be influenced by the choice to play either an individual or a team sport (Swindell, Marcille, Trofa, Paulino, Desai, Lynch... Popkin, 2019)

BMI equals 26.5 (just above the cutoff value of normal weight), and the mean ejection fraction equals 0.58. For both variables, there is a great deal of dispersion and thus variance. For learning purposes, think of the amount of variance as being represented by a circle, with larger circumferences representing greater variance. With this image in mind, the question now becomes, Is any portion of the total variance for BMI somehow linked, meaning shared in a systematic way that can be mathematically quantified, to the variance in the ejection fraction? **FIGURE 13.4** provides a handy visual about this concept of shared variance.

As you readily observe by looking at this figure, BMI has greater variance than the ejection fraction. What is important, however, is shown by the overlap depicted in the lower portion of the figure. In the language of science, this overlap would be explained as the amount of variance explained in the ejection fraction by BMI. Please take careful note of

the wording here. The variable being predicted is the one of interest; it is commonly referred to as the *outcome*. In this example, the ejection fraction is the outcome because BMI influences heart functioning rather than the reverse. With the ejection fraction as the outcome, we want to know what predicts the variance in this measure. Judging from the overlap shown in Figure 13.4, we can assume that a fair amount of the variance in the ejection fraction is explained by BMI. The word *explained* means the proportion to which a mathematical model accounts for the variance in a given data set. Thus, the greater amount of variance explained signifies that a statistical relationship exists, thereby giving us the ability to draw conclusions. For example, "People with a *higher* BMI are more likely to have a *lower* ejection fraction." At this juncture, we can depart from this rather philosophical approach to teaching you about variance and proceed to more practical applications.

▶ How Is Variance the Basis of Correlation?

Aside from the benefits of calculating variance covered in the previous chapter, another benefit or value of calculating a sample's variance is its use for determining the degree of association between two continuous variables. To refresh your memory, a variable is something that varies, and a continuous

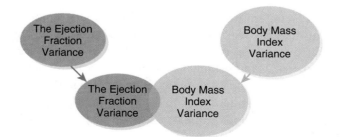

FIGURE 13.4 Depiction of Variance for Body Mass Index, the Ejection Fraction, and the Shared Variance Between These Two Variables.

variable is defined as a variable that can take on any value between a minimum and maximum value. Within a sample, you want the data values to have a certain degree of variability. You do not want a sample in which all of the values are too similar; that would equate with little to no variability and would be considered a constant. Variance is one type of variability that can be calculated from a data set of continuous variables, and correlation is a function of variance. Correlation is essentially viewed as the overlap or shared variance between two variables. In the absence of any variance, correlations will not occur. In fact, it is virtually impossible for a variable and a constant to be correlated. For example, suppose you want to know if income level is associated with the health behavior of contraceptive use among U.S. women not intending to have children. You happen to have a data set of 300 women, all of them part of a convenience sample recruited from a professional association. You find an absence of correlation between income and use of contraception. You conclude that income does not matter. The problem with this conclusion is that all of these professional women may have relatively high levels of income, thereby limiting the variance and consequently crippling the ability of this variable to be correlated with anything at all. Stated in simple terms, if everyone in one data set has nearly the same value for a particular variable (e.g., for income, $125,000), it is no longer a variable and will not be useful in a statistical analysis.

Building from what you learned previously in this chapter about shared variance (refer back to Figure 13.4), we now provide a more detailed example of how shared variance is the basis for correlation. **FIGURE 13.5** displays a new example depicting the overlap (shared variance) between "number of hours exercising" and "happiness." As you have previously learned, you will notice that the variance for the measure of happiness is somewhat less than for the number of exercise hours per week, and the area where the two circles overlap represents shared variance. To refresh you, this means

that increases or decreases from the mean go hand in hand for each variable, at least for the amount of variance in the shaded area.

To illuminate how this example of shared variance would be reflected in data, we refer you to the scores in **TABLE 13.2**. Without even using a computer, you can look at the values in Table 13.2 and ask, "Does there appear to be a relationship between each set of data points?" For instance, notice that persons number 2, 4, 9, and 13 all have high happiness scores (with 10 being the highest possible score on this scale measure). Notice also that these same four people report a greater number of hours per week

TABLE 13.2 Scores on Measures of Hours Exercised Per Week and a Scale Measure of Happiness

Person ID No.	Exercise Hours per Week	Happiness
001	10	7
002	12	9
003	6	4
004	17	10
005	3	5
006	7	6
007	8	8
008	1	5
009	9	9
010	4	3
011	7	8
012	6	5
013	15	9
014	12	8
015	11	7

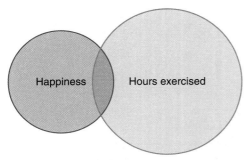

FIGURE 13.5 "Shared Variance" Between Happiness and Hours Exercised.

devoted to exercise than the other 11 people in the sample. Conversely, notice that persons 3, 5, 8, and 10 all have low happiness scores, with these same four people also reporting relatively low numbers of hours devoted to exercise each week. As an observation, you might conclude that as the number of exercise hours goes up, so does happiness. When scores on two variables rise or fall in connection with one another, this is known as a **positive correlation**. In the event that an increase in the score for one variable has a mathematical relationship to a decrease in scores for a second variable, the term used is **negative correlation** or **inverse correlation**.

Now that you have a philosophical understanding of correlation, the next step is to gain an understanding of how the Pearson product moment correlation coefficient is generated by a statistical software program (this can also be done in Excel). To begin, the term **bivariate data point** must be understood. The best way to understand it is to hand plot a graph of the intersections between the two variables shown in Table 13.2. Consider happiness as the y-axis (the vertical axis on a graph) and the number of hours exercised per week as the x-axis (the horizontal axis). Then, for the first person in the study (ID #001), locate the intersection in this graph for a score of 10 on the x-axis and a score of 7 on the y-axis; this is your first bivariate data point. Then simply repeat the process for the remaining 14 study participants. Now you have what is known as a **scattergram**—this should show a relatively discernible line of data points (as shown in **FIGURE 13.6**).

When lining up data points creates a left-to-right line that slopes upward, you have a positive correlation. And, of course, when this line slopes downward, you have a negative correlation. A *perfect* correlation would look like a 45-degree angle, bisecting the graph into equal portions; this would be a correlation of 1.0. It is highly unlikely you will come across a correlation coefficient of 1.0 in public health; instead, you will be lucky to find coefficients of 0.50—even 0.30 is considered good. So, as you might imagine, coefficients of 0.50 and 0.30, for example, will have much smaller slopes (that is, they rise or fall in a much less dramatic fashion compared with a 45-degree angle). The point here is that a software program will give you a value for what is known as the **Pearson product moment correlation**—this value will fall somewhere between −1.00 and +1.00. The Pearson coefficient (for short) is depicted by r and is an indicator of slope and direction, with slope being a matter of degree and direction being either negative or positive.

One final note about correlation is in order. The correlation coefficient (r) can be squared to become what is known as the **coefficient of determination** or as r^2. r^2 is a statistical measure of how close the data are to the fitted regression line. An r^2 value of 100% indicates that the model explains all the variability of the response data around its mean. For instance, the Pearson product moment correlation coefficient for the example in Table 13.2 is approximately 0.82, and squaring this value gives 0.67, meaning that 67% of the variance is explained. In the world of public health, however, correlation coefficients of 0.30, for example, are common and generally considered a medium effect. Squaring 0.30 would explain 9% of the variance. It is always wise when interpreting correlation coefficients, to square them and determine how much variance they account for regardless of the P-value.

Before preceding to the last two sections of this chapter, we need to make two warnings about correlation. First, correlation in no way can be considered a cause-and-effect relationship. Although exercise may lead to happiness, isn't it also plausible that people who are

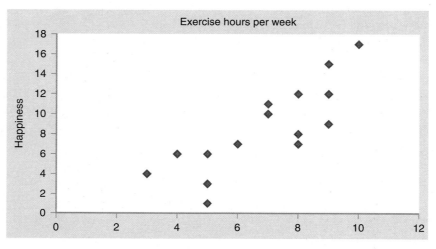

FIGURE 13.6 Scatterplot of Data Points of Happiness and Exercise Level.

A study of 188 obese children residing in China tested the proposition that physical activity and the consumption of vegetables and fruits would predict well-being and depression. Well-being was assessed by a validated five-item index, and depression was assessed by the Depression Self-Rating Scale for Children. Sufficient physical activity was as at least 60 minutes each day for 3 or more days per week. Sufficient vegetable and fruit intake was defined by consuming 5 or more servings each day over a 30-day recall period. Kids scoring higher on the physical activity and who had sufficient fruit and vegetable intake were significantly *less* at risk for depression and poor well-being, indicating fruit and vegetable consumption provides a protective effect. Although the study findings are intuitively appealing, there is a flip side to these cross-sectional findings: It could be that higher levels of depression lead to less exercise and a corresponding loss of desire to eat the right foods. These interpretations may have been neglected in this study design. In the United States, for example, the term *comfort food* is often used to represent the consumption of high-calorie, high-fat, and high-sugar foods that may bring some transient happiness to people experiencing depressed mood or actual depression. Whether this same phenomenon occurs in China (and among Chinese children) was not addressed as a possible alternate explanation of the study findings. Similarly, whether depression may have led to social disengagement in after school activities—including physical activities that produce exercise—would be a likely alternate explanation of the study findings.

Modified from Yu H, Li F, Hu Y, et al. Associations of physical activity and fruit and vegetable intake with well being and depressive symptoms among obese schoolchildren in Wuhan, China: a cross-sectional study. BMC Public Health 2018;18:986.

Consider the question of whether age is associated with a general measure of stigmatizing attitudes toward obesity. This brief scale measure uses a five-point response option ranging from 1 (Strongly Disagree) to 5 (Strongly Agree) to the nine stigmatizing statements. Suppose you administered this measure to 1000 people ranging in age from 16 to 66 years old. You calculate the Pearson product moment correlation to determine the association of age with scores on this measure; you obtain a Pearson r-value of -0.12. The computer output notes that this value is significant at $P < 0.01$. Thus, your first reaction is to conclude that as age increases, the level of stigmatized attitudes toward obesity decreases. Although this is a legitimate conclusion from a purely statistical viewpoint, it misses the point that squaring 0.12 gives 0.014—meaning that slightly more than 1 percent of the variance in this attitudinal measure is explained by age. So, you would be compelled to then ask yourself, is this an important finding? We trust that your answer would be "No."

Modified from Lewis RJ, Cash TF, Jacobi L, Bubb-Lewis C. Prejudice toward fat people: the development and validation of the anti-fat attitudes test. Obesity Research 1997;5:297–307.

happy tend to exercise more frequently than people who are not? It certainly is plausible. But, in this example, it is not possible to definitively say that one comes "before" the other; one would need a different study design that can examine the temporal ordering of happiness and exercise and to know whether exercise leads to more happiness or whether happy people exercise more. Nonetheless, the old saying applies in the current context: Correlation is not causation, but it is necessary to establish causation. **BOX 13.2** provides an example from the public health peer-reviewed literature.

As a second warning, and one that applies beyond correlation, output from a software program will automatically generate *P*-values for each correlation that is produced. These *P*-values do not indicate the strength of the correlation; instead, they simply inform you as to the basic question, Was this a chance finding? **BOX 13.3** provides an extensive example of why this warning is so crucial to comprehend.

▶ How Does Correlation Form the Basis of Regression?

Consider that you want to understand why teenagers begin to use opioids. You quickly decide to assess this outcome by a single-item measure that asks, How many times have you ever used opioids? For your explanatory variables (the *predictors* of opioid use), you might select *rural residence* (this can be assessed using a rating from 1 to 9 that is available through the U.S. government) as a top reason, but you may also want to consider the role of a scale measure capturing *sensation seeking* and perhaps a measure of *parental monitoring*. So, given that you collect these data from a representative sample, you can begin with what you know: correlation. Let's assume that you find that rural residence has a correlation with beginning opioid use of 0.16, sensation seeking of 0.35, and parental monitoring of 0.23. Again, staying with what you know, you can square each coefficient to see how much variance is explained in the outcome (opioid use) by the three individual predictor variables combined. That would equate with $0.16^2 = .03$, $0.35^2 = .12$, and $0.23^2 = .05$. The total is then $0.03 + 0.12 + 0.05 = 0.20$, explaining 20% of the variance in our outcome. Unfortunately, this method of ostensibly adding up the individual r^2 values is not an accurate way of assessing the total variance explained by the three variables. The reason the three r^2 values cannot simply be added together has to do with a concept known as **collinearity**. Collinearity is nothing more than intercorrelations among the predictor variables. As a result, the unique contribution of each predictor variable is less than its contribution alone. If two predictor variables are correlated somewhat, part of their influence is joint—that is, it cannot be assigned uniquely to one variable or the other. You can deduce then that some of the variance explained by rurality is also explained by the other two predictor variables because they also will have shared variance. To overcome this problem, the solution is **multiple linear regression**. Describing how multiple regression works is beyond the scope of this textbook, but its conceptual basis is simple. Instead of generating three separate regression equations, the multiple-regression equation includes all three predictors in one and takes into consideration the overlapping variance based on rules that can be set by the person doing the analyses. Regardless of the rules selected, shared variance is never double counted.

FIGURE 13.7 displays our example in the form of a path model. A path model uses multiple regression to evaluate causal models by examining the relationships between a dependent variable (or outcome) and two or more independent (or predictor) variables. In this example, the correlation coefficients in the brackets represent the multiple regression coefficients, also called *partial regression coefficients*, whereas the other coefficients in the parentheses represent the individual Pearson correlations between each predictor and opioid use. Collinearity is indicated as shown by the Pearson correlations between each of the three predictors.

The end product of a multiple regression equation is known as R^2; this is nothing more than the total amount of variance explained *collectively* by the predictor variables. For example, as you now know and can see, the combination of the three predictor variables shown in Figure 13.6 cannot possibly explain 20% of the variance as this would be inflated due to double counting of shared variance. In this example, if you add up the squared partial regression coefficients shown in the brackets ($.21^2$, $.29^2$, and $.14^2$) the total variance accounted for by combining the three variables is 14.78%. The variance accounted for jointly by the three predictors = 5.22%. Like the Pearson coefficient, R^2 ranges from 0 to 1 but cannot ever be a negative value. As a consumer of the public health professional literature, one habit you should develop is to look at the R^2 value in any journal article reporting the

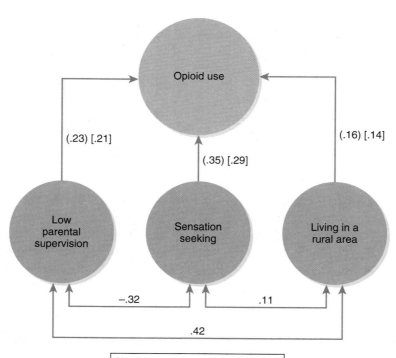

( ) = Pearson correlation coefficient
[ ] = Partial regression coefficients

FIGURE 13.7 A Path Model Demonstrating How Shared Variance Affects Coefficients.

use of multiple linear regression. **BOX 13.4** provides an example of a large, and nationally representative, study that used multiple linear regression to predict variance in two related outcomes. As you will see when you read about this study, many of the predictor variables were significant in the models that were constructed. However, we use this study to demonstrate to you why R^2 matters. It matters because predictor variables may have a significant relationship with an outcome, but that does not mean that large quantities of total variance are necessarily explained. Thus, we urge you to become a wise consumer of the professional literature and always look for and consider the size of the R^2 values.

Ultimately, we want you to understand how linear regression is used in the everyday world of public health. Consider, for example, the simple idea of how a clinician doing a checkup for an adult might assess how likely that person is to have a heart attack in the next 10 years. As you may know, people often go to a doctor and come back saying something like, "I'm good—my heart is okay for another 10 years or more." But have you ever wondered how doctors make this proclamation? To help you see behind the scenes, consider a recent study (one that used linear regression) that created an online

risk calculator that uses test results from various biological measures that can be easily assessed in a clinic setting and then entered into the calculator. **FIGURE 13.8** displays a screenshot of this risk calculator for a hypothetical 45-year-old male Caucasian. After taking a close look at Figure 13.8, the question that we would like you to consider is, How much weight does each one of the risk factors contribute to the overall risk score?

To answer this question, read the article by McClelland and colleagues (2015). In the event that you would like a preview of this, we have created a brief summary. To begin, you need to know that a standardized correlation coefficient is also referred to as a *weight* and is known specifically as a **beta weight**; it ranges from –1.0 to +1.0. So, given this knowledge, you can start to understand how beta weights calculated in the study were used to create an overall risk score. For instance, being a current smoker contributed a beta weight of 0.37 ($P = 0.005$), and having diabetes contributed a similar size beta weight of 0.38 ($P = 0.002$). Currently taking medications for diabetes contributed a beta weight of 0.23 ($P = 0.03$); perhaps as a marker of risk, currently taking medications for cholesterol contributed a beta weight of 0.12 ($P = 0.32$). Please notice

---

BOX 13.4 An Example of "Total Variance Explained"

A Canadian study of more than 7000 patients from 759 practices (for both physical and mental conditions) sought to determine the predictive value of five variables on the outcomes of (1) seeking care for *physical* health issues or conditions and (2) seeking care for *mental* health issues or conditions. The outcomes were assessed using the Responsive Care Scale (RCS), with one version being used for physical issues or conditions (RCS-P) and another being used for mental issues or conditions (RCS-M). The five predictor variables were:

1. Age
2. A single-item measure of attitude toward preventing illness
3. A single-item measure of trust in physicians
4. A single-item measure of perceived ability to "prevent problems with your health"
5. Whether study participants currently had a chronic disease

Each of these five variables was tested in four separate multiple linear-regression models. As the following shows, each model predicted only a tiny portion of the variance in the outcome, with model RCS-P predicting zero variance for males only.

Model Total Variance (R^2)

1.	RCS-M regressed on the predictor variables, for females only	2.7%
2.	RCS-P regressed on the predictor variables, for females only	1.0%
3.	RCS-M regressed on the predictor variables, for males only	3.6%
4.	RCS-P regressed on the predictor variables, for males only	0.0%

Based on these results, this national study concluded, "The variables were better predictors of healthcare-seeking behaviour in response to mental health concerns than physical health concerns, likely reflecting greater variation among those seeking mental healthcare." Although this conclusion is indeed "true," the underlying question to consider when thinking about the extremely low values of R^2 is, given the tiny amount of variance explained by the five predictor variables, is it truly possible to state that mental health issues are better predicted by this set of variables?

Modified from Thompson, A. E., Anisimowicz, Y., Miedema, B., Hogg, W., Wodchis, W. P., & Aubrey-Bassler, K. (2016). The influence of gender and other patient characteristics on health care-seeking behaviour: a QUALICOPC study. *BMC Family Practice, 17*(1), 38.

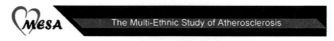

MESA 10-Year CHD Risk with Coronary Artery Calcification   Back to CAC Tools

1. **Gender**   Male ⦿   Female ○

2. **Age (45-85 years)**   48   Years

3. **Coronary Artery Calcification**   404   Agatston

4. **Race/Ethnicity**   **Choose One**

                                    Caucasian   ⦿
                                    Chinese   ○
                                    African American ○
                                    Hispanic   ○

5. **Diabetes**   Yes ○   No ⦿
6. **Currently Smoke**   Yes ○   No ⦿
7. **Family History of Heart Attack** Yes ⦿   No ○
   (History in parents, siblings, or children)

8. **Total Cholesterol**   190   mg/dL or   4.9   mmol/L

9. **HDL Cholesterol**   50   mg/dL or   1.3   mmol/L

10. **Systolic Blood Pressure**   150   mmHg or   20.0   kPa
11. **Lipid Lowering Medication**   Yes ○   No ⦿
12. **Hypertension Medication**   Yes ⦿   No ○

                    [Calculate 10-year CHD risk]

The estimated 10-year risk of a CHD event for a person with this risk factor profile including coronary calcium is 16.3%. The estimated 10-year risk of a CHD event for a person with this risk factor profile if we did not factor in their coronary calcium score would be 7.2%.

©2019 Collaborative Health Studies Coordinating Center | Risk Score API Help
Contact | Privacy | Terms

FIGURE 13.8 Hypothetical Results for Cardiovascular Heart Disease Risk Using an Online Risk Calculator.

MESA Risk Score Calulator, Multi-Ethnic Study of Atherosclerosis (MESA). https://www.mesa-nhlbi.org/CAC-Tools.aspx

in this last sentence that the beta weight of 0.12 is, of course, small and thus did not achieve significance. What this research team did find to be a strong predictor of future heart attacks was a variable known as coronary artery calcium (CAC). The beta weight for CAC was 0.25 ($P < 0.0001$). As you can see, the general health magazine article regarding the idea of how long someone will live actually has a mathematical basis, one firmly grounded in multiple linear regression.

▶ What Is Analysis of Variance?

One highly specific application of regression is known as **analysis of variance (ANOVA)**. This is best used when you want to compare means for three or more groups of study participants. For instance, let's say you have the privilege of being involved in a research project that uses a randomized controlled design to test a behavioral intervention designed to help people lose weight. The program uses random assignment to form three arms: a control group, an experimental group A, and an experimental group B. Your challenge is to determine if body mass index (the outcome variable or *dependent variable*, DV) has been substantially reduced 3 months following the intervention. More important, you want to know whether the DV was reduced differentially as a function of group assignment. One way to determine this—that is, to see if the program was effective—is to compare the means between:

- ▪ The experimental group A and the control group
- ▪ The experimental group B and the control group
- ▪ The experimental group A and the experimental group B

You might first consider conducting a *t*-test for each of these three comparisons. Unfortunately, there is a caveat to performing multiple statistical tests for one research question. For each test performed, you are essentially increasing the probability of finding an effect or a statistically significant result *by chance alone*. This probability increases exactly by the alpha level chosen for each test performed. Performing three different *t*-tests for this one research question would thereby increase your risk of finding a chance result (3 tests × 0.05) to 15%. To avoid this problem, ANOVA could be used instead because it compares all three means with one grand mean, taking into account their respective standard deviations. The result is expressed as an *F*-statistic. A significant *F* tells us that the means are significantly different from the grand mean, and a nonsignificant *F* tells us this is not the case (the intervention had no effect on BMI after 3 months). In the event of a significant *F,* however, you still are not sure how the three group means differ. Thus, there is one more step to this process. You will need to conduct what is known as a **post hoc test** to determine specifically how the means of the groups differ. For this example, post hoc tests would examine whether experimental group A is significantly lower than experimental group B, experimental group A is lower than the control group, and experimental group B is lower than the control group. However, doing this will bring us back to our initial issue of increasing the potential for Type I error. Thus, when performing these post hoc comparisons, now that we know that they do indeed differ, we can adjust for this. One specific type of post hoc test is called the *Bonferroni* and uses *t*-tests to perform the pairwise comparisons between the group means but controls the overall error rate or alpha level. To control the overall error rate, this post hoc test sets a new error rate for each individual *t*-test. This new error rate is equal to the original experiment-wise error rate (i.e., 0.05) divided by the total number of tests. In this example, alpha then would be set to 0.05/3 = 0.017. Thus, for the investigator to deem the test significant, the *P*-value needs to be less than 0.017. Hence, the Bonferroni adjusts or corrects the significance level for the fact that multiple comparisons are being made. Typically, we recommend that the only time you would change your alpha level during a study would be to make an adjustment that reduces the probability of making a Type I error as when doing a Bonferroni adjustment.

A final note is warranted before you leave this chapter. What this chapter has *not* done is teach you how to handle data that would be tested using nonparametric procedures. The types of data that typically fall into this category are described as categorical or nominal—for example, students who are stressed about college finances (strongly agree vs. strongly disagree), adult type II diabetes (yes vs. no), smoking cessation (yes vs. no), or effective use of contraception (yes vs. no). This mission, should you accept it, is waiting for you in the next chapter and will provide an overview of nonparametric tests.

Think About It!

So often in public health we are dealing with long-standing issues such as cancer, stroke, heart disease, and diabetes. Yet the public health workforce must be constantly alert and ready to respond to outbreaks of emerging threats such as Ebola, severe acute respiratory syndrome, and Hantavirus. A good example is captured by the annual potential of a *pandemic shift* in the protein composition of the flu virus because these shifts can lead to forms of the flu that rapidly spread and claim the lives of host organisms. Far from being theoretical, pandemic shifts have occurred in recent history. A good example is the 1918 Spanish Flu epidemic (see photo in **FIGURE 13.9**). The epidemic infected more than 500 million people worldwide and claimed the lives of more than 50 million people. It was not unusual for people to be infected in the morning and dead by evening.

Now, once again, let's return back to Figure 13.2 and that matter of the tiny overlap that precluded us from safely rejecting the null hypothesis. The word *safely* is the key here. The public health standard of an alpha equal to 0.05 and thus a 95% confidence interval is one that errs on the side of not being too quick to reject the null. The flip side to

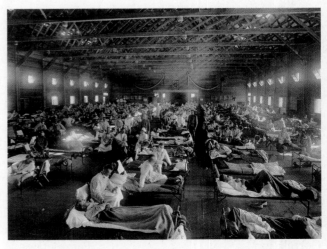

FIGURE 13.9 Battling the 1918 Spanish Flu Pandemic.
Courtesy of Centers for Disease Control and Prevention.

this for public health practice is that this standard results in practitioners being slow to adopt a new program practice or approach to prevention that showed no effects because the significance level was 0.052. Thus, the question we pose to you is whether this safety standard should ever be relaxed at all in the face of a public health emergency? Although some critics would say you should never relax your alpha level for fear of making a Type I error (see FIGURE 13.10), a practical and ethical way to think about this is to ask, Is it better to risk having a program in place that *may* not work or to risk *not* using a program that may work? This kind of question is precisely the intellectual acumen that we want you to have in the event of a public health emergency such as another pandemic shift in the protein structure of the flu virus.

DON'T MESS WITH THE ALPHA

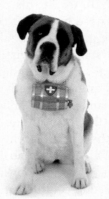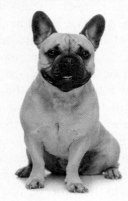

OR ELSE . . . .

FIGURE 13.10 Snow and Hamilton Public Health Mascots on Level of Significance.
© Eric Isselee/Shutterstock; © Svetography/Shutterstock

Take Home Points

- Parametric tests assume that data follow a normal distribution.
- The alpha level of a statistical test, also referred to as *Type I error*, signifies the probability of making a wrong decision and incorrectly rejecting the null hypothesis.
- The independent groups *t*-test is appropriate for when your only task is comparing the means of two groups.
- Correlation between two variables can only be determined if each variable has sufficient variability or variance among the scores.
- The Pearson product moment correlation coefficient is one measure and is appropriate when you want to know if two continuous-level variables rise and fall as a function of one another.
- Correlation does not indicate causation but is a necessary step for causation.
- Multiple linear regression is useful when you want to test the association of more than one predictor variable on a given outcome and accounts for the shared variance.
- Predictor variables that are intercorrelated suggest collinearity. When all predictors are in one regression equation, collinearity reduces the overall amount of variance accounted for by each individual predictor in isolation.
- ANOVA is used for comparing means when more than two groups are involved such as in the case of a three-arm randomized controlled trial.
- An overall significant *F*-statistic results from ANOVA and indicates that groups differ.
- Post hoc tests should be run following a significant ANOVA result with corrections to the alpha level to reduce Type I error.
- Running statistical tests requires setting a probability level that minimizes the risk of making a Type I error.

Key Terms

Alpha
Analysis of variance (ANOVA)
Beta weight
Bivariate data point
Coefficient of determination
Collinearity
Correlation
Critical region
Degrees of freedom

Grouping variable
Independent groups *t*-test
Inverse correlation
Multiple linear regression
Negative correlation
Nonparametric
Parametric
Pearson product moment
    correlation

Positive correlation
Post hoc test
Rejection region
Scattergram
Statistically significant
Test statistic
Type I error
Type II error

For Practice and Discussion

1. Compare and contrast parametric and nonparametric statistical tests. What are the characteristics of each?

2. Explain the purpose of a grouping variable within a public health context using a health topic of your choosing.

3. A researcher found that high BMI is correlated with lower socioeconomic status. Would this be an example of a positive or negative correlation, and why?

4. A postdoctoral fellow is conducting a study to examine whether alcohol use, drug use, and homelessness, are associated with sexual violence victimization. However, her three continuous predictor variables (alcohol use, drug use, and homelessness) are correlated with one another. What would be the best statistical test to use to conduct the data analysis for this study, and why?

5. Your research team would like to compare the differences between an intervention and control group in a randomized controlled trial. What would be the most appropriate parametric test to analyze the differences between groups?

References

Lewis, R. J., Cash, T. F., Jacobi, L., & Bubb-Lewis, C. (1997). Prejudice toward fat people the development and validation of the anti-fat attitudes test. *Obesity Research, 5,* 297–307.

McClelland, R. L., Jorgensen, N. W., Budoff, M., Blaha, M. J., Post, W. S., . . . Burke, G. L. (2015, October 13). 10-year coronary heart disease risk prediction using coronary artery calcium and traditional risk factors. *Journal of the American College of Cardiology, 66*(15), 1643–1653.

Schenker, N., & Gentleman, J. F. (2001). On judging the significance of differences by examining the overlap between confidence intervals. *American Statistician, 55*(3), 182–186.

Snedecor, G. W., & Cochran, W. G. (1989). *Statistical methods* (8th ed.). Ames, IA: Iowa State University Press.

Swindell, H. W., Marcille, M. L., Trofa, D. P., Paulino, F. E., Desai, N. N., . . . Popkin, C. A. (2019). An analysis of sports specialization in NCAA Division I collegiate athletics. *Orthopaedic Journal of Sports Medicine, 7*(1), 2325967118821179.

Thompson, A. E., Anisimowicz, Y., Miedema, B., Hogg, W., Wodchis, W. P., & Aubrey-Bassler, K. (2016). The influence of gender and other patient characteristics on health care-seeking behaviour: A QUALICOPC study. *BMC Family Practice, 17*(1), 38.

Yu, H., Li, F., Hu, Y., Li, C., Yang, X., . . . He, Q. (2018). Associations of physical activity and fruit and vegetable intake with well being and depressive symptoms among obese schoolchildren in Wuhan, China: A cross-sectional study. *BMC Public Health, 18,* 986.

For Further Reading

Gerstman, B. B. (2014). *Basic biostatistics: Statistics for public health* (2nd ed.). Burlington, MA: Jones & Bartlett.

Sullivan, L. M. (2017). *Essentials of biostatistics in public health.* Burlington, MA: Jones & Bartlett Learning.

CHAPTER 14

Nonparametric Data Analysis

LEARNING OBJECTIVES

1. Explain what nonparametric tests are and when they are appropriate.
2. Describe what the chi-square test does, when it is warranted, and how to calculate it.
3. Illustrate how to conduct a layered chi-square test and interpret the results.
4. Define the conceptual basis of logistic regression and how to interpret the results.
5. Distinguish between two methods of logistic regression analyses in the context of public health research.

▶ Overview

In Chapter 13, we described several parametric statistical analytic tools for analyzing data that are continuous in nature and also assume a normal distribution. But what do we do if our data are not normal? The parametric assumption of normality is particularly worrisome for small sample sizes ($n < 30$); and if the data deviate strongly from the assumptions of a parametric procedure, using parametric procedures could lead to incorrect conclusions. Also, parametric tests may not apply to many of the outcomes measured in public health research that are categorical rather than continuous in nature. Categorical data represent the quality of an outcome (e.g., disease or no disease) and are expressed in terms of percentages or proportions rather than means and standard deviations. Categorical data by definition are not from a normal distribution but are binomial, specifically when there are only two categories— that is, they are dichotomous. Fortunately, there are solutions for these problems. In fact, an entire set

of analytic methods has been widely adopted by the profession for application to data that are not normally distributed whether because of small sample sizes or the nature of the data. These analytic methods are deemed nonparametric procedures and are the answer if your data are not from a normal distribution and violate the underlying assumptions for parametric tests (see **FIGURE 14.1**). This chapter is devoted to helping you learn a few of the most basic nonparametric procedures. You will find that throughout your career in public health research and practice, each of these tools will be used on a routine basis. As such, we urge you to spend lots of time with this chapter and learn as much as possible.

▶ What Is a Chi-Square Test and How Does It Work?

A widely used nonparametric test that assesses whether an association exists between two categorical variables is the **chi-square** test of independence. At its

HAVE YOUR NON-NORMAL DATA GOT YOU QUESTIONING YOUR ASSUMPTIONS?

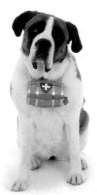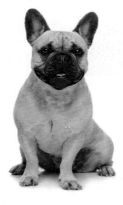

NON-PARAMETRIC TESTS ARE THE ANSWER

FIGURE 14.1 Public Health Mascots Snow and Hamilton Understand Non-Normality.

© Eric Isselee/Shutterstock; © Svetography/Shutterstock

TABLE 14.1	Example of a Contingency Table of Parental Monitoring and Binge Drinking Among N = 159 Teens		
	Binge Drinking		
Parental Monitoring (PM)	*No (0)*	*Yes (1)*	*Totals*
Low (0) Count % within PM	11	68 **86.0%**	79
High (1) Count % within PM	38	42 **52.5%**	80
Totals	49	110	159

essence, the chi-square test compares an observed pattern of responses with a pattern that would be expected if the variables were truly independent of each other. Calculating the chi-square statistic and then comparing it with a critical value from the chi-square distribution allows the researcher to assess whether the observed cell counts are significantly different from the expected cell counts. If they are significantly different, it signifies an association.

To put the chi-square test into its most basic terms, it first begins with a **contingency table** that is made up of two categorical variables of interest. A contingency table is also referred to as a *crosstabulation table* and involves crossing the frequency counts of each level of the categorical variables. For example, a study that involves determining whether biological sex is associated with having hypertension would create a table that crosses (1) the number of individuals who self-report male sex and who also have hypertension, (2) the number of individuals who self-report male sex and who do not have hypertension, (3) the number of individuals who self-report female sex and who also have hypertension, and (4) the number of individuals who self-report female sex and who do not have hypertension. If you can picture this 2 × 2 table, each intersecting row (biological sex) and column (hypertension) in the table is known as a **cell**, and within each cell, you will find the observed cell counts.

Although ostensibly easy, this first step in understanding the chi-square test can be confusing to students, but it can be mastered with the help of a visual.

TABLE 14.1 displays another contingency table that involves parental monitoring and teenage binge drinking. In this example, we are interested in knowing whether parental monitoring is associated with teenage binge-drinking behavior. The predictor variable or *exposure* variable in this study is a categorical measure of parental monitoring, and the outcome variable is a categorical measure of teenage binge drinking. It is customary and important to always set up a contingency table with the outcome variable being on the top (columns) and the predictor variable on the left-hand side (rows). Further, it is customary to assign numeric values of zero to represent low levels or absence of the construct, whereas a value of 1 is assigned to denote values representing high levels or presence of the construct. Thus, in this example, a value of 0 would equate with low parental monitoring and also no binge drinking, and a value of 1 would equate with high parental monitoring and also yes to binge drinking. As shown in Table 14.1, the predictor variable parental monitoring appears in the first row with the label "Low (0)" that corresponds to low values of parental monitoring and in the second row with the label "High (1)" that corresponds to high values. Teenage binge drinking appears in the first column with the label " No (0)", which corresponds to no binge drinking in the past 90 days and in the second column with the label "Yes (1)", which corresponds to binge drinking at least once in the past 90 days.

As shown in Table 14.1, 79 of 159 teens were classified as having low levels, and 80 were classified as having high levels of parental monitoring. The contingency table also shows that 49 teens had not engaged in binge drinking in the past 90 days while 110 had engaged in binge drinking on at least one occasion during this recall period. As you can see, there are four cells. Rather than considering all four cells, a streamlined approach is to focus only on the cells representing risk (i.e., the binge-drinking column). In this case, you can see that 68 teens were in the cell created by the intersection of low parental monitoring and binge drinking and that another 42 were in the cell created by the intersection of high parental monitoring and binge drinking. Before you jump to the conclusion that parental monitoring had an influence on binge drinking, bear in mind that the row totals are slightly different (i.e., 79 versus 80); thus, the percentages must be considered. On further inspection of the contingency table, you will see that 86.0% (68/79) of those with low parental monitoring reported binge drinking versus only 52.5% (42/80) of those with higher levels of parental monitoring. Mathematically, it appears that those with lower levels of parental monitoring were more likely to binge drink, but we must calculate the chi-square statistic to make sure. The formula for the chi-square statistic is straightforward if you care to calculate by hand, but most statistical software programs can run this with ease:

$$\chi_c^2 = \sum \frac{(O_i - E_i)^2}{E_i}$$

where c is the degrees of freedom that equal (# of rows − 1) × (# of columns − 1), O_i is the observed counts in the cells and E_i is the expected counts in the cells if no association exists. The expected frequency for each cell is based on its row and column totals. This expected frequency is then compared with the actual frequency (known as the *observed frequency*) to determine differences. As observed frequencies increasingly differ (either higher or lower) from the expected frequencies, the value of the chi-square test statistic increases. In the example of Table 14.1, after doing the math, the calculation of the chi-square statistic reveals that this difference in percentages is in fact statistically significant, $X^2 (1, N = 159) = 21.02, p < 0.001$. Following the point of only comparing those with and without the risk behavior (e.g., low versus high levels of parental monitoring) relative to having a "1" on the outcome variable (e.g., binge drinking at least once in the past 90 days), chi-square findings are easy to report in table form. A customary reporting format for chi-square results is shown as **TABLE 14.2**.

Although the chi-square statistic is the appropriate nonparametric test to use for associations between categorical variables, there are several important considerations. Because of how the chi-square value is calculated, it is extremely sensitive to sample size:

TABLE 14.2 Example of Chi-Square Results Reported in a Table

Risk Variable	Binge Drinking	P-Value
Low level of parental monitoring ($n = 79$)	86.0%	
High level of parental monitoring ($n = 80$)	52.5%	0.00001

When the sample size is large (~500), almost any small difference will appear statistically significant. The chi-square value is also sensitive to the distribution within the cells if cells have fewer than five cases. This can be addressed by always using categorical variables with a limited number of categories or by collapsing categories if necessary to produce a smaller table. **BOX 14.1** illustrates a research study that used chi-square to determine the barriers and facilitators of discussing HIV prevention with adolescents.

Before proceeding to the next section, we want you to understand a common statistical principle. The principle is that the "best" statistical test is the one that "best fits" the data and the purpose of the study. For instance, imagine that you design a study and, because you read Chapter 2 in this book carefully, you come up with the following statement of the study purpose.

> The purpose of the study was to compare college age females and males relative to drug use behaviors over the past 6 months.

Given this purpose, one of your variables (i.e., the predictor variable is sex of the student) is clearly nominal and dichotomous (please note, the statement refers to biological sex rather than gender because gender terms such as *man, woman, gender queer, transmasculine,* and *transfeminine* would not form a dichotomy). As it turns out, the survey questions used for this study involved a simple "yes versus no" response option; thus, the outcomes are also dichotomous. The purpose of the study calls only for a behavior-by-behavior comparison between females and males; nothing else.

If you have surmised that the chi-square test is a perfect fit for this study, you are indeed correct. Even so, you might have anxiety over the realization that "all that is needed is a chi-square" because the study is for an honors class, and you want to impress the professor with a more sophisticated statistical test. Fear not. Because you wouldn't want to cut a cake with a

This study examined conversations that HIV-infected parents had about HIV prevention with their uninfected adolescent children, and it used chi-square analyses to describe and compare the facilitators and barriers to communication. A total of 90 parents living with HIV or AIDS with children 10–18 years of age were recruited to participate in this study; participants completed interviews and a quantitative questionnaire assessing the frequency and content of these conversations, the parents' confidence level, and the perceived importance of discussing HIV prevention with their children. Data were analyzed using a variety of methods, including Pearson chi-square tests. Among 90 participants, 63.3% had disclosed their HIV status to their children. Results show that 81% of parents communicate about HIV prevention "sometimes" or "often" with their children, and 44% of parents found these conversations difficult and reported wanting support. Facilitators to communication included utilizing support (42.1%), focusing on the benefits of talking to their children about HIV prevention (43.9%), and having a previous relationship with their child (17.5%), though no significant differences were found between facilitators among those who did and did not disclose their status to their children. Barriers included living in denial (24.6%), fear of negative consequences (26.3%), and lacking a parental role model who discussed safer sex with them (14%); parents lacking a parental role model were less likely to disclose to their children than those who had a parental role model [$\chi^2 = 4.67$; df = 1; $P = 0.031$]. In addition, parents had varied views of how they believed their HIV status impacted communication, and those who did not disclose their HIV status to their children reported less frequent communication. Findings indicate that more interventions focused on building communication skills are needed for parents living with HIV or AIDS to facilitate healthy parent–child communication about HIV prevention and safer sex (Edwards, Reis, & Weber, 2013).

chain saw (see **FIGURE 14.2**), a smart professor will truly respect that you used only what was needed for your analyses and nothing more. In fact, you will find literally thousands of published studies that have used only a chi-square test.

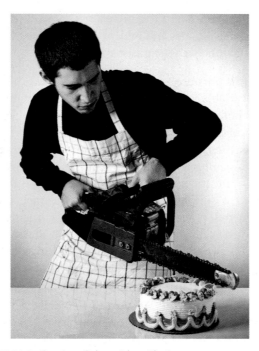

FIGURE 14.2 Cutting Cake with a Chainsaw.
© chang/E+/Getty Images

To give you an example of how this test is highly informative, **TABLE 14.3** provides some results. Notice in this table how the smaller chi-square values correspond with nonsignificant P-values and vice versa (larger chi-square values correspond with significant P-values).

▶ What Is a Layered Chi-Square and How Is It Interpreted?

In public health research, at a basic level, much of what we are interested in doing is identifying associations between two variables so that significant and modifiable risk and protective factors for different health outcomes can be identified and then subsequently targeted by public health interventions. Although this approach is intuitively appealing, reality is such that these observable but simple associations we may find between risk and health outcomes do not necessarily reveal a more complex picture. It is highly probable that other variables are involved and exert some type of influence. One such variable might be what is considered an **effect modifier**. Effect modification occurs when the magnitude of the effect of the primary predictor on an outcome (i.e., the association) differs, depending on the level of a third variable.

Going back to our example of parental monitoring and teenage binge drinking and the significant association we found, perhaps there could also be an effect

TABLE 14.3 A Sample Table Reporting Chi-Square Findings from 344 College Students Comparison of Recent (Past 6 Months) Drug Use Behaviors by Identification as Female or Male

Drug Use Behavior	Prevalence (%) Females (n = 177)	Prevalence (%) Males (n = 167)	χ^2	p
Used an opioid to deal with stress.	10.0	19.9	4.69	<0.001
Injected a drug to intensify the high.	7.2	7.9	1.53	0.62
Depended on a drug to wake up.	32.9	12.5	3.98	0.04
Used a drug to make sex better.	26.7	31.8	1.93	0.29
Got so high that I lost consciousness.	5.6	12.2	7.12	<0.001
Got so high that I missed school the next day.	2.3	3.1	1.82	0.34
Used a stimulant and became agitated.	5.4	8.5	1.32	0.44

modifier variable that under different levels would make the association differ. For example, perhaps gender could be an effect modifier such that the association of parental monitoring and binge drinking differs based on whether you are male or female: for females, the association is still significant, but there is no association for males. This information would be important to know and understand to ensure public health interventions are tailored and will be effective for all who are targeted. But how do you determine or look for potential effect modifiers? First off, the literature should at least provide you with clues as to which variables may be effect modifiers of the associations. Common ones in public health to look for include sociodemographic variables such as gender, biological sex, age, race and ethnicity, education level, geographic location, and socioeconomic status, although there could be others. To determine whether a variable is an effect modifier of your chi-square findings with data that are dichotomous, as in our example of gender, you simply run separate *two-variable* tests of independence for each group of the effect modifier variable (e.g., females and males). Note that in conducting this type of analysis, you can determine only the direction and strength of the association for each *level* of the effect modifier variable, but this type of analysis does not allow interpretation of the results for one group *relative* to the other group. To answer this latter question, you would need to create an interaction term based on the product of the predictor variable and the effect modifier variable and then test that term in a statistical model.

Consider our example of parental monitoring and binge drinking with gender as the effect modifier. Let's put this research question into practice. First, you could choose to do this calculation by hand by stratifying your sample by males and females and then calculating the chi-square test for each using the equation; however, most statistical software programs provide three dialogue boxes for you when a layered chi-square test is selected. The first is the row variable. In this example, you would enter the parental monitoring variable (High/Low). The second is the column variable. In this example, you would enter the variable representing teen binge drinking in the past 90 days (Yes/No). The third is optional; this is the one you select to conduct a layered chi-squared test. In this example, you would enter the variable representing sex (Male/Female). The resulting output from this layered chi-square test would then allow you to produce a table such as that shown as **TABLE 14.4**.

As you can see by close inspection of Table 14.4, the basic two-variable association does indeed look quite different, depending on the third variable (the layered variable) of sex. Specifically, the association is significant among female teens: χ^2 (1, $N = 79$) = 18.68, $p < 0.0001$. The correct interpretation here would be written as, "Among female teens, those who have low levels of parental monitoring are significantly more likely to binge drink (69%) than those with high levels of parental monitoring (20%). Among male teens, parental monitoring was not associated with binge drinking, χ^2 (1, $N = 80$) = 0.20, $p = 0.65$." We (the authors)

TABLE 14.4 Example of Layered Chi-Square Results Reported in a Table

	Binge Drinking	P-Value
Females		
Low level of parental monitoring (*n* = 29)	69.0%	
High level of parental monitoring (*n* = 50)	20.0%	<0.0001
Males		
Low level of parental monitoring (*n* = 54)	67.0%	
High level of parental monitoring (*n* = 26)	61.5%	0.65

also find it useful to reflect on findings such as this one and ask whether it makes sense from a public health viewpoint. That the association did not hold for male teens suggests that other factors such as peer influence may have more influence on binge drinking (see **FIGURE 14.3**). Conversely, female teens overall engage in lower levels of binge drinking compared with male teens, but an added protective factor for them is having parents who monitor them.

Given the contrasting results in Table 14.4, you would consider next what this means for public health practice. For instance, if you wanted to develop a program for high school students to reduce binge drinking that included a parent component, it may

be effective only for female teens. For male teens, this same program may not obtain the same results. Thus, gender-specific programming is warranted in this situation. These more nuanced findings often arise from the use of the layered chi-squared test and can help inform public health practice.

To give you a bit more practice regarding the concept of effect modification and the use of layered chi-square tests to detect this, we have developed a sample table for you (**TABLE 14.5**). Table 14.5 is a way for you to learn more and to practice what you are learning. We do not expect you to understand this table without guidance. So let's begin. First, think of this as a study of people who have been diagnosed with precancerous oral lesions (which are typically caused by smokeless tobacco, but other causes are not uncommon) and whether there were differences by gender. The study enrolled far more males than females because males use smokeless tobacco far more commonly. Second (and this is the key to understanding effect modification), this was a study that tested a hypothesis relative to whether immune compromise from HIV would "play out differently" in males versus females. Thus, you have six columns in the table: (1) the site of the oral lesion, (2) prevalence for females, (3) prevalence for males, (4) a *P*-value from a chi-square that compares the prevalence in females versus males, (5) a *P*-value from a layered chi-square test that shows the association of gender and oral cancer sites among those HIV-infected, and (6) a *P*-value from a layered chi-square test that shows the association of gender and oral cancer sites among those uninfected with HIV. Now begin by looking at the fourth column (i.e., the *P*-value from a chi-square that compares the prevalence in females versus males). What do you see in terms of significance? We hope your answer is, "I see there is an association between gender and lesions in the larynx and the posterior pharyngeal wall." (If so, well done!) Next, remember that this study is really about whether HIV affects the immune response for certain cancers and whether gender matters. Thus, the real question becomes, Do these significant associations differ by HIV status? At this point, we ask that you take one more look at the table (especially columns 5 and 6) and decide whether the hypothesis is supported and, if so, what is the appropriate conclusion? In case you are having a bit of trouble (or no trouble), we provide the following conclusion:

> Findings support the hypothesis that immune compromise has an effect. The association between prevalence of oral cancer in the larynx and posterior pharyngeal wall and gender

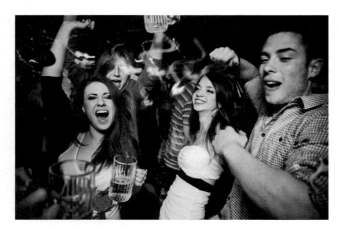

FIGURE 14.3 Teens Binge Drinking Alcohol.
© astarot/Shutterstock

TABLE 14.5 Comparison of Site-Specific Prevalence of Oral Precancerous Lesions Between Females and Males as Moderated by HIV Infection Status

Lesion Site	Prevalence		P	P-Effect Modifier[1]	
	Females	*Males*		*HIV+*	*HIV–*
Tonsils	1/29 (3.4%)	31/485 (6.4%)	0.52	0.74	0.48
Larynx	5/28 (17.9%)	20/469 (4.3%)	0.001	<0.001	0.46
Tongue	8/28 (28.6)	79/457 (17.3%)	0.13	0.03	0.59
Upper palette	1/29 (3.4%)	26/485 (5.4%)	0.65	0.26	0.29
Posterior pharyngeal wall	6/28 (21.4%)	44/469 (9.4%)	0.04	0.002	0.31
Lips	3/28 (10.7%)	63/456 (13.8%)	0.64	0.90	0.58
Oral Mucosa	7/29 (24.1%)	69/482 (14.3%)	0.15	0.13	0.69

[1]In each case where effect modification occurred, the association was only significant for HIV-infected study volunteers.

depends on HIV status. Among those living with some degree of immune compromise as a result of HIV infection, females had greater odds of lesions occurring in the larynx and posterior pharyngeal wall than males; among those uninfected with HIV, there was no difference in prevalence between males and females.

▶ What Is Logistic Regression?

So far in this chapter, you have learned about two-variable associations (these are more formally known as **bivariate associations**). Bivariate associations are the basis for thinking in more complex terms relative to the research question at hand. The real work of data analysis begins when you entertain multiple variables of interest as being "the cause" of any given outcome variable. You may recall from what you learned about multiple linear regression that these multiple variables of interest must be examined in a regression model to control for the fact that each is likely to have some degree of association with one another. That same process applies to research questions where the outcome variable is categorical. **Logistic regression** is the appropriate regression analysis to conduct when the dependent variable is dichotomous (binary). Like all regression analyses, the logistic regression is a predictive analysis. Logistic regression is used to describe data and to explain the relationship between

one dependent binary variable and one or more nominal, ordinal, interval, or ratio-level independent variables. When you have more than one independent or predictor variable in the same equation, it is considered multiple logistic regression and can be considered as the nonparametric counterpart to multiple linear regression.

To better demonstrate the basis for logistic regression, a new example may be worth a thousand words. Consider the public health problem of the use of electronic cigarettes (e-cigarettes) among adolescents (see **FIGURE 14.4**).

Also consider that you were informed by experts that adolescents who are high in the sensation-seeking personality trait are more likely to use

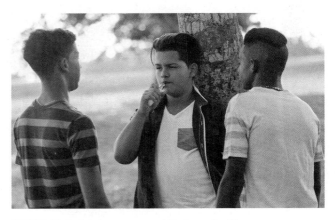

FIGURE 14.4 Adolescents and E-cigarette Use.
© Diego Cervo/Shutterstock

e-cigarettes. Thus, you want to test this bivariate association between sensation-seeking (assessed by a scale and then dichotomized at the recommended cut point to create a "low versus high" dichotomous variable) and e-cigarette use (Yes/No). Using a simple chi-square test, you find that of 93 adolescents who scored below the cut point on this scale, 67.7% indicated e-cigarette use at least once in the past 30 days. In contrast, among 63 being classified as above the threshold (high sensation seeking) by this scale, 85.7% reported e-cigarette use. Wisely, you checked the chi-square (χ^2) value and P-value before making the determination that the 18% difference was significant. You found the χ^2 value to be quite high (6.47) and the P-value to be quite low ($P < 0.01$), thus ensuring you that the difference was not the result of chance. You then wonder how this measure of sensation seeking might influence e-cigarette use when also considering parental monitoring and gender simultaneously. The use of multiple logistic regression now becomes your tool for solving this puzzle.

FIGURE 14.5 displays the output you obtain from a statistical software program that used multiple logistic regression to calculate two types of important values that apply specifically to nonparametric analyses. The first is the adjusted **odds ratio**, a measure of the association between an exposure and an outcome and represents the odds an outcome will occur given a particular exposure compared with the odds of an outcome occurring given the absence of a particular exposure. In this example, the odds ratio represents the odds of e-cigarette use given high sensation seeking compared with the odds of e-cigarette use given low sensation seeking. With the inclusion of other factors in the model such as parental monitoring and gender, this ratio is adjusted by these factors. The adjusted odds ratio is an estimate of how likely the outcome is given exposure to the variable of interest after controlling for the other variables. The numerical value of the odds ratio can range from close to zero (but cannot be zero) to numbers that exceed 1.0; however, adjusted odds ratios of more than 5.0 are relatively rare occurrences in the public health literature. When the value is close to 1.0 (or right at 1.0),

Classification Table[a]					
				Predicted	
	Observed		E-cigarette Use		Percentage Correct
			.00	1.00	
Step 1	E-cigarette Use	.00	0	39	100.0
		1.00	0	116	.0
	Overall Percentage				92.8

[a] The cut value is .500

Variables in the Equation									
								95% C.I. for EXP(B)	
		B	S.E.	Wald	df	Sig.	Exp(B)	Lower	Upper
Step 1[a]	Parental Monitoring	.041	.390	.011	1	.917	1.041	.485	2.238
	Sensation-Seeking	.998	.425	5.500	1	.019	2.712	1.178	6.244
	Gender	.016	.018	.806	1	.369	.984	.949	1.020
	Constant	1.253	.698	3.227	1	.072	3.502		

[a] Variable(s) entered on step 1: Parental Monitoring, Sensation-Seeking, Gender.

FIGURE 14.5 Statistical Output from a Multiple Logistic Regression Model.

the correct interpretation is that the odds of the outcome are the same for people regardless of their exposure to the variable of interest. Thus, having high or low risk makes no difference, and this would be a nonsignificant finding. However, let's say that the adjusted odds ratio is 2.72 (as is the case for the sensation-seeking variable shown in Figure 14.5). So, this would mean that the odds of e-cigarette use are 2.72 times greater for people classified as having high sensation seeking.

Now that you understand the value of 2.72 in Figure 14.5, the next question becomes, What do the numbers 1.18 and 6.24 mean in conjunction with that same variable (i.e., sensation seeking)? These numbers set up what is known as the 95% **confidence interval** for the value of 2.72. Remember that we have been calling the odds ratio nothing more than an estimate. So the question now becomes, How confident are we that the estimate is correct? The answer is that there is a 95% probability that the true odds ratio value lies somewhere between the range of 1.18 and 6.24. Please notice here that this is a relatively wide confidence interval. Also, from Figure 14.5, the one confidence interval that is significant also has a *P*-value of < 0.05. This observation is valuable in that the *P*-value is a confirmation that you are reading the confidence interval correctly (note also that the *P*-values for the other two variables are nonsignificant, which is consistent with their nonsignificant confidence intervals).

Further inspection of Figure 14.5 shows the value of parental monitoring in terms of e-cigarette use. As you can see, the adjusted odds ratio for this variable of interest is quite close to 1.0 (1.04 to be precise). Wisely, however (and clinging to your desire for this to be significant), you look for evidence that this is statistically significant. This brings up another learning point: A confidence interval that includes the value of 1.0 is always nonsignificant. Thus, as you see from the interval for parental monitoring, the values of 0.48 through 2.38 include the value of 1.0, so you are forced to abandon hope that parental monitoring matters relative to teens' e-cigarette use.

One final look at Figure 14.5 is warranted. Notice that the adjusted odds ratio for gender is less than 1.0. To explain this, let's first suspend the question of whether the value of 0.98 is significant. When an adjusted odds ratio is less than 1.0, it means that a negative outcome is actually *less* likely to occur. In this case, the odds are less than 1.0, which equates with a lower likelihood. A convenient way to think about this is to reverse the math by subtracting the odds ratio from 1. Once you do this, you can state that the odds of e-cigarette use are 2% (1.0 − 0.98 = 0.02) less likely for those who are female (female teens were coded as "1" versus male teens who were coded as "0"). Now, returning to the question of whether the 0.98 value is significant, the confidence interval tells us that the answer is clearly no (because it includes the value of 1.0). Thus, because the 0.98 value is nonsignificant, you would *not* be able to state that the odds of a negative outcome are 2% *less likely* for those who are female. **BOX 14.2** describes a study that used adjusted multiple logistic regression to determine associations between food insecurity, which is defined as "limited or uncertain availability of nutritionally adequate and safe foods, or limited or uncertain ability to acquire acceptable foods in socially acceptable ways" and poor mental health outcomes (Bergmans, Sadler, Wolfson, Jones, & Kruger, 2019, p. 264).

BOX 14.2   Example of a Study That Used Adjusted, Multiple Logistic Regression

Food insecurity is a psychosocial stressor with deleterious effects on mental health. This study examined whether the local food environment moderates the association of individual food insecurity with poor mental health. Cross-sectional survey data were collected from adult residents of Flint, Michigan (*n* = 291), in 2015. Multivariable logistic models assessed whether quality of the local food environment moderated the relationship of food insecurity with poor mental health. A binary indicator of poor mental health was created. Participants were asked to rate their overall "mental or emotional health" using a five-point Likert scale. Individuals were classified as having either good mental health (i.e., ratings of good, very good, or excellent) or poor mental health (i.e., ratings of fair or poor). In fully adjusted models, food insecurity was associated with 3.2 (95% confidence interval [CI]: 1.6–6.2) times higher odds of poor mental health. However, increased proximate access to vegetables and fruits moderated this association. For example, those in the bottom 25th percentile of access to vegetables had 7.4 (95% CI: 2.7–20.5) times higher odds of poor mental health. In contrast, for those in the top 25th percentile of vegetable access, food insecurity was only marginally associated with poor mental health (odds ratio = 2.2; 95% CI: 1.0–4.7). Greater proximate access to vegetables and fruits moderated food insecurity's association with poor mental health. Longitudinal evaluation of programs and policies that improve availability of nutrient-rich foods in food-insecure communities is needed to determine whether they yield a mental health benefit (Bergmans, Sadler, Wolfson, Jones, & Kruger, 2019).

▶ How Can Logistic Regression Be Used in Public Health Research?

The final objective of this chapter is to provide you with a brief introduction to the practical uses of logistic regression in public health research. The following two uses of this analytic method are common in public health research.

1. For only one main exposure variable and controlling for other variables, use a series of multiple logistic regression models to create a set of adjusted odds ratios for multiple health outcomes assessed dichotomously.

    For example, how does community violence exposure (Yes/No) influence risk behaviors such as (a) alcohol use, (b) interpersonal violence, (c) smoking, (d) drug use, and so on?

2. For only one dichotomous outcome, use as many applicable exposure variables to determine which best predicts the occurrence of the outcome.

    For example, does neighborhood cohesion, family violence exposure, single parent household, socioeconomic status, and gender influence bullying perpetration among middle school students?

Please notice that the two types of research are quite different and have only one point in common: The outcomes are both dichotomous. To illustrate the first example, we could conduct a study among a sample of older adolescents ages 17 to 23 years old. This span of 7 years would necessitate controlling for age; thus age would then be part of each logistic regression model. Further, it would be wise to also control for the effects of sex (i.e., female versus male) in these models. Consequently, each model would contain three predictor variables: (1) age, (2) sex, and (3) whether the person was exposed to community violence. The first model may test the outcome of "alcohol use" with the second and third models testing, respectively, "ever perpetrated dating violence" and "ever smoked cigarettes." The final model would test for the outcome of drug use. The result of this work would then become four adjusted odds ratios—one for each outcome—that inform you about the effects of adolescents' or young adults' exposure to violence. Each odds ratio is adjusted for the effects of age and sex, thereby implicating that any significant association with an outcome occurs independently from these two demographic measures.

In the second use of multiple logistic regression, we would recruit a national sample of middle school students to determine the multiple factors that are associated with bullying perpetration. We would assess these multiple exposures, sociodemographics, and the outcome of bullying perpetration with a survey and then run one multiple regression. **BOX 14.3** provides an example from the peer-reviewed literature of using a single multiple logistic regression model to determine the independent effects of numerous variables

---

BOX 14.3 Assessment of Multiple Predictors of Breast Cancer Using Multiple Logistic Regression

This study aimed to determine whether residential proximity to urban green areas, agricultural areas, and overall "greenness" surrounding residences were associated with the risk of breast cancer. Participants were drawn from MCC-Spain (i.e. the multicase-control study in Spain), which is a population-based multiple case-control study conducted from 2008 to 2013 of 5 types of cancer in 10 provinces of Spain. The current study used breast cancer cases and controls, with the final sample consisting of 1738 cases and 1910 controls, and data were collected via quantitative interviews. The authors assigned different indicators of exposure to green spaces in proximity to residences, presence of urban green areas, presence of agricultural areas, and surrounding greenness. Data were analyzed using logistic regression models, and the authors explored the effect of several potential effect modifiers. Findings indicated that the presence of urban green areas was associated with reduced risk of breast cancer controlling for age, socioeconomic status, education, and number of children [adjusted OR = 0.65 (0.49 – 0.86)]. Findings also indicated a trend between distance to urban green areas and breast cancer risk, with higher distance to green space indicating higher risk. However, presence of agricultural areas and surrounding greenness were associated with increased risk of breast cancer [adjusted OR (95% CI) = 1.33 (1.07 – 1.65)] and [adjusted OR (95% CI) = 1.27 (0.92 – 1.77)], respectively. Findings may reveal that the effect of green space and breast cancer risk depends greatly on how the green space is used, though more research is needed to fully understand this relationship (O'Callaghan-Gordo, Kogevinas, Cirach, Castano-Vinyals, Aragones, Delfrade, . . . Nieuwenhuijsen, 2018).

of interest related to green space on a single outcome: breast cancer. Please notice that only one regression model was used.

Now that you have a basic understanding of multiple logistic regression and its purpose in public health research, let us take you into one more example that would help in understanding a journal article that uses this all-so-important statistical tool.

BOX 14.4 displays an example of a study that used multiple logistic regression to fulfill the study purpose. As you read, we urge you to think about all that you have learned so far in this chapter. For instance, you will see in the table that some of the odds ratios are significant and below 1.0, while others are significant and above 1.0. Notice also that the findings are somewhat different for rural women than for nonrural women.

BOX 14.4 Description of a Study Designed to Understand the Uptake of Long-Acting Reversible Contraception (LARC) Among Low-Income Rural and Nonrural Women Addicted to Opioids

A clear and costly outgrowth of the national opioid epidemic involves neonatal abstinence syndrome (NAS). A potential public health response to the NAS epidemic involves averting unplanned pregnancy among women with opioid use disorder (OUD).

The Guttmacher Institute's most recent annual report suggests that 45% of the 6.1 million pregnancies occurring in that year were unintended.[1] Rates of unintended pregnancy appear to be substantially greater among women of the lowest socioeconomic levels. For example, in 2011, it was reported that ~112 pregnancies per 1000 were unintended among women living at or below 100% of the federal poverty level, in contrast, the rate among women living at or above 200% of the federal poverty level was ~20 per 1000.[1] The intersectional factors of extreme poverty being linked to unintended pregnancy, and far greater rates of OUD among rural women, combine to suggest that a responsible method of averting NAS in rural America is to avert unintended pregnancy via LARC implants. Yet, little is known about the factors that may predict LARC uptake among low-income rural women of reproductive age. Given the "spread" of OUD to suburban and urban America, the same question about promoting LARC is applicable. Consider, for instance, a hypothetical study that was designed to identify correlates of LARC use for averting unplanned pregnancy among both low-income rural and nonrural women with OUD. **TABLE 1** provides an example of how the hypothetical study findings would be presented, with six factors being investigated. Notice that the study findings are expressed in the form of adjusted odds ratios stemming from the use of multiple logistic regression.

TABLE 1 Correlates of Having a Larc Implant Among Low-Income Rural and Nonrural Women of Reproductive Age

	Rural Women (*n* = 399)			Nonrural Women (*n* = 406)		
	AOR	95% CI	P	AOR	95% CI	P
Age	0.92	0.84–0.99	0.04	0.94	0.86–1.02	0.14
Concurrent sex partners	1.56	0.87–2.82	0.14	2.70	1.48–4.95	0.001
Multiple sex partners	1.20	0.66–1.91	0.68	1.02	0.57–1.81	0.95
Has one or more living children	2.24	1.31–3.68	0.003	2.40	1.37–4.21	0.002
Married to a male	0.57	0.30–1.09	0.09	0.87	46–1.64	0.67
Has attended college	0.88	0.42–1.85	0.74	0.54	0.22–1.32	0.18

[1]Guttmacher Institute. (2019, January). Unintended pregnancy in the United States. Retrieved from https://www.guttmacher.org/fact-sheet/unintended-pregnancy-united-states

Data from Guttmacher Institute. Unintended pregnancy in the United States. Available at: https://www.guttmacher.org/fact-sheet/unintended-pregnancy-united-states.

Think About It!

A common problem in public health practice is that structured environments often have an undue influence in terms of sustaining unhealthy behaviors. A prime example involves the question of whether people will initiate exercise programs to strengthen the heart muscle after having survived a heart attack. As you might guess, dozens of cardiac rehabilitation programs have been tested to determine their value in helping people overcome what may have been a sedentary lifestyle (supported by their environment). Also, as you might guess, these types of programs are designed and implemented with varying levels of success. From a policy perspective, imagine that the question you have is, Are exercise-based cardiac rehabilitation programs worth funding?

Given this question, we suggest that you can locate the best possible answer by finding a journal article that reports a **meta-analysis**. Simply stated, a meta-analysis begins by locating journal articles according to a predefined set of criteria and proceeds to pool the findings from all of those studies that qualify for inclusion. The pooled findings are then used to calculate a summary statistic that represents the average effect of the type of program under study. Because logistic regression is a somewhat universal language of epidemiological studies (including intervention studies), reading about a pooled odds ratio as part of a meta-analysis is likely to be part of your future repertoire as a public health professional. In the case of the question "Are exercise-based cardiac rehabilitation programs worth funding?" we did a Google Scholar search and found a meta-analysis of 48 randomized controlled trials testing the effects of cardiac rehabilitation programs on subsequent mortality (Taylor et al., 2004). The following excerpt is taken from the abstract of that study.

> We included 48 trials with a total of 8940 patients. Compared with usual care, cardiac rehabilitation was associated with reduced *all-cause mortality* (odds ratio [OR] = 0.80; 95% *confidence interval* [CI]: 0.68 to 0.93)

and cardiac mortality (OR = 0.74; 95% CI: 0.61 to 0.96).

Looking closely at the first odds ratio reported by Taylor and colleagues (2004), you see that it is below 1.0 and significant. You know it is significant because the upper limit of the confidence interval excludes 1.0 (that is, the confidence interval does not cross the line of 1.0). Given its significance, you then think about the meaning of the 0.80 odds ratio. First, you realize that it is protective against the outcome of all-cause mortality, so this is good. Then, you remember from previously in this chapter to subtract the value of 0.80 from 1.0. Thus, you now know that the average program confers a 20% reduction in risk of mortality.

Looking next at the second odds ratio reported in the excerpt, you realize this is actually the one of more value to your question because, in this case, the outcome is highly specific: cardiac mortality. As a more specific measure, the protective value of this second odds ratio is somewhat better: 0.74 (translating to a 26% reduction in risk). You can also observe that the value of 0.74 is indeed (once again) significant.

This vignette provides you with a quick lesson in how to be responsive to questions regarding resource allocation (i.e., funding) in your career as a public health professional. The point here is that odds ratios can be combined in a meta-analysis, thus allowing you to quickly and easily answer literally hundreds of questions that essentially ask, Do the programs really work?

Finally, just to show you how easy it is to examine meta-analytic results when the test statistic is the odds ratio, we have constructed a hypothetical example (see **FIGURE 14.6**). As you inspect this figure, please notice the large diamond-shaped symbol near the bottom; this represents the average odds ratio. Notice also in this figure that the average of the odds ratios is nonsignificant—that is, the 95% confidence interval "crosses over 1.0."

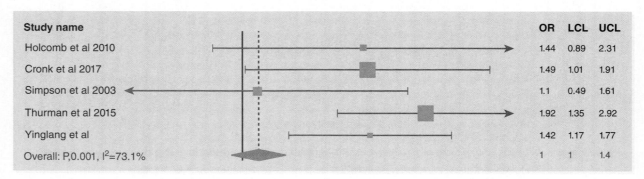

Study name		OR	LCL	UCL
Holcomb et al 2010		1.44	0.89	2.31
Cronk et al 2017		1.49	1.01	1.91
Simpson et al 2003		1.1	0.49	1.61
Thurman et al 2015		1.92	1.35	2.92
Yinglang et al		1.42	1.17	1.77
Overall: P,0.001, I²=73.1%		1	1	1.4

FIGURE 14.6 Hypothetical Figure of Meta-Analysis Results for Cardiac Mortality.

Take Home Points

- The chi-squared test of independence is a widely used nonparametric test that determines an association between two categorical variables.
- A layered chi-square test involves adding an effect modifier to the chi-square test and determines whether the independent test of association differs for each level of the effect modifier.
- Multiple logistic regression is a widely used nonparametric test in public health research that examines associations between exposure variables and categorical outcomes while controlling for other variables.
- Logistic regression calculates odds ratios that represent the odds of having an outcome given an exposure compared with the odds of having an outcome given no or low exposure.
- Confidence intervals for odds ratios are estimated in a logistic regression model and signify that there is a 95% probability that the true odds ratio lies within the range of the confidence interval.
- Confidence intervals for odds ratios signify statistical significance if they do not contain 1.0 within the range.
- Public health research commonly utilizes logistic regression in actual practice to inform interventions regarding what to target and who to target.
- The two most common types of logistic regression include using one exposure variable for multiple dichotomous outcomes and using multiple exposure variables as predictors of one dichotomous outcome.

Key Terms

Bivariate association	Confidence interval	Logistic regression
Cell	Contingency table	Meta-analysis
Chi-square	Effect modifier	Odds ratio

For Practice and Discussion

1. Explain when nonparametric tests are appropriate to use. What kind of data would you analyze using nonparametric tests and why? Describe a study that would be analyzed with nonparametric tests.
2. What is the chi-square test and what is it used to assess? Design a study that would use chi-square tests to analyze the data. Identify predictor variable(s) and outcome variable(s) and how you would measure them. What is the level of measurement of each variable—for example, nominal? ordinal? something else?
3. Set up a contingency table for a sample size of $N = 500$ with the following categorical predictor and outcome.
   a. Predictor: Alcohol use
   b. Outcome: Condom use

   Identify which variable goes in the row and which goes in the column. Of 500 people in your study, 75% reported alcohol use and 48% reported condom use. You also discover that there is a significant association between alcohol use and condom use such that those who consumed alcohol were more likely to *not* use condoms. Fill out the table so that these results are likely.
4. Explain what an effect modifier variable is. What effect modifier variable might influence the relationship between alcohol use and condom use? Explain why the variable you identified could influence the relationship between alcohol use and condom use.
5. A researcher is conducting a regression analysis to determine the effect of binge drinking (a dichotomous variable) on sexual aggression (also a dichotomous variable). What is the appropriate type of analysis to conduct and why? How do you determine whether the relationship is significant?

References

Bergmans, R. S., Sadler, R. C., Wolfson, J. A., Jones, A. D., & Kruger, D. (2019). Moderation of the association between individual food security and poor mental health by the local food environment among adult residents of Flint, Michigan. *Health Equity, 3*(1), 264–274.

Edwards, L. L., Reis, J. L., & Weber, K. M. (2013). Facilitators and barriers to discussing HIV prevention with adolescents: Perspectives of HIV-infected parents. *American Journal of Public Health, 103*, 1468–1475.

O'Callaghan-Gordo, C., Kogevinas, M., Cirach, M., Castano-Vinyals, G., Aragones, N., Delfrade, J., ... Nieuwenhuijsen, M. J. (2018). Residential proximity to green spaces and breast cancer risk: The multicase-control study in Spain (MCC-Spain). *International Journal of Hygiene and Environmental Health, 221*(8), 1097–1106.

Taylor, R. S., Brown, A., Ebrahim, S., Jolliffe, J., Noorani, H., Rees, B., ..., Oldridge, N. (2004). Exercise-based rehabilitation for patients with coronary heart disease: Systematic review and meta-analysis of randomized controlled trials. *American Journal of Medicine, 116*, 682–689.

For Further Reading

Corder, G. W., & Foreman, D. I. (2011). *Nonparametric statistics for non-statisticians*. New York, NY: John Wiley and Sons.

Gerstman, B. B. (2014). *Basic biostatistics: Statistics for public health* (2nd ed.). Burlington, MA: Jones & Bartlett.

Sullivan, L. M. (2017). *Essentials of biostatistics in public health*. Burlington, MA: Jones & Bartlett.

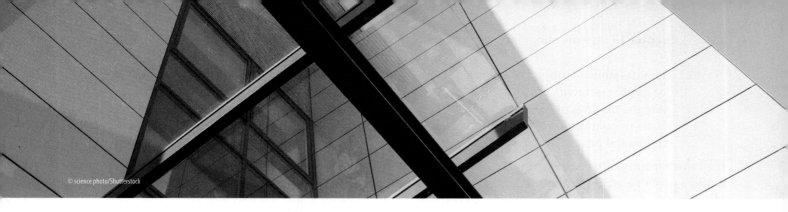

CHAPTER 15

Disseminating Findings and Informing New Research

1. Identify the key sections of a peer-reviewed research article.
2. Articulate the progression of disseminating findings through a series of strategies.
3. Describe the strategies to disseminate findings to practitioners of public health.
4. Describe the strategies to disseminate findings to public health researchers.
5. Describe strategies to disseminate findings to policy makers in public health.
6. Explain the "language of science."
7. Be able to compose a highly effective Introduction.
8. Understand how to effectively present study findings through the use of visuals.

▶ Overview

At this point, you have read and studied 14 chapters in this book. Your journey has been long. Assuming you wisely used all that you have learned in these preceding chapters to conduct the perfect research study, what comes next? The next step is to make sure your work is noticed. You may be familiar with the old saying that if something has been forgotten, is not being used, or no one is doing anything with it, then it is essentially "gathering dust on the shelf." This saying applies not only to old toys, books, and tools but also to research findings. Far too many people spend years and thousands if not millions of dollars working hard to produce research findings that never get past their computer screens and figuratively gather dust. The purpose of this chapter is to give you the skills

you need to avoid this awful fate. Indeed, this chapter is designed to give you the ability to escalate your research findings to the attention of colleagues in public health practice, others doing similar research, and even key members of the general public. This chapter will also teach you how to read and digest the research findings published in a journal article.

Before you begin mastering the objectives of this chapter, we have an informal assignment for you to complete. Please locate and carefully read a peer-reviewed journal article that describes findings from an **empirical research** study; this means it reports research based on actual observation or experiment in the field of public health. As you read the article, look for answers to three main questions:

1. Did the study findings have implications for public health practice?

2. Did the study identify next steps in terms of future research?

3. Are the findings of interest to policy makers, community leaders, or other influential people?

If all three features are present in the article, you have found a gem of a study. With most studies, if you can identify two of these three qualities, you can consider the findings of great value. However, we do not want to detract from or criticize those studies that perhaps have only one of these qualities because those can also make significant contributions and be highly valuable. We only want to make you aware of this trifecta of study attributes.

As you progress through this final chapter, please know that we wrote it to help you become a wise and savvy consumer of public health research in addition to helping you learns skills to disseminate your own research findings. Both functions are vital to being a professional public health researcher or practitioner.

What Are the Key Sections of a Peer-Reviewed Research Article?

To begin, let us define for you what is meant by **peer review**. To protect the rigor and integrity of research, all manuscripts are judged as suitable or not suitable for publication by a jury of colleagues with expertise in the subject matter of the submitted research manuscript. To expedite this review process (and to make life easy for readers when the manuscript matriculates into a published article), manuscripts are divided into seven primary sections. As a handy reference for you, **TABLE 15.1** presents these seven sections along with brief descriptions. Take time to familiarize yourself with the sections and their purposes because these descriptions will assist you when you write up results from your study as well as when you read through others' published research.

TABLE 15.1 The Seven Key Sections of a Research Manuscript	
Abstract	Typically, no more than 250 words that succinctly summarize the entire manuscript. The abstract is what people read first. Includes four sections: Objective or Purpose, Methods, Results, and Conclusion.
Introduction	Length varies greatly, but this section is where previous research is reviewed to show gaps in research. Filling the gap is then cast as the purpose of the study.
Methods	Every procedure involved in conducting the research such as the population targeted, recruitment of the sample, collection of data, the measures used, documentation of an institutional review board, and so on are described in addition to the data-analytic methods used. Enough information is provided for others to duplicate the study.
Results	The answers to the research questions are presented here, starting with a description of the sample relative to its characteristics and results of statistical analyses or qualitative analyses. Tables and figures are introduced to help tell the story more succinctly.
Discussion	This is the first section of the manuscript that is not written in the past tense. It provides a recap of the findings, congruency or not with previous research, plausible explanations for findings not in support of hypotheses, and description of implications for the field. It is interpretative and somewhat speculative.
References	Far from being a detail, this section should be considered much like evidence being shown to a courtroom jury. References support contentions from the introduction and decisions made relative to the study methodology and interpretation of results.
Tables/Figures	If a manuscript were like a television crew covering a sporting event, tables and figures would be the highlights shown on the nightly news. Both can tell a story in a highly efficient form.

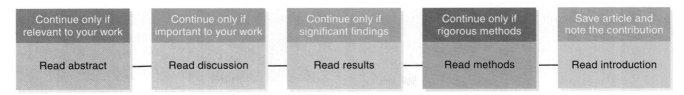

Continue only if relevant to your work	Continue only if important to your work	Continue only if significant findings	Continue only if rigorous methods	Save article and note the contribution
Read abstract	Read discussion	Read results	Read methods	Read introduction

FIGURE 15.1 Sequence in Which a Journal Article Should Be Read and Critiqued.

Now that you know the seven main sections of a manuscript, you are ready to read published articles. In fact, we suggest that you read at least one each day during your entire career. This is an excellent habit to develop and a vital obligation as a future public health professional, one that keeps you up-to-date on new developments and can inform your practice and research. We understand, of course, that time is valuable. Thus, let us provide you with a sequence of reading that may help. **FIGURE 15.1** provides a visual summary of this suggested sequence. The linear figure describes the order in which to review a journal article to judge the innovation and its contribution to what is already known. You may recall from an earlier chapter the idea of "filling in the gaps." Although the sequence is out of order in terms of reading the manuscript sections, we recommend you follow our sequence because it will save you time and energy from reading an entire manuscript, which may not be relevant or important to your work. By using our criteria to judge whether or not you continue with the article, you will actually reach the Introduction at the end of the sequence. It is a safe bet that if you reach the Intro, the article will be a keeper for your library.

How to Disseminate Your Findings

To begin, it is important to understand the term **dissemination**. This is a process of informing others about your research findings and is the first step in a larger process of translating research into practice that is commonly known as **translation science**. Translation science is defined as an effort to build on basic scientific research to create new therapies, medical procedures, or diagnostics (Noonan & Emshoff, 2013). In the absence of effective dissemination research, findings become nothing more than an academic exercise. More important, as described in Chapter 3, an ethical obligation exists to the people who volunteer for research studies because they are told that their participation will benefit science. This

GOT RESULTS?

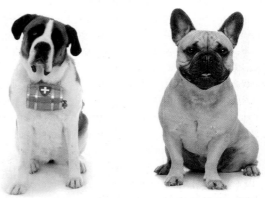

DON'T WAIT—DISSEMINATE!

FIGURE 15.2 Public Health Mascots Snow and Hamilton Get Behind Dissemination.
© Eric Isselee/Shutterstock; © Svetography/Shutterstock

promised benefit, of course, can only occur if the study findings are adequately disseminated. Thus, we strongly encourage you to disseminate once you have confidence in the results (see **FIGURE 15.2**).

Findings from empirical studies are typically disseminated through a defined sequence of events. This sequence begins with outreach efforts to public health practitioners, proceeds to researchers, and concludes with community leaders and people who can influence public health policy. Accordingly, you have three levels of dissemination to consider:

1. Dissemination to public health practitioners (i.e., people applying what we term *best practices* to everyday health-promotion efforts)
2. Dissemination to public health researchers who (like yourself) can continue the research trajectory and continue to expand the knowledge base by filling in the gaps identified in your research
3. Because public health relies on supporting policy, regulation, and even legislative changes, the ultimate step in dissemination involves reaching the people who can make the needed changes

Regarding the first point, we suggest several strategies to disseminate research findings to practitioners. The first involves your regional public health association. The United States is divided into 10 regions that group the many state and regional public health associations affiliated with the American Public Health Association (APHA, 2019). Joining your state association and being an active member implies that you will be attending annual meetings as both an audience member and a presenter. Thus, as soon as your research findings are completed and interpreted, your next step is to create an abstract that you can submit to your state association for presentation at the next annual (or biannual meeting). Be sure to read the "call for abstracts" carefully because this will provide a step-by-step set of instructions for preparing your abstract. If you have a travel budget, this same abstract can then also be submitted to the next annual meeting of the APHA. The annual meetings sponsored by this national organization of public health professionals are ideal in ensuring that your research findings will benefit public health practitioners. Typically, APHA releases its call for abstracts in early January of each year. In addition to APHA, there are countless numbers of professional organizations in the field of public health. We urge you to immediately begin thinking about which organizations you could join to optimize your professional connections (often referred to as *networking*). To help you get started, **TABLE 15.2** provides examples of the professional organizations you may wish to investigate, learn about in detail, and eventually join.

Once you have narrowed your options pertaining to which professional organizations you want to join, the next step is to check out their websites to learn more about the next conferences being held (these are typically promoted as many as 12 months in advance of the meeting dates). For example, as of

TABLE 15.2 Sample of Professional Organizations Relevant to Public Health Research and Practice

American Association for Health Education
American College of Epidemiology
American Nurses Association
American Public Health Association
American Society for Nutrition
American Society of Tropical Medicine and Hygiene
Association of Public Health Laboratories
Bill & Melinda Gates Foundation
Centers for Disease Control and Prevention
Doctors Without Borders
International Committee of the Red Cross
Kaiser Family Foundation
National Association of County and City Health Officials
National Association of Local Boards of Health
National Environmental Health Association
National Institute of Health
Pan American Health Organization
Society for Public Health Education
The Global Fund
UNICEF
US Public Health Service Commissioned Corps
US Public Health Service
World Health Organization

this writing (2019), the Centers for Disease Control and Prevention was promoting the next conference on sexually transmitted diseases to be held in 2020 (see **FIGURE 15.3**).

Regarding the second point—dissemination to public health researchers—submitting an abstract for oral or poster presentation to APHA is also an excellent way to disseminate your research findings. If the findings are significant, we recommend

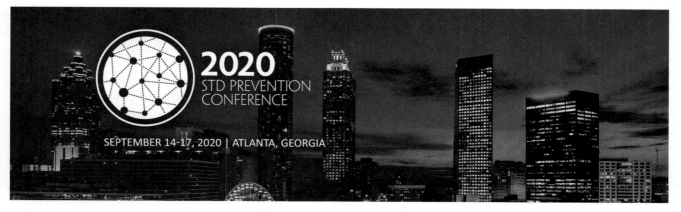

FIGURE 15.3 Actual Advertisement for a National Public Health Conference.

submitting the abstract as an oral presentation rather than a poster. This is because the abstract for an oral presentation is published in the conference proceedings (which does not occur with posters). The advantage of having it "published" is that even people who did not attend your session can still read and benefit from your findings. In the event that your oral presentation is a success, another potential and rewarding route of dissemination involves publication in a peer-reviewed journal. This, of course, is an option reserved for only the most rigorous and significant studies that fill a much-needed gap in the research literature. If you choose this method of disseminating your findings, many journals exist that publish research studies pertaining to public health. Of course, the flagship journal for the field of public health is the *American Journal of Public Health.* **TABLE 15.3** displays a few other select journals that publish research in the field of public health.

In addition to the journals shown in Table 15.3, please be aware that your options are nearly limitless

if you make the leap to a specific disease or condition (e.g., cancer, hypertension, HIV, or AIDS), or population (e.g., LGBT, transgender, etc.). For instance, if your findings pertain to a new method of promoting mammography, you will find dozens of journals devoted to cancer screening and prevention. Indeed, there is an abundance of journals devoted specifically to most content areas within public health. For instance, you will find numerous options related to: (1) HIV and AIDS, (2) adolescent health, (3) dietary health, (4) family planning and contraception, (5) diabetes prevention and control, and (6) infectious disease control.

Regarding the third point (dissemination to leaders who can leverage policy change), your dissemination options are centered less on conference and manuscripts and more on publications such as newsletters, newspapers, and even podcasts or press releases. The idea here is to place your findings in a strategic online location, one that will eventually attract community

TABLE 15.3 Sample of Journals That Publish Public Health Research	
Health Education and Behavior	Annals of Behavioral Medicine
American Journal of Health Promotion	Public Health Reports
Journal of Community Health	Frontiers in Public Health
American Journal of Preventive Medicine	Health, Culture and Society
Public Health Journal	Journal of Health and Social Behavior
Journal of Public Health Management	Journal of Epidemiology
Epidemiology and Community Health	The Lancet
BMC Public Health	International Journal of Public Health
Journal of Public Health Policy	American Journal of Epidemiology
Health Promotion and Health Behavior	Social Science & Medicine
Bulletin of the World Health Organization	Public Health Nutrition
Annual Review of Public Health	Canadian Journal of Public Health-Revue
European Journal of Public Health	Journal of American College Health
Public Health Nursing	Maternal and Child Health Journal
Salud Publica de Mexico	Ethnicity & Disease

To promote safety and avert traumatic brain injuries among bicycle riders, we tested a marketing program that sold bicycles with the price of a helmet built into the total cost. This study was done throughout calendar year 2017 in three bike shops in Oakland, California. The years 2018 and 2019 were used to conduct consumer surveys relative to bicycle accidents and head injuries. These data were then compared with similar consumer surveys conducted in Oakland during 2015 and 2016. Bicycle sales for 2017 were not significantly reduced from 2016 despite a $50 price increase to offset the wholesale costs of helmets. In 212 completed surveys conducted in 2018 and 2019, only three bicycle-helmet buyers suffered head injuries (including concussions) in 2017. In contrast, of 231 completed surveys in 2015–2016, seven head injuries occurred. For all 10 injuries, helmet use was not reported.

Findings suggest that coupling the sales of bicycles with protective helmets increased helmet use and thus reduces the number of reported head injuries. Making helmets a mandatory part (but at wholesale costs) of a bicycle purchase may be a promising public health policy.

leaders, policy makers, and even government officials who are influential in public health policy.

Your online posting (or even an old-fashioned off-line press release) may or may not gain traction, depending on how well you market it. Unlike conference presentations and manuscripts, the language here becomes that of the layperson. Words or terms such as *significance testing*, *P-values*, *hypothesis*, and *random selection* may not be understood by your targeted audience. Instead, your findings should be cast more in the language of a short story, one that has a clear conclusion and places that conclusion in the context of averting morbidity and mortality through prevention. **BOX 15.1** provides an example of an online posting that is worth mimicking with your own research findings.

As you might imagine, the sample online posting shown in Box 15.1 might not have much "traction" in most web locations. However, it may become quite popular in locations that are viewed by people who write articles for cycling magazines, by people who have experienced head trauma from bicycle accidents and have become activists who promote helmet use through policy, or by employees of government (state and national) agencies charged with averting head injuries, especially all-so-costly and debilitating traumatic brain injuries.

In thinking about dissemination of research findings to people who make or leverage public health policy, it is vital to understand a few basic points pertaining to this process. For instance, is there a strong connection between public health research and public health policy? Consider, for instance the ominous threat to public health of climate change. In 2017, the United States withdrew from the Paris Climate Agreement, despite overwhelming evidence that controlling carbon emissions is vital to protecting the future of the Earth and the health of all of its inhabitants (see **FIGURE 15.4**).

Other examples abound. For instance, at one point in our nation's history (under the Clinton administration) syringe-service programs (these are government-sponsored efforts to provide clean injection equipment to people who inject drugs) were simply not allowed to receive federal funds; thus, few programs existed. This policy decision was made in the face of voluminous research evidence showing that harm-reduction approaches such as syringe exchange have a net overall level of benefit in terms of cost savings and do

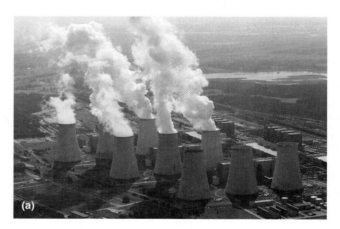

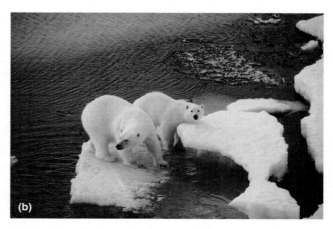

FIGURE 15.4 Climate Change: Cause and Effect.

BOX 15.2 Summary of a Policy-to-Practice Study in the European Union

To understand what promotes or hinders the uptake of research evidence in the policy-making process, a European-based study assessed health-enhancing physical activity (HEPA) policies in six countries. The study investigated policy development in the Netherlands, Italy, Romania, the United Kingdom, Denmark, and Finland. Although the countries varied on certain contextual levels, the researchers solely focused on assessing policies related to HEPA at the national and local levels.

Semistructured interviews were conducted with 86 stakeholders who were directly involved in the policy-making process. Interviews were specifically designed to gather in-depth information about the stakeholder's experience of potential barriers or catalysts pertaining to using research evidence as a method of informing policy development. The respective country's research team reviewed responses using a previously constructed guideline for analysis.

The overall results were categorized into three domains. The first focused on organizations, systems, and infrastructure. The most frequently identified facilitators of making new policy included having a supportive administration with managers who held largely positive attitudes and closely monitored the policy-making process. Media were also frequently mentioned as a facilitator of policy-making decisions. A lack of connections between research and policy making was frequently mentioned as a barrier.

The second domain focused on access and availability of relevant evidence. Several barriers were identified. For instance, one barrier was the inapplicability of evidence based on its complexity or lack of relevance or a lack of information on the potential economic impact of the corresponding policy.

The third domain to emerge focused on networking and collaboration between policy makers and researchers. Stakeholders believed that greater personal contact with other stakeholders could increase the likelihood of creating a liaison between "knowledge" institutes and "policy-making organizations" that would, in turn, facilitate the translation of research into public health policy. Indeed, one study recommendation was that research should focus on bringing policy makers, researchers, and other stakeholders together into a shared effort to improve evidence-based public health policy decisions (van de Goor, Hämäläinen, Syed, Lau, Sandu, Spitters, ... & Aro, 2017).

---

not promote increased use of injectable drugs. Similarly, and even today, U.S. states endorse so-called abstinence-only education for adolescents despite decades of research showing that comprehensive sex-education programs (and their derivatives) are the only effective method of reducing teen pregnancy rates.

All too often, public health policy may be driven by factors other than evidence derived from public health research. To give you a "closer look" at what may be a large gap between research and policy in public health, **BOX 15.2** summarizes a recent study in six European countries that describe this phenomenon in more detail using data collected from six countries in the European Union. Please note as you read this box that criteria other than research evidence were commonly used to inform policy decisions.

▶ What Is the "Language of Science"?

With the exception of dissemination efforts prepared specifically for the lay public or for policy makers, you will need to learn a few basic rules pertaining to the language of science before you prepare the abstracts or manuscripts. **TABLE 15.4** summarizes these rules.

For each rule in Table 15.4 we will provide some guidance relative to clear and accurate writing. Starting at the top, consider the bicycle and helmet set study described in Box 15.1. Whereas the writing style for the conclusion to the online posting may be okay, it would most likely not pass the test of peer review. Notice that the conclusion lacks words such as *may*, *might*, or *could*. The rather definitive statement saying that pairing helmets with bicycle sales "increases" safety ignores the fact that this was a study done in one U.S. city without a control city as a comparison. It is, of course, quite possible that the findings could have been less positive in East Coast cities, for example.

Moving to the second rule, a primary goal of science is comparison. Simple comparisons (e.g., "7 is greater than 3"), however, are not acceptable. Again, using Box 15.1 as our example, a difference between seven injuries before the program and three after the program is not only clinically meaningless but also assuredly not statistically significant. Thus, any comparison with corresponding terms such as *greater than*, *more likely*, and *increased likelihood* must be supported by a significant statistical test of some sort. This burden on the writer to provide "statistical evidence" is precisely what distinguishes scientific writing from ordinary writing.

TABLE 15.4 Cardinal Rules for Scientific Writing

Rule	Reasoning Behind the Rule
Absolute words should not be used.	Words such as *prove, definitive,* and *demonstrate* suggest too much confidence in findings from a single study.
Always provide test statistics.	When making statements that involve comparisons, you are obligated to show the corresponding test statistics.
Conclusions must align with the stated study purposes.	The study aims are the only fair game for a study conclusion.
Avoid jargon.	Terms that are not common in the dictionary limit the appeal of the writing to people in your own discipline
Write with parsimony in mind.	As a rule, if five words can have the same meaning as 10, go with the five. Strive for simple (not compound) sentences and do not repeat things.

Next, regarding the rule about aligning conclusions with the purpose of the study, we recommend that the conclusions drawn should not fall outside the specific objectives of the study. Consider, for instance, a study of adolescents and teen pregnancy. Imagine that as part of the study you find that male adolescents specifically and those of a lower socioeconomic status were more likely to have experienced child sex abuse. Although you may be personally interested in this finding and have a desire to write something like, "Experiences of child sex abuse were experienced by lower-income male teens as compared with male teens of other socioeconomic status or female teens," we caution you that a study on risk factors for teen pregnancy should report on the conclusions related only to this topic. Other conclusions drawn may be spurious and should be interpreted with caution.

Turning to the subject of jargon, consider the following sentence: "From a biopsychosocial standpoint, the findings suggest that theory amalgamation is essential to primary prevention." Although this sentence may be clear to your immediate colleagues, it most certainly leaves other readers in a haze regarding the word *biopsychosocial* and the term *theory*

amalgamation. Instead, the sentence might be written as follows: "Considering the roles of biology, psychology, and the social system, the findings suggest that combining two or more theories into a single intervention approach is essential to primary prevention." In this amended sentence, you can see that the meaning would be clear to people in any profession that involves itself with disease prevention. Thus, rather than being easily understood only by biopsychologists, the revised sentence becomes easily understood by healthcare practitioners, epidemiologists, public health policy professionals, and even persons yet to receive an academic degree that places them in a given discipline.

Regarding the final entry in Table 15.4, here we will rely on the philosophical principle called **Occam's razor** (or *Ockham's razor*). William of Ockham, a 14th-century Franciscan friar who studied logic (see **FIGURE 15.5**), first made this principle well known. In Latin, it translates to "the law of briefness," and the concept behind this principle is that simplicity is always the best policy, or, as is often said in the modern world, "Less is more."

To illustrate this principle, consider the following sentence from the concluding paragraph of a research manuscript:

> Albeit a study conducted with modest limitations to rigor, the findings are intriguing and highly suggestive of a causal association between daily dietary consumption of wheat-based products (including those in breads and pastas) and early-onset adult diabetes, as defined by standard criteria.

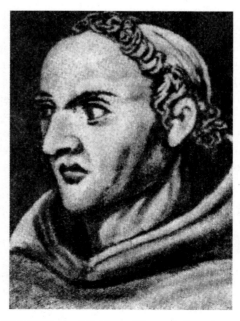

FIGURE 15.5 William of Ockham (Occam's Razor).
© Interfoto/Alamy Stock Photo

Now, let's apply Occam's razor. First, in the Discussion section of a manuscript, the "Limitations" section always precedes the "Conclusion." Thus, the opening phrase "Albeit a study conducted with modest limitations to rigor" can be cut entirely. Second, the words *intriguing* and *highly* are editorial and do not belong in the world of scientific writing, so more can be cut. Third, is the word *daily* critical here? The word *consumption* encompasses the point that diets are indeed consumed on a daily basis, so one more word can be deleted. Fourth, the parenthetical phrase about breads and pastas is certainly redundant with "wheat-based products," and that information was already provided in the Methods section. Finally, it appears that "early-onset adult diabetes" is the outcome variable of the study; thus, it would have been defined previously and does not warrant the phrase "as defined by standard definition." The revised trimmed and more parsimonious sentence looks like this: "Findings suggest a causal association between consumption of wheat-based products and early-onset adult diabetes." In case you are wondering, applying Occam's razor to this sentence trimmed 28 words from the initial sentence of 42 words. Bear in mind that most readers do not want to read long sentences, so this writing principle may improve your writing and ultimately your ability to get published.

▶ What Makes an Effective Introduction?

Although your findings are the most important aspect of what you disseminate, even professionals who are highly dedicated to public health issues require of bit of "coaxing" before they are likely to read what you have written. The coaxing takes the form of a formalized section of the article (or report) known as the Introduction. Think of writing the Introduction as occurring from a "wide lens" starting point that progressively becomes more narrow until it reaches a highly specific research question; this is the question you originally formulated before the research began (see Chapter 2). **FIGURE 15.6** displays this "funnel model" of writing an effective Introduction.

In our experience of teaching students, a frequently asked question goes something like, "How many past studies should I cite and what else should be in the introduction of my manuscript?" Much to the dismay of many students, the answer here is one of our favorite refrains: "It depends." Following the principles of Occam's razor, an important aspect of writing an effective Introduction is the judicious use of references. By *judicious*, we mean that you need to provide the readers with the basic and most relevant background information that highlights your public health issue and the gap in the literature, bearing in mind that the things you do cite give readers a gateway into learning more if they want. As you may imagine, this *gateway principle* works far better when the journal articles that you cite are relatively recent. As a rule, you should keep your citations as recent as the preceding 5 years (this also keeps the Introduction at a succinct length). Although we understand the temptation to over-reference your Introduction (thinking "more is better"), citing a litany of articles is discouraged because it detracts from the overall quality and relevance of the reference list. We typically tell our students that a good reference list is a product of restraint in selection. In essence, only those articles that are key to the research question should be cited. At this juncture, you should know that one good review article could be cited rather than citing dozens of articles that were reviewed.

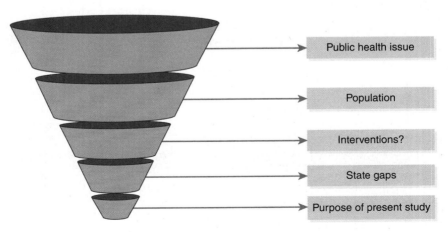

FIGURE 15.6 Funnel Model of an Effective Introduction of a Journal Article.

▶ How Should Results Be Presented?

Ultimately, think of your study results as being comparable to a brand new product that the inventor (you as the researcher) wants to bring to market and amass sales. For this to happen, the new product requires packaging that will help sell it. The packaging process in this case, rather than consulting with a packaging engineer and manufacturers, is about constructing easy-to-follow tables of the results and constructing visually appealing (and easy-to-follow) figures. Tables are used to display results that can be presented as lists, whereas figures are used to capture more complex findings such as a trend in a dependent variable over long periods of follow-up or a test of a complex theoretical model. The act of balancing text with these visuals, however, can be extremely challenging. On the one hand, the text must tell a complete story (some readers will not look at the visuals). On the other hand, the visuals must also tell a complete story that enhances and simplifies the story told in words. This seemingly complex task can be achieved by following a few helpful rules:

- Tables are the place to report test statistics, confidence intervals, and *P*-values
- Tables should be intelligible without reference to the text
- Titles should be brief but clear and explanatory
- Explain all abbreviations except for standard ones
- Always identify units of measurement

- Figures are best to show trend lines, dramatic differences between groups, and simple descriptions of a single variable (such as a pie chart to show the race or ethnicity of a study sample)
- Tables and figures should have footnotes when these are needed to complete "the story"; footnotes also preserve white space in visuals (leaving ample white space is important to the overall aesthetics and easy-to-follow nature of an effective visual)
- Visuals should always augment rather than duplicate text
- Visuals should be referenced and explained in the Results section; this gives readers a sense of what to look for and how to best understand the visual

To help you appreciate and better understand what we mean by effective visuals, we have provided two samples from our own work. **FIGURE 15.7** displays an example of two trend lines relative to binge drinking over a 90-day recall period. The two lines are shown in contrasting colors because one represents study participants randomized to the intervention group and the other represents study participants randomized to the control group. Notice that even though the figure does not give highly specific information, it does provide a quick and easy-to-follow visualization of the two trends over a 12-month period.

TABLE 15.5 provides a sample of how to easily report 20 statistical findings in what appears to be a

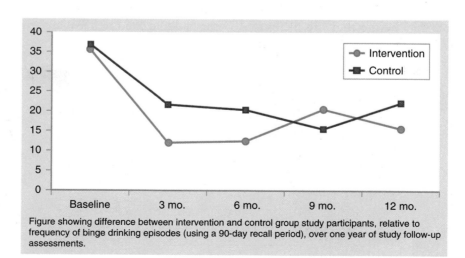

Figure showing difference between intervention and control group study participants, relative to frequency of binge drinking episodes (using a 90-day recall period), over one year of study follow-up assessments.

FIGURE 15.7 Figure Graph of Study Results.

TABLE 15.5 Results of Five Paired Samples *t*-Tests

Outcome	Mean 1[a]	Mean 2[b]	t	P
Frequency of binge drinking[c]	26.4	3.9	3.81	0.001
Barriers to sobriety[d]	15.10	14.69	1.01	0.32
Attitudes toward intoxication[e]	17.96	16.46	2.43	0.027
Self-efficacy to avoid alcohol use[f]	22.93	16.60	3.57	0.001
Situational avoidance of alcohol use[g]	15.71	16.25	1.18	0.25

[a]Mean score at baseline assessment.
[b]Mean score at the 6-month follow-up assessment.
[c]Assessed by a single item with scores ranging from 0 to 72.
[d]Assessed by a scale measure with scores ranging from 7 to 35 (high = more).
[e]Assessed by a scale measure with scores ranging from 9 to 45 (high = attitudes supporting binge drinking as "normal").
[f]Assessed by a scale measure with scores ranging from 7 to 35 (high = more self-efficacy).
[g]Assessed by a scale measure with scores ranging from 5 to 25 (high = more likely to avoid drinking in social circumstances where this is not a "normal" behavior).

simple layout. In this case, test results for each of five variables are presented over a 6-month time span (i.e., baseline and again 6 months later). A mean is reported for each time point. For each test, you also will see a *t*-value (the test statistic for the *t*-test) and *P*-value. Thus, each variable has four corresponding statistics.

Please note that inspecting the mathematical difference between means is only possible here because the table footnotes provide guidance on how to read these scores. In looking at the table, you can see that even without the accompanying text, you would be able to understand the results and what they mean.

Think About It!

The related U.S. epidemics of type II diabetes and obesity are largely caused by physical inactivity and processed sugars such as those used to produce mass quantities of soft drinks (known as sweetened beverages). Although seemingly oversimplistic, a highly effective public health approach to curtail the "sugar side" of these epidemics lies in taxing sweetened beverages (see **FIGURE 15.8**). As you may know, this type of public health action is known as a *structural-level intervention*. In addition to curtailing the consumption of sweetened beverages, this type of approach has been applied to other public health issues such as alcohol consumption, for example (Elder, Lawrence, & Ferguson, 2010). As you learn more and more about public health practice, we suspect you will come to realize that the interventions delivered at the structural level are quite different from those delivered at the individual level. One key difference in this regard is the speed of translating

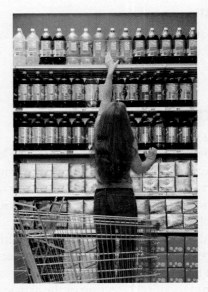

FIGURE 15.8 Woman Shops for Sugar-Sweetened Beverages in Grocery Store.
© Paul Burns/Stockbyte/Getty Images

research into practice. A prime example is found in a sweetened-beverage tax recently passed by the city of Philadelphia, Pennsylvania. Without having to conduct a time-consuming, costly, and cumbersome randomized trial, the evidence reported in an article in the *Journal of the American Medical Association* by Roberto and colleagues (2019) indicates a net decline of 38% in sales (and thus consumption) of sweetened beverages as a consequence of this public health intervention. Given this overwhelming evidence from 2019, the questions to you become, "How long will it take for other U.S. cities to begin passing similar tax-based intervention programs?" and "Should people who like sugar-sweetened beverages have to pay more even if they are not overweight or have type II diabetes?" We suggest that other cities will follow suit and pass their own taxes, and certainly people will complain; however, we also realize that in the United States, the profit motive of industry frequently wins out over the prevention motive of public health. If you are at the start of your public health career, we encourage you to think in terms of intervention programs like this one that will transcend the "17-year lag period" (Morris, Wooding, & Grant, 2011) and can benefit entire populations even if they are not popular with the public at large or with the industry that will be affected financially.

Take Home Points

- Dissemination of research findings is a central obligation of all empirical studies.
- Abstracts have four key sections: Objective or Purpose, Methods, Results, and Conclusion
- Manuscripts have seven main sections: Abstract, Introduction, Methods, Results, Discussion, Figures or Tables (or both), and References
- Presentations at conferences can assist with dissemination by reaching attendees in person and those who later read the conference proceedings
- Manuscripts submitted to peer-reviewed journals are instrumental in disseminating research findings to public health practitioners, researchers, and policy makers
- The use of the media via an online press release or other format can also help disseminate research findings
- Scientific writing follows set rules for style, content, and language
- The principle of Occam's razor should be applied to the write-up of research findings

Key Terms

Dissemination
Empirical research

Occam's Razor
Peer Review

Translation Science

For Practice and Discussion

1. You were asked to conduct a literature review of peer-reviewed journal articles on e-cigarette interventions to inform e-cigarette smoking-prevention programs on college campuses. How can you disseminate findings to highlight implications for health promotion?
2. Find a journal article on a public health area of your choice. Using the seven key sections of a research manuscript, write a one-sentence summary of each section of the article.
3. A researcher conducts a major study on cancer screening and has breakthrough results that she thinks can significantly affect the field. She wants to make sure her study findings are available to other researchers and healthcare professionals in her field. What would be the most effective way for this professor to disseminate study findings to a wide audience, and why?
4. You are reading a peer-reviewed journal article of an observational research study on alcohol use and its relationship to condom use, and the results show that binge drinking is associated with lower condom use among

study participants. You notice the article states, "Binge drinking causes lower condom use." Using the five cardinal rules for scientific writing, explain why this sentence is a red flag.

5. While you are writing up the results of the research study mentioned in the previous question, you think back to Occam's razor and ponder how you should explain the results of your study. How can you write up these findings so they will be understood by researchers and practitioners alike?

References

American Public Health Association (APHA). (2019). State and regional public health associations. Retrieved from www.apha.org/apha-communities/affiliates/state-and-regional-public-health-associations

Elder, R. W., Lawrence, B., & Ferguson, A. (2010). The effectiveness of tax policy intervention for reducing excessive alcohol consumption and related norms. *American Journal of Preventive Medicine, 38,* 217–228.

Morris, Z. S., Wooding, S., & Grant, J. (2011). The answer is 17 years, what is the question: Understanding time lags in translation of research. *Journal of the Royal Society of Medicine, 104,* 510–520.

Noonan, R. K., & Emshoff, J. G. (2013). Translating research to practice: Putting "what works" to work. Pp. 309–334 in R. J. DiClemente, L. F. Salazar, & R. A. Crosby (Eds.), *Health behavior theory for public health.* Burlington, MA: Jones & Bartlett Publishing.

Roberto, C. A., Lawman, H. G., LeVasseur, M. T., Mitra, N., Peterhans, A., Herring, B., & Bleich, S. N. (2019). Association of a beverage tax on sugar-sweetened and artificially sweetened beverages with changes in beverage prices and sales at chain retailers in a large urban setting. *JAMA, 321*(18), 1799–1810.

van de Goor, I., Hämäläinen, R. M., Syed, A., Juel Lau, C., Sandu, P., Spitters, . . . , & REPOPA Consortium. (2017). Determinants of evidence use in public health policy making: Results from a study of six EU countries. *Health Policy, 121,* 273.

For Further Reading

Crosby, R. A., Salazar, L. F., & DiClemente, R. J. (2015). Introduction to scientific writing. Pp. 493–524 in L. F. Salazar, R. A. Crosby, & R. J. DiClemente (Eds.), Research methods in health promotion (2nd ed.). San Francisco, CA: Jossey-Bass, 2015.

Ioannidis, J. P. (2006). Evolution and translation of research findings: From bench to where. *PLoS Clinical Trials, 1*(7), e36.

Eslava-Schmalbach, J., & Gilberto Gómez-Duarte, O. (2013). Scientific writing, a neglected aspect of professional training. *Revista Colombiana de Anestesiología, 41*(2), 79–81.

Klingner, J. K., Scanlon, D., & Pressley, M. (2005). How to publish in scholarly journals. *Educational Researcher, 34*(8), 14–20. Retrieved from https://doi.org/10.3102/0013189X034008014

Vintzileos, A. M., & Ananth, C. V. (2010). How to write and publish an original research article. *American Journal of Obstetrics and Gynecology, 202*(4), 344–e1.

Glossary

A

Adaptation The adaptive changes to a stimulus that lead to a change in outcome.

Alpha Represents the odds of making a wrong decision, meaning that you reject the null hypothesis.

Analysis of Variance (ANOVA) Best used to compare means for three or more groups of study participants.

Attrition Also referred to as *mortality*, attrition is the loss of participants from the research study and can bias results.

Autonomy A principle in research ethics that all volunteers must be fully aware of all possible risks and benefits associated with participation and that volunteers are allowed to end their participation at any time without penalty.

Autoregressive Integrated Moving Average A statistical analysis model that uses time-series data to either better understand the data set or to predict future trends.

Average Interitem Correlation Involves assessing the interitem correlations among all items in a scale measure and then taking the average.

B

Bar Chart A graph that is useful for depicting categorical, nominal, or ordinal data in quantitative scales.

Baseline Assessment Conducted immediately after enrollment, this is the first assessment or observation conducted before any treatment.

Beneficence A principle in research ethics that states that researchers should have the welfare of the research participant as a goal of any clinical trial or other research study.

Beta Weight Standardized correlation coefficient.

Between-Subjects Factor In an experimental design, refers to using more than one group for which comparisons are made on the dependent variable.

Biomarkers Typically, some type of chemical, antigen, hormone, or metabolite that will fluctuate as a function of changes to a given system in the human body.

Bivariate Association An association between two variables in which one variable is defined as the outcome and its values are compared based on the values of the explanatory or predictor variable.

Bivariate Data Point Data on two variables in which the value of one variable is paired with a value of the other variable on a graph.

Blended Approach
Blended Approach An approach that uses any and all aspects of community-based participatory research (CBPR) that will improve the value of the final research findings.

C

Carryover Effects Occurs when exposure to the first treatment affects the subjects' subsequent performance.

Case-Control Design A type of observational design in which participants are selected on the basis of whether they have (case) or do not have (control) the disease or other health-related outcome of interest.

Case-Crossover Design A type of observational design in which each participant serves as both a case and a control.

Case-Exposure Window The transitory period of time when a person is considered a "case" as part of a case-crossover design and is compared with the control window and relates to the time period (e.g., hour before, day of, etc.) right before the onset of an acute outcome.

Case Study A research method involving an up-close, in-depth, and detailed examination of a subject of study (the case), as well as its related contextual conditions.

Cases Those who have the outcome of interest in a case-control observational study.

CBPR *See* Community-Based Participatory Research.

Cell The point at which a row and a column intersect on a table.

Central Tendency A descriptive summary of a data set through a single value that reflects the center of the data distribution.

Chain of Knowledge Emphasizes the current knowledge about a given subject while also indicating gaps in understanding of that given subject.

Chi-Square A nonparametric statistical test that compares an observed pattern of responses with a pattern that would be expected if the variables were truly independent of each other.

Children Persons younger than 18 years of age.

Clarification Probe A neutral probe that avoids introducing bias into the answering process.

Climate Change Occurs when changes in Earth's climate system results in new weather patterns that remain in place for an extended period of time.

Cluster Defined as a geographically distinct collection of organizations, businesses, or entities that serve a particular region of a city.

Coalition A board or organization that may sponsor and support the research.

Code Descriptive word or short phrase that is used as a label and is attached to units of data.

Codebook Book that provides a key to naming study variables and, more important, to assigning a numerical value to each possible response to a given questionnaire item.

Coefficient of Determination A statistical measure related to accounting for variance and indicates how close the data are to the fitted regression line.

Coercion Undue influence on research participants to take part in a research study.

Cohen's Kappa Takes into account agreement in coding that can occur from chance and is a more stringent measure than percent agreement.

Collinearity The intercorrelations among the predictor variables.

Community Advisory Board (CAB) Advisory board that is key to ensuring principles of ethical research are upheld; composed of community members who share a common identity, history, symbols and language, and culture.

Community-Based Participatory Research (CBPR) A concept that suggests to achieve full success in recruiting, retaining, and intervening; a partnership must exist between the researchers and the community; only through this partnership can the research agenda be carried out.

Community-Based Research Research at the community level via partnerships with community leaders and their respective communities.

Community Empowerment The process of enabling communities to increase control over their lives.

Comparative Case Study When a case is investigated across geographically distinct areas.

Comparison Group A method used to control for many threats to internal validity that is created through randomization and involves an additional group that receives either no TREATMENT or an alternative treatment.

Complete Observer Involves the researcher observing without ever becoming part of the setting.

Complete Participant A covert role in research that allows people to see the researcher as a participant, not as a researcher.

Computer-Assisted Self-Interview (CASI) A programmed computer tool used to allow respondents to complete surveys that reduces the researcher's survey burden.

Concept Refers to an idea or notion that is suggestive of the data.

Confidence Interval A range of values so defined that there is a specified probability that the value of a parameter lies within it.

Confidentiality The duty given to anyone or any organization to keep the information of study participants private.

Confounding variables Variables other than the independent variable that are not of interest in a research study but may affect the dependent variable.

Constant Comparative Analysis Uses data to generate a theory; subsequent data are then compared against the initial theory.

Construct An indicator variable that represents a hidden characteristic or a trait.

Construct Validity A form of validity related to a measure that indicates your measure indeed measures what it is supposed to as evidenced by its correlation with another scale measure of the same construct.

Contingency Table Also known as a *cross-tabulation table*, it involves crossing the frequency counts of each level of the categorical variables.

Control Phase In a quasi-experimental design, the time that elapses between the start of the research study and the start of the intervention phase.

Control Window The transitory period of time when a person is considered a "control" as part of a case-crossover design and is compared with the case-exposure window and relates to a chosen time period (e.g., day, week, month, year, etc.) well before the onset of the acute outcome.

Controls Those who do not have the outcome of interest in a case-control observational study.

Convenience Sampling A preexisting group of people who represent the pool of recruitment opportunities for the sample.

Correlation A statistical measure that indicates the extent to which two variables are related.

Counterbalancing A technique used in experimental designs to control for carryover effects that involves randomizing each group to receive each level of the independent in different or varying order.

Criterion Validity A form of validity that indicates how well a scale measure predicts an outcome it should be associated with.

Critical Region Total area under the normal distribution curve representing the level of alpha, or probability of rejecting the null hypothesis; also known as the *rejection region*.

Cronbach's Alpha A measure of internal consistency that takes into itself the number of items in the scale, the average covariance between item pairs, and the average variance.

Cross-Sectional Design A type of observational design in which measurements or observations are collected at only one time point.

Crossover Trial A within-subjects experimental design in which each subject is randomized to study arms consisting of a sequence of two or more treatments given consecutively with a washout period between treatments.

D

Deception Occurs when investigators provide false or incomplete information to participants for the purpose of misleading research subjects.

Decision Points Represents opportunities to realistically adopt a given aspect of the CBPR approach to conducting research.

Degrees of Freedom The number of observations used to calculate a test statistic that are free to vary, meaning they are not fixed.

Demand Characteristics An experimental artifact in which participants form an interpretation of the experiment's purpose and change reports of their behavior to fit that interpretation.

Demographic Indicators Information about a population such as age, education level, socioeconomic status, sex, gender, race, and ethnicity that is related to health outcomes.

Dependent Variable (DV) The variable of interest to the researcher that is measured in an experiment; also known as the *outcome variable*.

Differential Attrition Difference in attrition levels between two or more groups.

Differential Selection A potential threat in nonequivalence groups—specifically, that prior differences among groups may affect the outcome of the study.

Dispersion The distance, in units of measure, that scores or observations deviate from a midpoint.

Dissemination Process of informing others about research findings or other information.

E

Echo Probe A strategy interviewers can use in which they paraphrase what an interviewee has just said.

Ecological Momentary Assessment (EMA) A method of assessment that involves repeated sampling of subjects' current behaviors and experiences in real time in subjects' natural environments.

Effect Modifier The magnitude of the effect of the primary predictor variable on an outcome variable differs, depending on the level of a third variable.

Effect Size Quantitative measure of the magnitude of a phenomenon.

Effectiveness Trial Measures the degree of beneficial effect under real-world circumstances, not under the researcher's control.

Efficacious In the context of an experiment, the treatment or intervention worked as expected.

Efficacy Trial Determines whether an intervention produces the expected result under ideal controlled circumstances.

Element A basic unit that defines the study population.

Emic Perspective An insider's perspective meaning *insider participant*.

Empirical Research Reports based on actual observation or experiment.

Epidemiology Study of the distribution and determinants of health-related states or events.

Error Variance In statistics, the portion of the variance in a set of scores that results from extraneous variables such as individual differences and measurements.

Ethnography Social scientific description of a people and their cultural beliefs, values, and traditions.

Etic Perspective An outsider's perspective meaning *outsider researcher*.

Expected Frequency A subject's reported usual frequency over a specified time period *before* the occurrence of a specific outcome.

Experimenter Expectancy A form of reactivity in which a researcher's cognitive bias causes him or her to subconsciously influence the participants in an experiment.

Exposure Refers to experiencing or engaging in a certain risk factor such as lead poisoning, poor air quality, poor diet, drug use, or tobacco use.

External Validity The extent to which the results of a study can be generalized to a population but only as a function of the researcher and the design of the research.

Extraneous Variables Variables that may have influence on your outcome but are not of interest to the research.

F

Fatigue Deterioration in performance from being tired from the first treatment.

Fidelity Degree of exactness with which something is copied or reproduced.

Focus Group A form of interviewing that conducts a session in a group setting, often allowing for stimulating, thoughtful discussion; varied opinions; experiences; beliefs; and so on.

Follow-Up Assessments An assessment that provides contrast to baseline assessments and is normally conducted at regularly scheduled intervals for the duration of the study.

Formal Needs Assessment A systematic process for determining and addressing needs or gaps between current conditions and desired conditions or wants of a targeted community or organization.

G

Generalizability The extension of research findings and conclusions from a study conducted on a sample population to the population at large.

Geographically Defined Population A population that is defined by a location parameter.

Grounded Theory A general methodology that has been described as marriage between positivism and interpretivism.

Grouping Variable Variables used to group or categorize observations.

H

Habituation The effect of repeated exposure to a stimulus that leads to reduced responsiveness.

Hazard Period A period of risk exposure.

Health Disparities Preventable differences in the health, violence, or disease burden experienced by socially disadvantaged groups.

Histogram A diagram consisting of rectangles whose area is proportional to the frequency of a variable and whose width is equal to the class interval.

History An extraneous event that could have affected the internal validity of a study.

Homogeneous A sample in which participants have similar characteristics that are chosen based on the research question, such as gender, age range, socioeconomic status, education level, or race or ethnicity.

Hypothesis A proposed explanation, assumption, or idea made on the basis of limited evidence that acts as a starting point for further investigation.

I

Impact Factor Measure of the frequency with which the average article in a journal has been cited in a particular year.

Imputation Process of replacing missing data with substituted values.

Independent Groups *t*-Test A parametric test that compares the means of two independent groups to determine whether statistical evidence shows that the associated population means are different.

Independent Variable (IV) The variable manipulated by the researcher in an experiment.

Index A set of questionnaire items that independently adds to the measure of something that may, in fact, be tangible.

Informal Needs Assessment Using existing data to identify salient health disparities.

Institutional Review Board (IRB) An administrative body established to protect the rights and welfare of human research subjects recruited to participate in research activities conducted under the auspices of its affiliated institution.

Instrumentation Process of constructing research instruments that could be used appropriately in gathering data in the study—for example, a questionnaire, an interview, or an observation.

Intercoder Reliability In qualitative data analysis, each coder's codes attached to the data are compared to determine the level of agreement.

Internal Validity A degree of confidence in the results, depending on the level of rigor in a study's design and methods.

Interpretivism A philosophical view of reality as being a function of individual perceptions where each person finds meaning of their reality in different ways.

Interrupted Time-Series Design (ITSD) Considered by many as the strongest quasi-experimental approach for evaluating longitudinal effects of interventions because it involves collecting a series of data points over time before and after some kind of intervention has been implemented.

Intersectionality The interconnectedness of social categories such as race, gender, sexual orientation, and so on that applies to individuals or groups and is regarded as creating overlapping and interdependent systems of discrimination or disadvantage.

Intervention Phase The step in a stepped-wedge design where researchers implement the intervention following the control phase.

Interviews A qualitative research technique that involves a researcher engaging respondents in a conversation and asking questions to explore their perspectives on a particular idea, program, or situation.

Inverse Correlation Also known as a *negative correlation*, when the increase in the score for one variable has a mathematical relationship to a decrease in scores for a second variable.

J

Justice A key ethical principle pertaining to the moral imperative to conduct research studies with the same populations for which intended benefits are sought to occur.

K

Key Words A set of words in nonsentence structure that highlights the focus of a research article.

L

Learning A carryover effect in which performance is enhanced after the second treatment, a result of the first treatment.

Likert Scale A type of rating scale used to measure constructs such as attitudes, beliefs, perceptions, and so on.

Listwise Deletion In statistical models, an approach to missing data that drops all cases from the analysis when at least one value is missing from one of the variables in the model.

Literature Review A search and evaluation of the available literature on a given subject or chosen topic.

Logistic Regression A statistical method for analyzing data in which one or more variables determine an outcome that is dichotomous or binary, meaning there are only two possible values.

Longitudinal Cohort Study A study design in which the same participants are followed over a period of time and interviewed more than once during the time period; also called *prospective cohort design*.

M

Manipulation Process by which researchers purposely change, alter, or influence the independent variables.

Matched-Pairs Group Design A type of between-subjects design in which participants are matched on a particular subject characteristic strongly associated with the intended outcome and then participants from each pair are randomized into treatment and control groups.

Maturation The process within which subjects act as a function of the passage of time.

Maturational Trend A change in observable behavior because of the aging of human subjects over time.

Mean Arithmetic average of all recorded scores or observations.

Median The data value that divides the distribution of scores into equal halves.

Meta-Analysis A statistical analysis that combines the results of multiple scientific studies to determine an overall or pooled effect.

Methodology Techniques required to fulfill the conditions of any given study design.

Mindfulness Purposefully paying attention in a particular way in the present moment and without judgment.

Missing at Random (MAR) In examining a data set, when the probability that missing responses are unrelated to its value.

Missing Completely at Random (MCAR) In examining a data set, the probability that missing data are not related to its value or to the value of other variables in the study.

Missing Not at Random (MNAR) In examining a data set, when the probabilities that missing data are related on unobserved values.

Mode The data value that is the most frequent in the data set.

Mortality The loss of participants from a longitudinal research study, which can bias the results.

Multiple Case Study Multiple-case design is a research methodology in which several cases are examined using multiple data-collection methods.

Multiple Linear Regression An equation that combines multiple predictors and then considers the overlapping variance based on rules that can be set by the person doing the analysis.

Multistage Cluster Sampling A form of sampling that divides a targeted population into groups or clusters and then draws a random sample of clusters; all elements from each cluster are selected.

N

Negative Correlation A relationship between two variables in which one variable increases as the other decreases and vice versa. In a statistical model, a perfect negative correlation has the value of –1.

Negative Skew A continuous distribution of scores on a histogram with a preponderance of scores on the right-hand side.

Noise Random error in measurement resulting from unknown or unpredictable causes.

Nominal Group Process A form of consensus building in which each member of a group offers a solution to a given problem and redundant solutions are then collapsed.

Nonequivalent Groups Posttest-Only Design A quasi-experimental research design in which the dependent variable is measured only after exposure to the treatment (posttest) in one group and is similarly measured in another group that does not receive the treatment.

Nonequivalent Groups Pretest–Posttest Design A quasi-experimental research design in which the dependent variable is measured before (pretest) and after exposure to the treatment (posttest) in one group and is similarly measured in another group that does not receive the treatment.

Nonparametric Statistical Test A test that assumes nothing about the underlying distribution of data.

Nonprobability Sampling Sampling method that yields weak levels of generalizability.

Normal Distribution Curve A bell-shaped curve that represents values from a data set and is symmetrical around its center so that the side right of the center is a mirror image of the left side. The mean, median, and mode are equal to each other.

Null Findings Outcome in research that does not show an otherwise expected effect.

O

Observational Research Type of research in which participants are only assessed or observed and no treatments are implemented.

Observer as Participant Status in which the investigator's main role is that of observer, although it allows the investigator to enter the setting periodically with limited interaction.

Occam's Razor A logical principle stating that simplicity is always the best policy.

Odds Ratio A measure of association between an exposure and an outcome. The ratio represents the odds that an outcome will occur given a particular exposure compared with the odds of the outcome occurring in the absence of that exposure.

Oppression When a minority member (whether racial or ethnic, sexual orientation, gender, gender expression, or living below the federal poverty level) is substantially more likely than nonminority counterparts to experience a riskier environment for any given disease or condition.

Outcome Variable In observational research, the main variable of interest in a research study.

P

Pair-Matched Interval A statistical comparison of the case window with the control window.

Pairwise deletion In statistical models, this approach to missing data allows more use of data and involves using cases that contain missing data. Only cases relating to each pair of variables with missing data involved in an analysis are deleted.

Parametric Statistical Test A test that makes assumptions about the parameters of the population distribution from which data are drawn.

Participant as Observer This role allows the investigator to be overt in that it identifies him or her as a researcher.

Participant Observation A type of naturalistic observation in which researchers have little knowledge of a culture or the people but want to study and immerse themselves in that culture.

Participation Rate A rate calculated by setting the number of people who enrolled in a study as the numerator and the number asked to join the study as the denominator.

Pearson Product Moment Correlation A value that falls between −1.00 and +1.00 to depict correlation.

Peer Review When a jury of colleagues with expertise in the subject matter evaluates a submitted research manuscript for quality; an evaluation of scientific, academic, or professional work by others working in the same field.

Percent Agreement Measures the number of times that two coders agreed or disagreed in the coding of a text segment.

Periodicity A cyclical order of elements that can lead to bias when random or systematic sampling is used.

Placebo A neutral substance without any related biological effects.

Placebo Effect The positive physiological or psychological changes associated with the use of inert medications, sham procedures, or therapeutic symbols.

Population The defined segment of people that the research targets, which can be based on geography, group, or other factor.

Population Health Health and wellness of a particular town, area, or country.

Positive Correlation A relationship between two variables in which one variable increases or decreases as the other increases or decreases. In a statistical model, a perfect positive correlation has the value of +1.

Positive Skew A continuous distribution of scores on a histogram with a preponderance of scores on the left-hand side.

Positivism The view that scientific inquiry should be confined to the study of relations existing between facts that are directly observable.

Post Hoc Test Meaning "after this," a test that analyzes results for the probability of a Type 1 error.

Potential Risk The negative consequences a research participant might experience as a result of participating in a study.

Predictor Variable In observational research, the variables that are hypothesized to be associated with the outcome variable.

Preexposure Prophylaxis (PrEP) The use of antiretroviral drugs to prevent HIV infection in people who have not yet been exposed to the virus.

Principal Investigator The holder and lead researcher of a grant project, usually in science-related studies.

Privacy A right given to study participants to limit the distribution of their personal information.

Probability Sampling Sampling method in which a sample from a larger population is chosen using a method based on the theory of probability.

Probing During the conducting of an interview, the interviewer makes an effort verbally or nonverbally to elicit more details, guide dialogue, or elaborate on the meaning of something said.

Prospective Cohort Design A study design in which the same participants are followed over a period of time and interviewed more than once during the time period; also called *longitudinal design*.

Publication Bias A type of bias that occurs when the null outcome of an experiment or research study influences the decision of a publisher to publish or distribute it.

Purposive Sampling A nonprobability sampling technique that selects participants based on characteristics of a population and study objectives.

Q

Qualitative Research Research focused on understanding the meaning of phenomena rather than documenting their quantity.

Quasi-Experimental Design An empirical study used to estimate the causal impact of an intervention or policy on a target population without using random assignment.

Quota Sampling A sampling method that requires that representative individuals are chosen from a specific subgroup.

R

Random A sample or method in which all people or things involved have an equal chance of being chosen.

Randomization The hallmark of a true experimental study design, a method that involves assigning study participants to different groups based on chance and minimizes the differences among groups by equally distributing people with particular characteristics among all trial arms.

Randomized Controlled Trial (RCT) A type of scientific experiment that aims to reduce bias when testing the effectiveness of an intervention; it is accomplished by randomly designating subjects to two or more groups.

Recall Bias A form of systematic error that occurs when a participant is asked about events, behaviors, and so on that occurred in the past.

Rejection Region Total area under the normal distribution curve representing the level of alpha, or probability of rejecting the null hypothesis; also known as the *critical region*.

Reliability The degree to which an instrument consistently measures a construct across items and time points.

Replacement When a sampling unit is drawn from the sampling frame or population and is returned, after its characteristic(s) have been recorded, before the next unit is drawn.

Respect for Autonomy The guiding principle of research study that provides people with full disclosure about their enrollment, including all possible risks and benefits that may possibly be associated with their participation.

Rurality A condition shared by people with common ancestry and who reside in culturally or geographically defined areas recognized to be rural.

S

Sample A proportion of a study population rather than all of the people or elements of that population.

Sampling The process of selecting individuals within the target population.

Sampling Frame A formal and often exhaustive list of the elements or units that make up the target population.

Sampling Technique The process of selecting a representative portion of the population.

Saturation A commonly used concept in qualitative research that refers to when no new information or findings have been found thus indicating the exhaustive exploration of the phenomena being studied.

Scale A selected set of correlated questionnaire items created to assess a specific construct that has been operationally defined.

Scattergram A graph depicting bivariate data points.

Seasonal Trend When observations are influenced by the season in which data are collected.

Secondary Research The use of a preexisting data set for a study that was not planned at the time the data were collected.

Security The active defense measures to protect private information.

Seed A randomly selected starting point in the sampling frame.

Selection History When a historical event affects one group but not the other.

Selection-instrumentation Any differential change made to the test or instrument used from pretest and posttest for the groups.

Selection-maturation Differential rates of normal growth between pretest and posttest for the groups.

Selection-regression Different rates of regression to the mean in the two groups.

Self-Efficacy An individual's confidence in the ability to exert control over his or her own motivation, behavior, and social environments.

Self-Reported Measures Survey items that ask people to report their behavior, including knowledge, intentions, attitudes, perceptions, beliefs, and so on.

Semistructured Interview An interview that involves asking a series of questions that are open ended but in a predetermined order.

Sensitization Stronger responses to stimuli stemming from initial exposure to a different stimulus.

Simple Random Sampling Sampling method in which each element has an equal probability of being chosen and is the most common and user-friendly method of selecting a probability sample.

Single Case Study A research method based on an in-depth investigation of a single individual, group, or event.

Snowball Sampling A sampling method that recruits qualifying participants through its initial participants, creating tan ever-expanding number of people who may be recruited for a given study.

Social Desirability Bias A form of systematic error occurring when people want to avoid embarrassment and project favorable images to others so they appear better than they really are.

Spurious Finding A false finding that can stem from not being able to establish a temporal order between two variables.

Stakeholder People or organizations who have an interest in the research project or are affected by its outcomes.

Standard Deviation A statistic that measures the dispersion of a data set relative to its mean; calculated as the square root of the variance.

Statistical Power The probability that a statistical test will correctly reject a false null hypothesis. Power is partly a function of sample size.

Statistically Significant A result obtained that indicates it was very unlikely to occur by chance alone.

Step Length The length of time between successive crossover points in a stepped-wedge design.

Stepped-Wedge (SW) Design A study design that involves random and sequential crossover of clusters from control to intervention until all clusters are exposed.

Stratified Simple Random Sample A method of probability sampling that involves the division of a population into smaller groups or *strata* that are formed based on members' shared attributes or characteristics.

Study Arm Commonly known as the *treatment condition* or *treatment group* in randomized controlled trials.

Study-inclusion Criteria Defines who is eligible for study participation.

Study Protocol A guide for conducting the actual study, training staff, and developing assessments, as well as any other functions of the study.

Successive Independent Samples Design A hybrid research design that combines a cross-sectional design with a prospective cohort design in that it incorporates a series of cross-sectional studies conducted over a period of time.

Sustainability Implies that the program being designed and tested will become an ongoing part of the public health structure in the community.

Switching Replication A further step that can be taken in quasi-experimental design studies; allows for the control group to receive treatment intervention, thus overcoming the ethical issues of withholding needed programs.

Systematic In the context of measurement, refers to the nonrandom causes of error.

Systematic Error Any kind of measurement error that leads to systematic (i.e., nonrandom) differences between an observed measurement and its true value.

Systematic Random Sampling A method of probability sampling involving the selection of elements from an ordered sampling frame in which the first element is selected at random and each additional element is selected using a sampling interval equal to the sampling frame size divided by the targeted sample size.

T

Test–Retest A way to assess reliability of an instrument over time and involves administering the scale measure on two occasions separated by days or weeks.

Test Statistic Random variable that is calculated from sample data and used in a hypothesis test to determine whether to reject or accept the null hypothesis.

Testing Effects The effects observed in a research study that may be related to taking the test more than once rather than to the treatment.

Themes Part of qualitative data analysis in which concepts emerge from the data during the analysis process and represent the underlying meaning attached to the data associated with a particular code.

Timeline Follow-Back Method A data-collection method that facilitates recall in studies that may not have the advantage of using ecological momentary analysis.

Translation Science The practice of translating research into practice.

Trend A general direction in which something is developing or changing.

Triangulation A method to facilitate validation of data through cross-verification from more than two data sources.

Type I Error Error that occurs when the null hypothesis is rejected when it should have been accepted; also known as a *false positive error*.

Type II Error Error that occurs when the null hypothesis is accepted but should have been rejected; also known as a *false negative error*.

U

United States Office for Human Research Protections (OHRP) Governing body that oversees the protection of participants in human subject research and sets rules and guidelines for all studies conducted in the United States.

Unstructured Interviews A qualitative method of data collection involving an informal conversation rather than a formal interview.

Usual Frequency Approach In a case-crossover study design, this approach is used to create the control period and is calculated as the average frequency and duration of reported transient risk exposures in the month before the acute outcome.

V

Validity The degree to which an instrument measures what it is supposed to measure.

Variance A measurement of spread in a dataset and equals the average of the squared differences from the mean.

Venue–Day–Time (VDT) Sampling Nonprobability sampling that adds an element of randomness by counting the number of places (*venues*) where recruitment might reasonably occur, the days each week when those venues are available for use as a recruitment site, and the times (assessed in blocks of 4 hours) when recruitment may occur.

Verbatim In the context of transcription, converting spoken words into text so that a message is captured exactly the way it was spoken.

Vulnerable Populations Refers to but is not limited to children, minors, fetuses and neonates, pregnant women, prisoners, and other demographically disadvantaged populations.

W

Within-Subjects Factor In an experimental design, refers to comparing scores on the dependent variable within the group over time.

Written Informed Consent Obtaining written consent involves informing the subject about his or her rights, the purpose of the study, the procedures to be undergone, and the potential risks and benefits of participation.

Index